Praise for
You Can Fix Your Brain

"If you are feeling foggy, please read *You Can Fix Your Brain* today! Use Dr. Tom O'Bryan's new book to draw a clear road map to healthier, more vital, and clearer cognition."

—Jayson Calton, PhD, and Mira Calton, CN,
bestselling authors of *The Micronutrient Miracle*

"Dr. Tom is always ahead of the health curve, connecting the dots in unique and insightful ways. In *You Can Fix Your Brain*, he brings together both the autoimmune and toxicity angles into optimizing brain health, which is scientifically solid and easy-to-follow with just a 1 hour a week time investment. He traverses the continuum from body to mind to environment with thoughtful techniques and quick tips. Follow the health pack with this incredible book!"

—Deanna Minich, PhD, FACN, CNS, IFMCP,
author of *Whole Detox* and *The Rainbow Diet*

"This book is a must-read if you want to improve your memory and clear brain fog, have amazing sleep, reduce anxiety and ADHD, be productive, and even feel happier."

—Trudy Scott, CN, author of *The Antianxiety Food Solution*

"Once again Dr. Tom O'Bryan has crafted a resource that is equal parts inspiring and practical in helping people take action toward changing their health trajectory."

—James Maskell, founder and CEO of Evolution of Medicine

"Dr. Tom O'Bryan's new book gives you all the tools to 'fix it,' and perhaps take your brain age back several decades. What he proposes is easy to read and understand, even if your brain is not working well right now! There is hope as this book takes you on the journey toward revitalization. The commonalities of brain function, dysfunction, and treatment are very similar to cardiovascular disease, which is my specialty, and I know that these treatment recommendations will work for both. I strongly recommend this book to you."

—Mark C. Houston, MD, MS, associate clinical professor of
medicine at Vanderbilt University Medical School

YOU CAN FIX YOUR BRAIN

Just 1 Hour a Week to the Best Memory, Productivity, and Sleep You've Ever Had

DR. TOM O'BRYAN

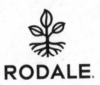

RODALE.

Copyright © 2018 by Dr. Tom O'Bryan

All rights reserved.
Published in the United States by Rodale Books, an imprint of the Crown Publishing Group, a division of Penguin Random House LLC, New York.
crownpublishing.com
rodalebooks.com

RODALE and the Plant colophon are registered trademarks of Penguin Random House LLC.

Library of Congress Cataloging-in-Publication Data is available.

ISBN 978-1-62336-702-2
Ebook ISBN 978-1-62336-703-9

Printed in the United States of America

Illustrations by Mapping Specialists
Jacket design by Jessie Sayward Bright
Jacket illustration by Lorelyn Medina/Shutterstock

10 9 8 7 6 5 4

First Edition

As I write this dedication, tomorrow happens to be my granddaughter Mia's second birthday. Her birth and early-life experiences *stacked the deck* against her for survival. Multiple brain-bleeds and other complications of a premature birthing which not that long ago would have been the sentence for a very short or very limited life. Every day, I thank God for the medical technology that gave her a fighting chance to survive. And today, she is a thriving, feisty, top-of-all-performance-scales, 2-year-old that leaves no corner unexplored, no book unopened (as long as it has colorful graphics), and who does not accept "no" for an answer! Mia models living life with a brain that will not stop for any boundaries, wanting to learn everything, processing information, continually building new neural circuits into an ever-expanding network of brain fibers whose results are visible every day as a happy, playful, engaging child continuously modeling the "joy of life."

Whenever we go on a road journey, it's helpful to have a map (or program GPS) that gives you the options of the quickest route, or the most scenic route, or where there may be construction ahead that will slow you down (with alternative routes).

This book is dedicated to my granddaughter and to you, the Reader, that your brain can lead you forward instead of holding you back and you once again can experience your own "joy of life."

CONTENTS

PART II: THE LADDER: CREATING BETTER BRAIN HEALTH

A NOTE FROM THE AUTHOR: PROGRESS, NOT PERFECTION

DEAR FRIEND,

I want to talk to you about this exciting journey you are about to embark on. I know that many people feel intimidated by the massive amount of health information that is out there—so much data, so many experts who often contradict each other, so much advice. It's no wonder we find ourselves immobilized with minimal results, or not getting better at all. There is so much information at our fingertips that it can be extremely difficult to know which recommendation to believe in. We jump from one expert to another, one concept to another, in search of what is "right." We put our toes in the water of each expert's opinion and then feel disappointment when we're not better in 2 weeks.

However, your journey to better health and vitality—and better brain function—doesn't have to be difficult and confusing. There is an easier way to approach this information, adopt and integrate it into your lifestyle, and then share what you've learned with your loved ones. I call it "Progress, Not Perfection," and in this book, you'll learn that doing the right thing is as individualized as you are. What works for your best friend may not work for you. What works for your son may not work for your daughter. My goal is to make it easy for you to do the right thing. And that means discovering exactly what's right for you—what will move the needle to get you to better health.

We live in a society that wants everything right now, including healing. We have been trained that if you have pain, you take a pill and the pain is gone, like that—poof—instant gratification. The problem is that instant gratification does not apply when you're dealing with uncovering the mechanisms that have caused bodily or brain imbalances to develop over years or even decades and eventually produce symptoms.

So let's reset our expectations. If I can show you a process by which in 6 months you will have made substantial progress in your quest to better mental and physical health, to a point at which your friends are saying, "Gee, you look different, what are you doing?" would you give me 1 hour a week of your time?

I think of the number one as a very powerful number. I was once in the Galileo Museum in Florence, Italy, and walked over to a peculiar exhibit: A marble display with a glass dome held one of Galileo's fingers. Just one, but it is meant to represent the whole man and everything he created. When I saw it, I realized that I couldn't possibly learn everything about Galileo in one sitting. But, if I could remember just one out of the many, many things that I learned that day in the museum, and it could stay with me, the trip was worthwhile.

So now, I'm asking you for just 1 hour a week. That's the key to success when you're going to change the underlying mechanisms that have caused, over time, the symptoms you are currently dealing with. Over time, 1 hour a week will lead to great changes.

So relax a bit before you turn the next page. You don't have to take in all the information in this book in one sitting. And you don't have to adopt all of the strategies at the same time. I tell my patients, "It's the base hits that win the ball game." This week, set a goal to learn one thing, and apply it.

Here's an easy one: You know that smell that overtakes you when you're pumping gas? That's benzene, and it's a strong carcinogen (something that can cause cancer) and a neurotoxin (something that affects the function of your brain). As you breathe it in, the benzene goes through your permeable lungs, into your bloodstream, and right up to your brain, where it initiates an immune response producing inflammation, which damages your nerve cells. Well, most of us can't totally avoid gasoline, but we don't have to breathe this stuff in. Next time, look where you're standing. If you're smelling benzene, that means you're standing downwind. All you have to do is walk around to the other side of the hose. Now you're upwind. That one simple maneuver every time you pump gas, over a lifetime, dramatically reduces the amount of benzene you're exposed to. See? A very easy fix to what really does add up to be a big problem.

Next week, you'll grasp something else and apply that. The following week, you'll implement yet another small teaching—always a step or "one base hit" at a time. Before you know it, you'll have made lasting, permanent changes that lead us to winning the ball game of healthy living.

My next suggestion is going to be a game-changer for most of us. As you read this book, remember to be kind to yourself. A good friend of mine shared his opinion of the difference between being kind and being nice. Being "nice" is speaking or acting in ways that are sensitive so as to not hurt someone's feelings (including ourselves). Being "kind" is recognizing/speaking the truth from a non-blaming point of view.

When I was going through a particularly difficult time in my life, I came across a book called *When Things Fall Apart*. The author, Pema Chödrön, shares a Tibetan term, *maitri*, which means loving-kindness and an unconditional friendship with oneself. That concept hit me between the eyes. It never occurred to me to be kind to myself or periodically let myself off the hook. I was always the guy who charged after goals, whose efforts were never good enough, without realizing that it's all about the journey and never about perfection.

Suppose that after reading this book and following my suggestions, you're doing quite well, until you momentarily forget what you've learned and eat something you know you shouldn't, skip a day of exercise, or stop working on your mind-set. You wouldn't be the first: We all occasionally suffer from what I call the Christmas Cookie Syndrome.

It took me 8 years to give up Christmas cookies, even though I lived completely gluten-free otherwise. Eight years! Every time I went home at Christmas, my mom would make all these different, delicious cookies. Have you ever noticed that when you are back home as an adult, you sometimes revert to old, familiar behaviors, which have become the automatic responses to your family? Year after year I told myself: *"I'm not having the Christmas cookies. I'm just not going to do it. I always feel lousy later, and the temporary benefits are not worth the long-term price."* And then I'd wake up in the morning and there would be plates of all of my favorites, just staring at me as I sipped my coffee. In comes the devilish thought: *"Oh, I'll make Mom happy; maybe I'll just have one."* Or there would be no thought at all—just an automatic response, and before I knew it, I'd swallowed a cookie! Then I'm having two or three each day over my vacation, and all of a sudden, my energy goes down. My vitality lags and my brain feels foggy. Then I would return home and feel terrible, both physically and about myself. I'd be back up to speed within a week, and I would vow that I was never doing that again. And the following year I'd go back and have my Christmas cookies.

Was I being ridiculous—or just human? Eventually, I got the message. When you suffer long enough or frequently enough, you get motivated to make the needed change. I got to a point where I couldn't ignore the message my body was sending me. But before I learned to stop eating the cookies, I learned to stop beating myself up. I've cultivated *maitri*—that loving-kindness. I realized that the unrecognized patterns of old relationships reactivated a side of me that I thought I had long since improved on, triggering my Christmas cookie binge. Instead of feeling guilty, I could talk to myself from a place of kindness: *"I did my best; let's see if I can do better next time."* Just that internal conversation dissipated the strength of an unhealthy habit. And you know what? Within a year or two, even Mom got the message, and she made me some gluten-free cookie options.

What's your Christmas cookie trigger? For some of you it may be other foods; for some of you it may be cigarettes, or alcohol, or drugs, or toxic relationships, or . . . You get my message. Most of us beat ourselves up for something, blaming ourselves, or telling ourselves we have to do better—

our efforts are not good enough. Yet for any task, especially one as important as improving our health, we can only do our best. If we can be truly kind to ourselves, we can evaluate our actions at the end of each day and say, *"I'm trying my best, and it's certainly better than how I was living last month, or last year. Now, what action can I take to make the next effort even better?"* That's a great deal kinder than *"I messed up again. I should have done this better."*

No matter how you are feeling right now, don't expect miracles tomorrow. Look forward to change from what your current situation is, but look toward that change with loving-kindness, adapting the "base hits win the ball game" approach. With loving-kindness and an unconditional friendship with yourself, and the lessons in this book, you will get there. You will experience vibrancy and much better health.

And in the meantime, if you are tempted by a Christmas cookie along the way, enjoy it. Don't feel guilty while you're eating it. Know that it's all right, you'll survive, you're on a journey, and in the moment, that cookie tastes great. In so many ways, that, too, is another form of loving-kindness. Remember, it's about progress, not perfection.

With Loving-Kindness,
Dr. Tom

FOREWORD

Since I wrote *The UltraMind Solution* back in 2009, science's understanding of the brain and how it functions has changed. In just 10 years we've seen huge advancements in imaging technology, and study after study has pointed to the success that lifestyle changes, including nutrition and exercise, can have over brain function. Yet sadly, so many people continue to suffer from what I call a "broken brain."

Doctors refer to broken brains by many names: depression, anxiety, memory loss, brain fog, chronic fatigue, and even attention deficit. Broken brains can include psychotic disorders such as schizophrenia, as well as neurodegenerative diseases like dementia, Alzheimer's, and Parkinson's. And while these conditions seem wildly different, we now know that there may be an underlying mechanism that connects them all: inflammation caused by a highly responsive immune system.

If you are one of the many millions of people who find that their mood or memory is off, aren't getting a good night's sleep or feel tired all the time, or are beginning to suffer from symptoms that affect your thinking, you may have a broken brain. Don't despair, even if you've been to the doctor and have been told that these are normal signs of aging, or "nothing's wrong; it's all in your head," or worse, that "there's nothing you can do." These responses are inappropriate at best and dangerous at worst. The truth is, your health and the way you live your life is almost always within your power to change.

Luckily, you've taken the first step to regain your health just by picking up this book. I've known Dr. Tom O'Bryan for years. He is one of the world's preeminent experts in autoimmunity—the mechanism in which your immune system attacks the organs and tissues in your body and brain in its attempt to protect it. In fact, he trains tens of thousands of doctors and health practitioners across the globe every year about the autoimmune spectrum, and how it affects both the brain and the body's overall health. His functional medicine approach of addressing the root cause of disease, along with his understanding that the body and brain comprise one integrated system, are the key pieces of information you'll need to move from fatigue to boundless energy, and from brain fog to enhanced memory and cognition.

The information you're about to read takes you outside of the traditional health-care system that has not provided the answers that you are looking for. Instead, you'll learn how to begin to implement strategies to change your everyday behaviors. His instructions are simple and sound: by choosing the right foods and avoiding the wrong ones—including environmental toxins—you can "stop throwing gasoline on the fire," and lower inflammation in a natural and healthy way. Then, by paying attention to your body and mind, you can begin to think better, and feel better, and improve your quality of life.

—*Mark Hyman, MD, director of Cleveland Clinic Center for Functional Medicine, board president of Clinical Affairs for the Institute for Functional Medicine, and 11-time* New York Times *bestselling author*

INTRODUCTION

THIS BOOK HAS been written with one overarching purpose in mind—to help you and your family obtain optimal brain health. No matter what your current brain health state may be, the lessons on these pages will enable and empower you to take concrete steps that will make an immediate difference in your brain's vitality, clarity, and energy. Your memory will improve. Fogginess will disappear, you'll be less tired all the time, and much more. And you'll learn that these aren't empty promises. I know how to create lasting changes in health, and I'm here to share them with you.

Throughout my entire career as a health practitioner, I've been a catalyst for change. I've learned to initiate a different way of communicating with my patients and the doctors I teach as I introduce new concepts. I'm known for making really complex science easily understandable in a variety of media. When I created *The Gluten Summit* in 2013, an online seminar that more than 118,000 people attended, nothing like that had ever been done before. Today, there are hundreds of summits online, on almost every subject.

Then I created a Web-based docuseries called *Betrayal: The Autoimmune Disease Solution They're Not Telling You*. It includes interviews with 85 of the world's top researchers in autoimmune diseases, the doctors who applied these principles, and the patients who followed these clinicians' recommendations and reversed their rheumatoid arthritis, multiple sclerosis, lupus, and many other autoimmune diseases.

My first book, *The Autoimmune Fix*, offered a really deep dive into the causes of the autoimmune response, with easy-to-implement lifestyle changes to reverse disease or prevent it from happening in the first place. That preventive model, and the introduction of predictive autoimmunity, was groundbreaking, and I'm proud to have brought it to readers like you.

This book is also meant to highlight something completely new and unique. In it, you'll learn exactly how the autoimmune response affects your brain. You can replace almost every organ in your body, except your brain. You can, however, regenerate healthier brain cells. And if you are like me, I bet that's one organ you'd like to keep in tip-top shape for as long as possible.

The fix for brain health comes down to lifestyle changes, and I have plenty to share inside. But what's even more important is understanding why there is a problem in the first place. I always tell my patients, by the time you go to see a doctor with symptoms, it's like you've fallen over a waterfall and you've crashed into the pool below. At first, you're simply glad that you're still alive, so you start to swim to the surface. But the waterfall keeps crashing down into the pool, and the water is really turbulent; it's splashing everywhere. All you can do is try to stay afloat.

If you have brain fog, or you can't get a good night's sleep, or you are experiencing seizures, or your child has been diagnosed with Attention-Deficit/Hyperactivity Disorder (ADHD), I completely understand if you're mainly concerned with staying afloat in this pool of symptoms. We're all looking for a better life jacket (usually in the form of a better quick fix, such as a better drug) to keep us alive in these turbulent waters. And this is not to say that life jackets are unimportant: Sometimes, you can't live without them. If you have a disease, you may have to calm down the symptoms by reaching for one of these life jackets; so if you need medication to get your high blood pressure down, or to reduce your sky-high cholesterol, or to alleviate migraines, please, take the meds. However, a life jacket won't stop the water from crashing down on you. If you can't sleep, a prescription for Ambien and maybe the supplement melatonin will provide short-term results. But the reason why you can't sleep isn't an Ambien deficiency! We need to know where the problem is really coming from.

If you want to get better, you're going to have to look for a ladder and get yourself out of the turbulent water (your symptoms). Then you have to go back upstream and find out why you fell in the water in the first place. In this book, you are going to learn how to think differently about your health, and your family's health, and why you fell in the river that eventually took you downstream and over the waterfall, into the pool of your unique symptoms. And here's the secret: If you have a brain that's not functioning very well, you don't focus on treating only the brain, because that would be like staying stuck paddling in the turbulent waters with a life jacket on that's keeping you afloat. You may need to treat the brain, but you will also have to go upstream and find the source, which most often is elsewhere in your body. Once you do, you can get out of the pool and, often, throw away the life jacket. (You'll want to do this with your doctor's permission, of course. Never stop your meds without your doctor's approval, but don't be surprised if your doc is startled to see that you're doing better without as much medication.)

The promise of this book is to give you information, the ladder to get out of this pool. We can't promise to shut off the waterfall. Some of the underlying triggers are out of our hands, at least for now. We can't clean the air you breathe, or remove the chemicals from your food. But we can give you the tools you can use to protect yourself and avoid chronic offenders. For instance, one of my new heroes and good friend Dr. Dale Bredesen (whom you'll be hearing a lot about) has identified five types of Alzheimer's disease, and one of them is called inhalational Alzheimer's, meaning that the polluted air we breathe is literally robbing us of our memory.

For instance, the children of Mexico City have an extremely high percentage of the earliest signs of Alzheimer's, and the reason is that their air quality is so bad.[1] My heart breaks for them, because there's nothing I can do about their air quality to change their lot. However, I can demonstrate why air pollution is just as great a problem here in the United States. Ever notice the pervasive film of crud on your windshield that reappears just a few hours after you've had the car washed? That's sediment in the air settling on the windshield, and we're breathing that sediment into our lungs with every breath. It's the reason you need to have the best air filtration system that you can find in your bedroom, because that is where you spend at least 6, 7, or 8 hours breathing, every single day. We can't change the world overnight, but we can certainly minimize the impact of the world on us.

WE'RE ALL ON THE JOURNEY TOGETHER

Getting out of the pool is not that hard to do, but I'm constantly perplexed as to why more health professionals don't impart this critical information to their patients. When I was 44, I was diagnosed with a cataract in my left eye. I went to three different eye doctors who measured my vision before I got the right diagnosis. Finally, my internist asked me the most general question, "Are you having any problems with your health?" And I said, "Well, you know, my vision's getting a little off, but my ophthalmologist says that my vision test still looks okay."

My internist was just as confused as I was, so he took a look in my eye and saw the cataract. I then went back to the ophthalmologist, who confirmed the finding. The ophthalmologist was embarrassed but told me that it's extremely rare for someone my age who is in good health to have a cataract. It's even rarer that the evidence is in only one eye. I asked, "Why is that?" And he had no idea. He told me, "We don't know. It just happens."

Well, as a functional medicine practitioner, I knew that his answer wasn't good enough. Nothing "just happens" to the body or the brain. So

I started doing my own research, and I learned that lead poisoning can cause cataracts. I couldn't imagine that I had lead poisoning, but just to be sure, I did a provocative heavy metal test. Wouldn't you know, it came back that I had the highest level of lead of anyone I had ever tested. And I've done hundreds of heavy metal tests over the course of my career.

I was born and raised in Detroit, right across the river from the Ford River Rouge Complex, which was the largest assembly line that Ford had in the 1950s. It's hard to believe, but back then, there were no, or very minimal, air pollution guidelines. I was exposed to lead every day of my childhood from the chemical by-products produced by the auto plant. Every day. We are all affected by environmental exposures, and we have to go back upstream to see why we fell in the river that eventually created problems wherever the weak link in our chain is (in my case, my eyes), especially for our brain health.

Here's another story: Just as I was writing this introduction, a woman named Leona came in to see me. She had been diagnosed 12 years earlier with an autoimmune disease, scleroderma (a chronic hardening and tightening of the skin and connective tissues that can occur throughout the body and the brain), and had previously seen eight other doctors, but no one could help her. She came in with a folder of 84 pages of test results. No one had ever asked her anything about her life history. These were chairs of departments at the best universities, world experts in scleroderma. Her symptoms of brain fog, short-term memory lapses, and brain fatigue (where her brain wasn't generating the necessary energy to get her up and moving) required a life jacket—powerful steroid medications meant to slow down the progression of the disease. However, the best that the meds were able to do was suppress her physical symptoms a little; they didn't address the issues she was having with her brain.

I explained to Leona the concept of the waterfall, and that every patient is looking for a better life jacket. Then I told her that together, she and I were going to find the reason she fell over the waterfall in the first place and figure out, "What the heck happened here?"

So we started at the beginning. She worked through the Living Matrix timeline with me (which you'll also learn how to use in Chapter 5), and she told me a story her mother had told her about her birth. When her mother was in the recovery room and Leona was in the nursery, her mom said to the nurse, "I can hear a baby who won't stop screaming. Please tell me that's not my baby." The nurse responded, "I'm sorry, that is your baby, but we don't know why she's so distressed."

I remembered a conversation I had with my good friend Dr. Steven Masley, who told me about a presentation he had heard at the American College of Nutrition conference. A researcher from Norway was discussing PCBs and breastfeeding. Norwegians are notorious for having extraordinarily high levels of polychlorinated biphenyls, or PCBs, in their blood, which has been traced to their high-fish diet (the fish in the fjords are exposed to tremendously high levels of PCBs from agricultural runoff into the water). When a mother is exposed to PCBs, and she has crossed a threshold where there are too many toxins in her system and she cannot clear all of them through the body's elimination process, many of these toxins are stored in estrogen-loving cells, like breast tissue. With childbirth, the mammary cells of the breast begin to produce milk. If those mammary cells are loaded with years of accumulation of PCBs, the concentration of PCBs in the breast milk will be very high. We know that PCBs are just one type of neurotoxin among many that can transfer from mom to baby through the breast milk, with the risk of inhibiting normal brain development and function. I personally wonder if this is one of the reasons why the incidence of autism is so high today.

I explained this to Leona, and she thought about it for a minute. Then she started crying and said, "Well, I was definitely breastfed. Plus, we lived on the outskirts of a steel mill and coal-mining town. No one wants to live there anymore because the air and soil are so toxic. My mom was born and raised in that town, so she could easily have had high toxin levels in her body. We had a small farm, and as a child I used to go out and play in the cornfields with other kids, and the crop duster planes would fly overhead. We would run around and dance in the crop dusting stuff, what was coming from the planes. Could those exposures be affecting me now, for the first time? No one's ever asked me anything about this. Could these be the environmental toxins, Dr. O'Bryan, that you talk about in your book that are a trigger in the development of autoimmune disease?"

I held her hand and said, "Absolutely. Absolutely. Your mother may have been carrying a very high toxic load in her body, and during her pregnancy and your development in utero, you could have absorbed these chemicals that are toxic to your nerves and your brain. Her breast milk would have been highly loaded with these chemicals." I told her that we would do our best to get to the bottom of her problem. Yet at the same time I was angry about the time she lost on her journey. No one had ever checked Leona for heavy metals, toxic chemical exposures, or even food sensitivities. And just like I had toxins building up in my body for 40 years, which eventually caused the development of a cataract, Leona may have been affected by toxin accumulation that manifested as systemic scleroderma that was affecting both her body and her brain.

HOW THIS BOOK WORKS

Now, together, let's see what's been cooking in your body that may be affecting your brain health. First, you'll learn how your brain works, and how the autoimmune cascade can affect its function. Then you'll learn about different mechanisms that affect any health condition, and we'll focus on the way they affect the brain. The first and the most important system is the gut, and particularly important is the health of your microbiome. You'll learn how imbalances in the gut directly affect the function of your brain. Then you'll see how our toxic environment affects the way you think. You'll learn how to determine which of these mechanisms you have to focus on for your particular symptoms, and then learn the best ways to reverse problems or address potential ones even before they occur.

You'll also learn about the leaky brain. Everyone knows about leaky gut and its relationship to gluten sensitivity (and if you don't, you'll learn about it now), but most people don't know that you can experience the same kind of breach in the blood-brain barrier. I'm going to refer to this

throughout the book as "B4": a breach of the blood-brain barrier. One of
the big breakthroughs you'll learn about is the latest testing to see if you
have B4, and then how you can repair this tear-in-the-cheesecloth that
protects the brain. This is critically important, because if you don't, an
inflammatory cascade (which you'll learn about in the next chapter) continues every day. It doesn't stop. And it creates a problem that builds upon
itself until you have symptoms you cannot ignore.

Throughout the book you'll learn about Dr. Dale Bredesen's work,
and how he is redefining the way we look at Alzheimer's disease. I know
that more people are afraid of getting Alzheimer's than of getting cancer,
and frankly, I don't blame them. The good news is that Dr. Bredesen has
treated more than 100 people with Alzheimer's who have experienced
complete reversals of their brain health. What's more, he has identified
more than 100 mechanisms that may be contributing to Alzheimer's, and
very few of them are in the brain. You have to look at your environment.
You have to look at your mechanical structure: your bones, your ligaments,
your muscles, the way you stand, sit, and sleep. You have to look at your
mind-set, exercise routine, and diet. Together, we'll explore his research
and see how it pertains to you.

I'm also going to introduce the concept of the Triangle of Health, first
developed by George Goodheart, DC, the founder of applied kinesiology.
Dr. Goodheart was one of my first mentors, and he taught me that you
have to look at any health condition from three perspectives. Whether it's
the gut, the cardiovascular system, hormones, the brain, or the musculoskeletal system, for example, you have to look at the condition from all
three sides of a triangle:

- Structure: Approaching health from a chiropractic, massage, physical therapy, or exercise point of view means looking at the muscles, bones, and joint movements (or lack thereof). This includes
  how you sit in your car, what positions you use to sleep, what kind
  of pillow you have, and the wear and tear of your shoes—all affect
  the mechanical aspects of your health. There are literally tens of

millions of people who have received dramatic benefit from chiropractic care. If your recurring headaches are due to poor posture, no medication will bring permanent relief: You must go upstream and correct the structural trigger, which will then restore both body and brain function.

- Biochemistry: This includes what you eat, drink, and otherwise consume, including the air you breathe. You'll learn why certain foods, such as gluten, dairy, and sugar, are toxic to the brain, how your immune system reacts to them, and how to successfully replace them.

- Mind-set: This encompasses the emotional and spiritual aspects of your life that may be affecting your health and brain function. Have you ever heard of "stinking thinking"? It's a real phenomenon that's been identified in the research that shows how our attitudes, and how we handle the stress of life, can be the primary trigger in the development of many different diseases.

By the early 1990s, I realized that there is a fourth component to the triangle of health that has begun to substantially affect our lives over the last 20 to 30 years. As a matter of fact, there are hundreds of studies now documenting the impact of this new arena with brain deterioration diseases (Alzheimer's, Parkinson's, schizophrenia . . .). As a result, when you look at the diagram on page 10, you'll see the shape actually has a fourth side, turning the triangle of health into a pyramid. The base is the structure. The three remaining sides include biochemistry, mind-set, and electromagnetics. This last side is as important as the other three sides, which most of us are unaware of and take for granted.

The fourth component of health is the effects of exposures to electromagnetic fields, or EMFs. The constant bombardment of EMFs is a new category in the last 20 years of immune system assault, particularly to our brains. This is an unintended side effect of technology, but make no mistake: EMFs are potentially as damaging as any other toxic assault on our bodies. To see what I mean, just go into a restaurant and check for wireless access on your smartphone. Many times, there are 6, 8, even 10 different networks available. That means there are 6, 8, or 10 different electromagnetic frequencies pulsing through the air, hitting your brain, with the potential of negatively affecting its function. It's a minor impact, but a cumulative one. In this book, you will learn all about these EMF exposures, how they can be a primary culprit affecting brain function and a detriment to your health, and what you need to do to stop their harmful effects.

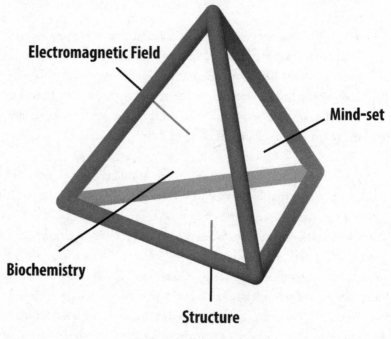

The Pyramid of Health

Let's start our journey out of the turbulent pool together. The first step up the ladder is to understand the basic principles of autoimmunity and how your body's best defense can wreak havoc on your brain health.

PART I

THE WATERFALL: THE TRIGGERS IMPACTING BRAIN FUNCTION

AUTOIMMUNITY: HOW IT AFFECTS BRAIN FUNCTION

AUTOIMMUNITY REFERS TO the mechanism in which your immune system attacks the organs and tissues in your body and brain. Whenever we are exposed to any environmental toxin that triggers an immune response (foods such as gluten, or toxic chemicals, or infections), that substance is now categorized as an *antigen,* something that our immune system is activated to protect against. This immune response can occur at any time, day or night, and it's designed to work in the background of our lives so we don't notice it happening. You don't feel it, see it, taste it, smell it, or experience it in any way, yet your body is silently protecting you. If this initial immune response is not strong enough, then the immune system releases *antibodies,* a more powerful weapon for dealing with an antigen. If this mechanism continues long enough, damage to body or brain tissue will occur, and wherever the damage occurs, that organ can no longer function as it's meant to. This usually begins with the mildest of irritations, like a runny nose, sore muscles, or brain fog. If the antigenic response continues, damaging the tissue, eventually you will develop a disease related to that tissue. It doesn't matter what tissue we're talking about: This mechanism occurs in every and any tissue in your body, including the brain. Now you've developed a disease.

There are more than 70 recognized autoimmune diseases and more than 300 autoimmune conditions. Common autoimmune diseases include Alzheimer's, Parkinson's, cardiovascular ailments, strokes, diabetes, multiple sclerosis, psoriasis, rheumatoid arthritis, lupus, scleroderma, and dementia. You may be wondering how it is possible that these diseases run such a gamut, and why so many affect the brain. The reason is that all of these diseases are linked to the same by-products of an autoimmune response: elevated antibodies and inflammation.

IMMUNE SYSTEM BASICS

Your immune system acts like the armed forces in your body—it's there to protect you. It's composed of five different branches that work together. There is a metaphorical army, navy, air force, marines, and coast guard (which are referred to by doctors as autoimmune responses, or the antibodies IgA, IgG, IgE, IgM, and IgD), each of which has a distinct role. There are also four different immune systems in the body. Each of these systems operates separately, but all follow the same owner's manual and communicate with each other. The largest one is found in the gastrointestinal tract (the gut), where 70 to 85 percent of your immunity resides. There is another immune system in the liver called the Kupffer cells. The third comprises the white blood cells found in the bloodstream.

Finally, the most potent immune system in the body is in the brain and made of glial cells. These cells act as sentries standing guard with high-powered rifles just inside the blood-brain barrier, which is the filtration system of what gets into the brain. Glial cells are the most powerful immune response in the body: These guys don't walk around with just six-shooters; they have bazookas. Any foreign matter that gets into the brain activates the glial cells to fire chemical bullets.

From an evolutionary perspective, humans thrive as the dominant species on the planet because we can reason and other species cannot. The "thinking" area of the brain, the cerebral cortex, allows us to reason, and as a result, it's most important to our survival. We know this because there are 60.84 billion glial cells protecting the cerebral cortex, making sure that if anything gets past the blood-brain barrier, there is an army there to address it. There are only 16.34 billion neurons that comprise the cerebral cortex, giving this large region a glial-to-neuron ratio of almost 4 to 1 (actually it's 3.72 to 1—sorry, I am a geek!). These thinking cells need to be protected at all costs. It's the reverse in the cerebellum, the more primitive muscle and motor command center in the brain, where there are more neurons than glial cells. This may be why so many autoimmune diseases that affect the brain affect your motor function, as is the case in Parkinson's, multiple sclerosis (MS), and others.

Each of the four immune systems has at least two arms: the ancient arm of the immune system, found in all living creatures, called the cellular, or innate, immune system, which acts as the protective handguns firing chemical bullets and creating inflammation to destroy a threat; and the humoral, or adaptive, immune system, which is the heavy artillery that's called in when you need to produce even stronger inflammation as a backup support system.

When faced with an environmental exposure, whether it is bacteria, a virus, a parasite, offensive dietary proteins and peptides, or even chemicals or medications, the innate/cellular arms produce *cytokines*, the biochemical bullets I refer to as the first responders. These cytokines recognize and then destroy whatever they consider threatening. There are a number of different types of cytokines, and the immune system determines which one to launch depending on the threat.

If the cellular arms' defensive strategy cannot get the job done, the immune system calls up the big guns. This is when the humoral/adaptive immune system kicks in and its soldiers launch targeted missiles called *antibodies*. Antibodies work like trained assassins; they go after a specific target. Anywhere the antibodies find an invader, they fire their missiles at that specific invader. If you've ever received blood test results with the words "elevated levels of antibodies," or an "H" next to the antibody marker, this refers to the fact that the basic immune system is overwhelmed, and now the big guns are working overtime to contain a perceived threat. These antibodies circulate in the bloodstream looking for the environmental exposures they've been trained to attack.

And here's the kicker: Even after the offending bug or food has been destroyed, along with the damaged cells, antibodies continue to inhabit your bloodstream for an additional 2 to 6 months. Even when you have no symptoms, elevated antibodies are a signal that the immune system is working with its last option to respond to a perceived threat before the development of disease.

Elevated antibodies can also occur when our innate immune system (the first responders) becomes depleted and ineffective. Our immune system can get worn out just by responding to the way we live our hectic lives and the food choices we make. Whether the continued unrelenting antigen is biochemical (food sensitivities, environmental toxins, etc.), structural (poor posture, intestinal permeability), emotional stress (stinking thinking), or electromagnetic, it can deplete our first responders (the innate immune response) so that they are no longer effective. How many years did you smoke, or drink soda, or eat sugary foods? The damage from those habits, or others, might now look like recurring colds ("I get the flu once or twice a year, and I'm out for a week"), or forgetfulness ("Where did I leave my keys?"), or a 3:00 p.m. energy crash. These subtle but annoying health problems are suggestive of a worn-out innate immune system.

CONTROLLING INFLAMMATION IS THE NAME OF THE GAME

When the innate immune system is worn out, the big guns are called on more frequently, resulting in higher levels of antibodies (which will show up on a blood test) that attack and destroy antigens in a process that creates *inflammation:* Additional blood containing immune-enhancing white blood cells and antibodies is directed to the areas of the body or brain that require healing. In some instances, like when you get a small cut on your hand, you can see and feel the inflammatory barrier: You may notice tenderness, redness, and swelling. However, inflammation mostly occurs inside the body and the brain. If you didn't go looking for inflammation with highly sensitive blood tests, you wouldn't even know it's there. And you won't have any symptoms from excess inflammation until your immune system has killed off so many cells that the organ or tissue can't function normally anymore. Symptoms are usually mild at first and progressively increase in intensity over time. Autoimmunity is a notoriously misdiagnosed condition because the symptoms are at first so benign. That's why the average person who is eventually diagnosed with an autoimmune disease suffers for 3 to 7 years before they get the right diagnosis. For example, we know that Parkinson's patients suffer for years with inflammation causing chronic constipation, but most don't think to see a neurologist to check on their brain health.[1]

Don't get me wrong—inflammation is also the primary way your immune system keeps you healthy. This is critical to remember, because inflammation gets a bad rap. The truth is, inflammation is not bad for you. *Excessive* inflammation is bad for you. Once the antigen is destroyed and the damage to your body is repaired (like when the cut on your finger heals), the inflammation response subsides and the cellular (innate) branch's immune response goes back to a resting state. However, if the inflammatory process recruited the big guns, the adaptive immune response with antibody production, the antibodies can continue for months even after the threat is contained. This might occur when the ammunition in your innate immune response wasn't powerful enough to successfully contain the antigen and the big guns had to be called in, or when we continue to expose ourselves from unknown sources, such as lipsticks that contain gluten, or orthodontic retainers that may contain gluten, or when we keep eating the wrong foods.

When inflammation in the brain gets out of control, you might notice subtle symptoms, like when you can't remember things the way you used to and chalk them up to "getting older." You might feel confused or depressed, or you might be overly anxious. No matter what you hear from "experts," it is not normal to have a poorly functioning brain in your forties and fifties. It is common, but it is not normal. It means that something's not working right. And that something is likely the result of an autoimmune response in your brain. That's what this book is about. If you understand this, then you have a very good chance of being sharp-witted well into your eighties and nineties.

Creating excess or chronic inflammation is like throwing gasoline on a fire: It adds to the problem instead of resolving it. This is when the inflammatory cascade begins. Inflammation beyond the normal range will cause cellular damage. Continued cellular damage will cause tissue damage. Continued tissue damage will cause organ inflammation. Continued organ inflammation will initiate elevated antibodies to that organ and trigger small, annoying dysfunction of that organ. Continued inflammation with elevated antibodies and small, annoying dysfunction becomes increased compensatory dysfunction causing noticeable signs and symptoms. Continued inflammation with elevated antibodies creating compensatory dysfunction causing noticeable signs and symptoms leads to organ or tissue damage. Continued inflammation with elevated antibodies and ongoing organ or tissue damage eventually creates stronger symptoms that get the person worried. Now you go to a doctor and describe the symptoms you've been feeling. At this point, you have fallen over the waterfall and are trying to stay afloat in the turbulent waters of the symptoms you're experiencing. The doctor prescribes a medication that is hopefully the right life jacket for you to stay afloat. And now you're at risk of all those crazy side effects that we hear about in the television commercials for the latest and greatest drug being promoted.

And why is the inflammation out of control? Why are the big guns activated, causing all of this mess? You have to go upstream to find out what fell in the river. Just staying afloat with a pretty good life jacket for your thyroid problem, or your diabetes, or your brain problems, or your arthritis, or, or, or . . . is why we have such poor results from our healthcare system today.

Chronic inflammation is like having a light switch on all the time. Ever go into a bathroom that has an automatic switch that turns on the lights when you walk in? My favorite breakfast restaurant has one just like that. It is activated by motion and then stays on for a specified amount of time. That's what your immune system is doing. Keep moving around in the bathroom and the light will stay on all the time you're in there and for a few minutes afterward. Keep exposing yourself to the environmental toxins your body is sensitive to, whether they are new exposures or if the amount of chemicals stored inside your cells is large enough, and the inflammation will continue to be produced in high amounts to protect you. It's not "out of control"; it's trying to protect you.

The light switch of inflammation will also stay on when you get hit in the head every once in a while because you're taking boxing or martial arts classes or playing sports such as soccer or football. (Shockingly, 99 percent of all NFL football players have severe, life-altering, and life-threatening inflammatory damage to the brain called CTE, or chronic traumatic encephalopathy. Yes, 99 percent! College football players are not much safer; 91 percent experience CTE. And even 21 percent of high school players are affected.[2]) The light switch could even stay on because you're eating foods that you're sensitive to (like wheat or dairy). My point is we have to go upstream to figure out what is activating the light switch of inflammation. We don't necessarily want to try to shut off the inflammation with a better life jacket.

Excess inflammation affects the weak link in your health chain—the part of your body or brain that fails first or most often. This location is determined by your genetics (your family's health history) and your antecedents (the environmental exposures you've accumulated in your body from how you have lived your life so far; e.g., eat tuna every week, and you're likely to have a mercury problem). Your weak link can be joint pain, or it can be poor attention, or fatigue. If it's your thyroid, you may notice that you are more chilled or have trouble losing weight. If it's your liver, you may find that alcohol has a stronger effect on you than it did before. If it's your brain, you may forget simple things, like where you've left your keys, or have trouble with your memory in general. If someone has a gluten sensitivity, it may manifest as chronic constipation. In the next person, it may manifest as liver disease or acne. In the next person, it might be attention-deficit disorder. What's more, practically every degenerative disease is linked to excessive inflammation, including cancer, heart disease,

Alzheimer's, Parkinson's, diabetes, multiple sclerosis, psoriasis, rheumatoid arthritis, and lupus.

If the weak link is your brain, inflammation may compromise brain function, leading to headaches, memory loss, seizures, anxiety, depression, or schizophrenia. As a matter of fact, scientists tell us that inflammation in the brain trumps any other brain function. Inflammation is a survival mechanism protecting us from a perceived threat: It becomes the top priority.[3] How your brain function is affected depends on where the inflammation occurs. For instance, forgetfulness occurs when inflammation in your brain affects the nerves that carry messages. Depression is an example of inflammation often occurring in the frontal lobes of the brain. Seizures result from inflammation in the back of the brain, in the occipital lobes.

Every brain disease or dysfunction that I have researched features inflammation as the trigger as well as a primary cause of the symptoms. This is why we need to be particularly concerned about inflammation in the brain. In truth, almost all of us have some level of brain inflammation, and you'll learn how it is created in the next chapter. This inflammation can stem from any one of the four sides of the new shape of health. And it's why even 35-year-olds claim to feel old and can't remember where they put their keys or where they parked their car.

We must treat the underlying inflammation causing the symptoms before they progress into a brain-related disease or disorder. It's so much easier to address a downward spiral before it crashes into the turbulent pool of a diagnosis. Thousands of clinicians have found that an anti-inflammatory approach to health care, like the one you'll learn about in this book, can arrest and even in some cases reverse these brain health problems and degenerative diseases.

As baby boomers like me get older, the incidence of Alzheimer's and dementia will only continue to skyrocket. According to the Alzheimer's Association, by midcentury, someone in the United States will develop the disease every 33 seconds.[4] We all know someone who has recovered from a heart attack and is now thriving, but very few of us know someone with a brain-deteriorating disease who is now thriving. Since almost all of us have unnecessary brain inflammation, that's why I chose the brain to be the focus of this book. The science is now clear: You can arrest the development of brain-deteriorating diseases. Read on.

Collectively, our brain is on fire, and we have to put the fire out. How do we do that? We have to identify where the fire is, where the "gasoline" is coming from, and then stop both. First, you stop throwing gasoline on the fire, then you rebuild the damage. You must let your brain rest and regenerate by removing the environmental antigens that are creating chronic inflammation.

UCLA's Dale Bredesen, MD, who runs the Buck Institute for Research on Aging at the Alzheimer's Research Center, is now reversing Alzheimer's. The first paper he wrote, in November 2014 in the medical journal *Aging*, outlined how 9 out of the 10 Alzheimer's patients in his study completely reversed their condition in 5 years. Patients went back to work. They moved out of institutions and back home with their families. They became fully functional again—almost miraculously.

What did he do? He looked at the mechanisms that caused the disease and fixed them. In essence, he followed the principles of functional medicine and put the fire out in the brain. He figured out 37 things that cause inflammation and put the fire out. You'll learn exactly how he did it as you read on.

ANOTHER PIECE OF THE AUTOIMMUNE PUZZLE: MOLECULAR MIMICRY

There are two types of antibodies you need to know about: the antibodies to antigens we are exposed to that we just discussed (outside invaders), and *autoantibodies:* antibodies that are produced inside your body that attack your own tissue. The body experiences some cellular damage every day, just in the course of life, from aging cells to the hormones we produce or the chemicals we're exposed to, or a little too much sun. In fact, we generate a whole new body's worth of cells every 7 years. Some of those cells turn over very quickly: The inside lining of your gut turns over every

3 to 7 days. Other cells, like the ones that make up your bones or your brain, turn over much slower.

The body removes old and damaged cells to make room for new cells to develop. One of the ways it accomplishes this cellular replenishment is with autoantibodies. There is a normal level of autoantibodies that we are supposed to have. Every day, the immune system creates the exact right number of autoantibodies to get rid of specific damaged cells. But when you are exposed to a toxin (food that you are sensitive to, mold, stress, hormones, bugs, etc.), the inflammatory cycle begins by activating the innate immune system (the first responders). As we discussed above, if the exposure continues and the demand of the innate immune system is greater than it can manage, your adaptive immune system (the big guns) come in to help. These antibodies to toxins are powerful but not as precise as autoantibodies.

Imagine a "terminator" wildly firing a machine gun out the window of a moving car while chasing a bad guy in the bloodstream. This is how antibodies react to a perceived toxin. He might shoot down the bad guys he's chasing, but he's creating lots of broken glass and debris along the way. This is what happens with antibodies to gluten or any other toxin we're exposed to. In the body, this debris is a mix of your damaged cells as well as the remnant bits and pieces of the antigens your immune system was working so hard at destroying. I call this mess the *collateral damage* of the immune response.

The body responds to the collateral damage by making autoantibodies to get rid of the damaged cells. This is normal; however, when antigen exposure is ongoing (as when you're eating wheat every day), creating excessive collateral damage, the body has to make an excessive amount of autoantibodies to the damaged cells.[5] Now we have elevated autoantibodies to our own tissue, creating even more inflammation. Having elevated autoantibodies puts us on the autoimmune spectrum. If this process continues, you create more damage to your tissue, and now you begin having symptoms from sluggish, damaged tissue. Eventually, the damage is so excessive, and the dysfunction is so pronounced, that you go to the doctor and will be diagnosed with a full-blown autoimmune disease. Remember, the mechanism started years earlier. And the disease will continue wherever the weak link in your chain is.

Now I'm going to tell you about a very important concept, *molecular mimicry*, that is one of the most common causes of brain dysfunction (including Alzheimer's disease, depression, anxiety, seizures, and schizophrenia), yet most doctors were not taught about this in medical school. Both antibodies and autoantibodies can easily mistake and destroy other molecules that look very similar to toxins. Infectious agents, food, or bacteria may confuse the body's immune system, because they are structurally similar to human tissue.

For instance, think of proteins like a pearl necklace. The job of our digestive system is to produce enzymes, chemicals that act like scissors that snip the necklace into individual pearls called *amino acids*, which are absorbed into the bloodstream. The body then uses these amino acids to build each and every one of our cells. However, the problem with wheat is that as humans, we do not have the enzymes to break down the necklace into individual pearls. The best we can do is to snip the wheat proteins into clumps of pearls called *peptides*.

These wheat peptides have a signature that every person's immune system recognizes as a threat, and will produce antibodies against this signature. The most common peptide of wheat that the immune system fights is called alpha-gliadin, which is a signature of 33 amino acids.

Let's call the peptide amino acid sequence of alpha-gliadin A-A-B-C-D. Each of the letters represents different amino acids. When alpha-gliadin molecules enter the bloodstream, your immune system starts making antibodies to A-A-B-C-D. That's a good thing, because the immune system is protecting you from a foreign substance. These antibodies travel through the bloodstream, looking for A-A-B-C-D, firing missiles wherever it finds A-A-B-C-D. The problem is that the surface of your brain contains a protein signature that looks similar to alpha-gliadin's A-A-B-C-D. The antibodies produced to attack alpha-gliadin may then attack your brain tissue. Your body is attacking wheat, but now it starts attacking your cerebellum or your myelin (the plastic wrap around your nerves) or any other brain tissue that is the weak link in your genetic chain. This *molecular mimicry* mechanism is the most common immune trigger in brain antibody production.

Molecular mimicry increases inflammation in the tissue, eventually damaging the tissue, and, if continued unchecked, will damage the organ. The body now starts to produce autoantibodies to get rid of the damaged organ cells. That's not a problem, unless the original antibodies (in this example, alpha-gliadin) continue to be produced as a result of toxic exposure, e.g., toast for breakfast, a sandwich for lunch, pasta for dinner, day after day after week after month after year. If this continues, the antibodies continually damage the organs, resulting in damaged organ tissue, resulting in autoantibodies to the damaged organ tissue to get rid of the damaged organ cells until eventually the production of the autoantibodies to the organ is self-perpetuating. Now not only have you developed symptoms, but you have a full-blown autoimmune response.

This is theoretical in numbers, but I hope the example is clear for you. Imagine that you're a teenager with a sensitivity to wheat. You eat it multiple times a day every day, and you inadvertently kill off 500 of your 20 million brain cells per day. Five hundred cells doesn't seem like much out of 20,000,000, but if this happens every day, in a week you've lost 3,500—still nothing compared to 20 million cells. Yet in a year, 3,500 cells lost per week times 52 weeks equals 182,000 cells. After 20 years, you will have killed off 3,640,000 cells. Now you are in your midthirties and have lost 18.2 percent of your brain cell function. That's almost one-fifth of your brain. Without those cells, brain function is impaired: less thinking, less sleep, less resiliency to mood shifts, and more anxiety. While you're constantly producing new brain cells, if you are killing off extra beyond normal loss, due to the wheat you're eating, or the other environmental toxins you're exposed to, you are killing off more cells than you are making, and that deficit is what creates poor function. This is the mechanism that creates 35-year-olds who can't find their keys.

Back in 1997, I ran a study in my practice in which every one of my 316 patients participated; they ranged in age from 2 to 92. We did a very sophisticated blood test that checked antibodies for a number of different tissues. We were looking for antibodies to wheat, dairy, corn, soy, and egg, and autoantibodies to brain tissue. What we found was astonishing. Of those participants who had any elevated antibodies to wheat, 26 percent of them also had elevated antibodies to the area of the brain called the cerebellum. This means they were on the autoimmune spectrum with the risk of developing gait ataxia (an autoimmune disease that affects your balance, which is controlled by the cerebellum). Of those patients who had elevated antibodies to wheat, 22 percent had elevated antibodies to myelin basic protein, which is like a plastic wrap protecting your nerves. Elevated antibodies to myelin basic protein is the primary mechanism in the development of the autoimmune disease multiple sclerosis. Obviously, for almost 25 percent of the study participants, the brain was the weak link in their chain, and it was affected because of elevated antibodies to wheat.

Those are horrible numbers. Your cerebellum controls muscle movement and coordination. How many people do you know who are in their seventies and can go up and down the stairs with grace and ease? Not many. This is why. The problem is not with the muscles; it's with the brain, and specifically the cerebellum, which controls muscle movement. When older people walk with apprehension, it's often because their cerebellum has been shrinking due to the constant attack of elevated autoantibodies creating damage and killing off tissue over many years. This is a classic example of molecular mimicry—wheat sensitivities causing brain damage.

ARE YOU ALREADY ON THE AUTOIMMUNE SPECTRUM?

No one wakes up one morning and all of a sudden their pipes plug up and they have cardiovascular disease and are at risk of a heart attack. The truth is, poor health is a slow, insidious process: In this example, blood vessels plug up over time, caused by an autoimmune mechanism that slowly deposits "crud" into the walls of the blood vessels. In the same way, no one wakes up one morning with Alzheimer's. Just like heart disease, it's a decades-long process with many steps along the way before you eventually have such severe brain dysfunction that you qualify for a diagnosis.

Autoimmunity, and all of its associated diseases, develops over time. There is a spectrum from a minor imbalance that eventually, over a number of years, becomes a major problem.

As I've said, we all have a normal level of antibodies and autoantibodies that are there to protect us from threats and to clear away dead cells. But when you have elevated antibodies to your own tissue, you are killing off more cells than you're making. This is the beginning stage of *organ deterioration,* caused by losing more cells than you can make. When this happens, even before symptoms occur, you are on the autoimmune spectrum. When any organ or tissue in your body has lost a significant number of cells, that organ or tissue can no longer work properly. As the autoimmune mechanism continues, you move further along on the spectrum of dysfunction, until eventually you have symptoms that are strong enough to make you go see your doctor. Without the right care, you will eventually get a diagnosis of an autoimmune disease, which simply means you are further along the spectrum.

The way you can definitively tell if you are on the autoimmune spectrum is to have your antibody levels tested, and we'll discuss that more in Chapter 2. Note that when there is a slight elevation of antibodies, some people may have noticeable symptoms, while others with tremendously high levels of antibodies may have no symptoms. Yet both types of people are on the autoimmune spectrum. This is why it does not matter whether you notice symptoms or not: If you have elevated antibodies, they are fueling tissue degeneration and disease. And unfortunately, the vast majority of us are moving toward the dangerous, far end of the autoimmune spectrum as a consequence of our immune system trying to protect us from the increased exposures of a toxic environment.

When is the optimal time to find out if you are on the spectrum of autoimmunity? Would you wait until you had enough organ damage to have noticeable symptoms, or would you try to catch early deterioration of tissue before there is so much damage that the symptoms demand medical attention? When it comes to the brain, I think it's a fairly easy question to answer. On one end of the spectrum are the annoying symptoms we deal with every day: anxiety, depression, forgetfulness, and fatigue. On the other end are diseases that will kill us or dramatically affect our daily life: multiple sclerosis, Parkinson's, and Alzheimer's.

We all want and expect perfect brain health. I'm here to show you that it's possible to not only arrest brain deterioration but regenerate a healthier brain and develop enhanced brain function. This just requires that you understand and apply the protocols to wear the life jackets you need when you're in the turbulent waters of symptoms, and then get out of the water, go upstream, and find out what it is that your immune system is trying to protect you from.

As we age, the brain literally slows down: We lose 7 to 10 milliseconds of processing speed every year past the age of 20. This loss of processing speed affects the ways you pull up memories and pay attention, but given that there are countless examples of elders learning new languages, it is not normal for your brain to slow down to such an extent that you experience brain health symptoms that are obvious and diagnosable. If you have any symptoms of brain dysfunction that are impacting your life, you are most likely on the autoimmune spectrum.

Using the antibody blood tests you'll learn about in Chapter 5, you can identify your *positive predictive value*—your current vulnerability that a disease is developing—and approximately when there will be enough tissue damage for you to get a positive diagnosis for that disease. We call this ability the science of *predictive autoimmunity*, and even though I've been reading research papers and talking to functional medical practitioners about this since 2007, traditional medicine is just getting on board. In fact, the study of predictive autoimmunity is now being recognized as a subcategory of immunology: Doctors are now focusing more on the world of autoimmunology.[6]

Recurring symptoms such as fatigue, lack of energy, memory lapses, or mood shifts might be messengers from your immune system letting you know that something's out of balance—you're being poisoned and your armed forces are trying to protect you. Even these brain symptoms occur on a spectrum. You can have mild fatigue, meaning that you just have to rev yourself up to get going in the morning, and it may progress to the point where you're completely dysfunctional and can't get out of bed.

FOCUSING ON THE BRAIN

Brain disease is frightening—maybe even terrifying. Most of us know someone who has had a heart attack and made it through and may even be thriving today after changing their diet and beginning to exercise. Most of us know someone who suffered from cancer and survived. Hardly anyone knows of anybody with a diagnosis of a brain disease whose condition stopped or improved. That is about to change. In this book, you'll learn more about the remarkable work of Dr. Dale Bredesen, who is now teaching functional medicine practitioners how to arrest and reverse cognitive decline and Alzheimer's disease. Yes, you heard that right. Alzheimer's is an immune-response disease that we now know can be stopped in its tracks and in many cases reversed.

Now that you have a good understanding of the autoimmune response, you're ready to take your next step on the ladder. My goal in this chapter was to give you a big-picture overview of how autoimmunity can impact your brain. Personally, I think much more detail on this topic would empower you, and for that I suggest you read my first book, *The Autoimmune Fix*.

In the next chapter, you'll learn more about the structure and function of the brain, so that you can begin to understand exactly why you may be experiencing the symptoms you have, and see how they relate to the foods you eat, or the chemicals you are exposed to, or even the lifestyle you are leading. All of these "fixes" are the base hits that can direct you to the low end of the autoimmune spectrum. By doing the work outlined in Part II of this book, you'll be able to restore your health.

ACTION STEP WEEK 1: START LISTENING

Pay attention and listen to what your body and brain are telling you. Body language never lies. Some people are fluent in French along with English, others understand Spanish, yet very few people are fluent in body language. That's one of the goals of this book: to teach you how to listen to your body so that you can notice changes that occur before they turn into health hazards. Even if you're having symptoms that just annoy you and aren't stopping your daily living, they still need to be taken seriously.

Have you noticed any of the following incidences? They are scaled in order of appearance, from early impairments of thinking to more severe dysfunction.

- Do you forget where you placed familiar objects, such as your keys?
- Do you forget names you formerly knew well?
- Do you walk into rooms and "forget" why you walked into the room?
- Have you gotten lost when traveling to an unfamiliar location?
- Have family or coworkers become aware of your relatively poor performance?
- Is it becoming evident to those close to you that you're having problems with word and name finding?
- Do you read a passage of a book and retain relatively little material?
- Do you have a decreased ability to remember names upon introduction to new people?
- Have you lost or misplaced an object of value?
- Have you been tested for failing concentration?
- Do you find yourself experiencing mild to moderate anxiety?

2

THE LEAKY BRAIN

IMAGINE THAT YOU'RE in your kitchen, preparing your favorite meal that you've cooked a thousand times before. You know exactly what it's supposed to look like, taste like, and smell like. But this time, you notice that it's not as aromatic, so you adjust the seasonings. It smells the same afterward. You chalk it up to getting older, and the next time you see your doctor, you tell him that there's something wrong with your nose. Your doctor gives you a cursory once-over and says it's normal (but you'll learn the difference between "normal" and "common" very soon). Or, if he's more thorough, he might refer you to an ENT (ear, nose, and throat specialist), who takes a longer peek and finds that there is nothing wrong.

Both doctors would in fact be right: There's nothing wrong with your nose. The truth is actually a much bigger concern: Your loss of smell is caused by brain deterioration, not your nose. Your body is trying to tell you something by sending you a signal when you notice that "things don't smell the same." It's a temperature gauge on your dashboard, telling you to check out what's under the hood long before the "hot light" comes on.

In this case, we know from the latest research that if you are 70 or older and you lose your sense of smell, you have a 48 percent increased risk of death *from any cause* in the next 5 years.[1] Loss of smell is actually a biomarker, much like a blood test, that exposes "underlying physiologic processes or pathology," which means that your brain has been wearing down slowly and surely for years. The biomarker shows up as a warning bell before an actual disease diagnosis. The olfactory cortex is linked to the area in the brain that is affected by Parkinson's and Alzheimer's diseases, the *substantia nigra*. It definitely is not normal for you to lose your sense of smell, but it sure is common. It's just one example of the thousands I could choose from that show how the brain is involved in all bodily functions.

However, here is some surprisingly good news. In a 2017 study, researchers found that even those subjects who lost their sense of smell, and on autopsy had the physical markers of Alzheimer's, never developed the symptoms of dementia if they were healthy overall.[2] This is why I say when you fix your body, you'll fix your brain.

In order to understand the deep connection between your brain and your body, you need a little primer. First, you'll learn about the brain's anatomy, how it works, and which "temperature gauges" or biomarkers you need to be aware of so that you can measure your own brain function (and dysfunction) years before the imbalance is so bad you now have a disease. If you want to reduce your risks of a brain disease as you age, these are the concepts you need to be familiar with.

DR. TOM'S TIP
TRY A SMELL TEST

Have your doctor order a smell test. One easy, four-item pocket smell test that you can even do at home comes from Sensonics International. A smell test measures your ability to identify a particular smell. Most use "scratch and sniff" technology, and you are rated as either "yes, can smell the item," or "no, you cannot." This particular screen is inexpensive and comes out of research from the University of Pennsylvania, longtime leaders in smell research. If your doctor can't get the test, or is reluctant to order it, go to my Web site, theDr.com/smell, where you can order the test yourself.

THE ANATOMY OF THE BRAIN

The brain is composed of three distinct parts: the cerebrum, the cerebellum, and the brain stem. The cerebrum, which is also known as the cerebral cortex, is the largest part of the brain. This is where the highest level of brain function, the "thinking" that we humans do, occurs. When we visualize the brain, what we see in our mind's eye is the cerebrum. The cerebrum is where the collection of folded bulges—known as gray matter—is located. These bulges enable us to fit a larger volume of surface area into a tight space, similar to the way the intestines work.

The cerebrum plays a key role in memory, attention, awareness, thought, language, and consciousness. It's the evolutionary development that allows humans to be the alpha species on the planet. The cerebellum is a ball of tissue located below and behind the cerebrum. It decodes sensory information (such as our sense of touch and balance) and integrates it with the muscles to coordinate movement. It's the part of the brain that sends the

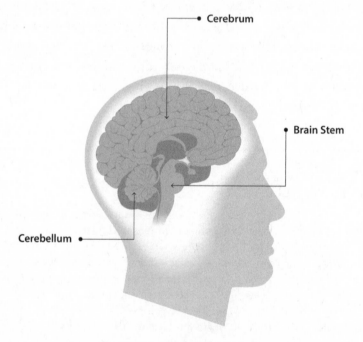

The "Big Picture" Overview of the Brain

DR. TOM'S AT-HOME BIOMARKERS

If you want to test the function of your cerebellum:

1. Stand up.
2. Lift your right knee toward your chest, and hold it for 10 seconds.
3. Lift your left knee toward your chest, and hold it for 10 seconds.
4. Now, close your eyes.
5. Lift your right knee toward your chest, and hold it for 10 seconds.
6. Lift your left knee toward your chest, and hold it for 10 seconds.

Did you have any trouble with your balance? Many people will lose their balance when they have their eyes closed, and some will even lose their balance with their eyes open. If you had any difficulty, it suggests that your cerebellum may be impaired due to a long-term autoimmune mechanism killing off your cerebellar tissue. Ask your doctor to confirm your findings with a blood test for cerebellum antibodies, which you'll find more information on in Chapter 5.

messages that enable us to bend and twist in ways few other species can. I remember a forest ranger once telling me that humans can run straight across the side of a hill, while bears can only run up and down (which is important to know when you are running away from a bear). Finally, the brain stem links the brain to the spinal cord. It controls bodily functions such as heart rate, blood pressure, and breathing.

Beneath the cerebrum lie several small structures that form the *limbic system,* the most primitive part of the brain, which is involved in decoding our emotions and motivations, including fear, anger, and pleasure. Certain structures of the limbic system are involved in creating and maintaining memory. The first is the *amygdala,* which is responsible for determining how and where memories are stored in the brain. The *hippocampus* is where short-term memories are stored, and it's one of the primary areas of the brain affected by Alzheimer's disease.

The *hypothalamus* controls emotions, eating, and sleeping. The *thalamus* transfers messages from the spinal cord into the brain. These regions will be important to remember when you read the next chapter, where you'll learn how bacteria in the gut can influence different areas

---

DR. TOM'S AT-HOME BIOMARKERS

Close your eyes. Try to remember what you had for lunch yesterday. What time did you go to bed the previous night? Can you remember what you did last Monday evening? When was the last time you forgot where you placed your keys or where you parked your car?

   If you can't remember any of these, your brain may be inflamed due to being on the autoimmune spectrum. You'll learn more about testing for brain autoimmunity in Chapter 5.

---

of the brain. For example, out-of-balance bacteria in the gut equals out-of-balance emotions, or poor sleep, or short-term memory loss. But more on that later.

Each of these brain regions is made of nerves. Nerves are made of *neurons*. The neuron is the basic working unit of the brain, a specialized cell designed to transmit information to other nerve cells, muscle, or gland cells. There are 100 billion individual neurons in the brain, and we are constantly adding new ones and removing old and damaged ones. Neurons process and transmit information to one another through *neurotransmitters*, or brain hormones. Damage to any part of this system limits or prevents the neuronal message from transferring from one cell to the next. This will be important to remember when we talk in the next chapter about foods that enhance the flow of neurotransmitter information.

The nerves are protected by a type of plasticlike wrap called the *myelin sheath*, an insulation barrier much like the material surrounding an electrical wire. The myelin sheath helps the nerve hold on to its chemical message until it's delivered to the next nerve. Think of the wire that goes from the battery of your car to the headlights. If you take some of the insulation off the middle of the wire, the wire is now exposed. If the exposed wire touches the frame of the car, the lights start flickering off and on. There may be nothing wrong with the wire, nothing wrong with the lights, but without the right insulation, it causes a problem—the lights are flickering. When that happens in the brain, you're on the spectrum heading toward multiple sclerosis (MS). That's why biomarker tests for antibodies to myelin basic protein (MBP) and myelin oligodendrocyte glycoprotein (MOG) are so important: These tests are the earliest way to check the mechanism of destruction for the insulation of your nerves, and when elevated, you're on the autoimmune spectrum heading toward MS.

The brain is surrounded by cerebrospinal fluid, blood, and blood vessels that continuously nourish it. The blood vessels, called *capillaries,* are connected to each neuron. Laid end to end, the capillaries would cover 400 miles.[3] Some of the blood vessels are so small that only one red blood cell at a time can get through. Blood circulates throughout your body 24/7 and travels everywhere, from the tips of your fingers and toes to the top of your brain. In fact, 20 to 25 percent of all the blood in the body at any one time can be found in the brain. This large concentration is necessary because your brain is processing tens of thousands of messages every second, and it needs blood to fuel its activity.

B4: BREACHING THE BLOOD-BRAIN BARRIER (theDr.com/B4)

This next topic (B4) is one of the most important takeaways in this book. Even though we're talking about the brain, this story begins in your gut (you'll learn all about this relationship between the brain and the gut in the next chapter). The contents of our blood are determined by what we take in through the air we breathe; by what is absorbed through our skin, eyes, and ears; and by the foods we eat. Anything on your fork that comes

DR. TOM'S AT-HOME BIOMARKERS

Do you have numbness and tingling in your hands and feet, in your cheek, on your tongue? Does one of your legs give out on you, even once in a while? These may be signs of *neurodegeneration*, a breakdown of nerve flow from the brain to body tissue, and may be the first noticeable signs of MS. Again, antibody tests for myelin basic protein (MBP) and myelin oligodendrocyte glycoprotein (MOG) would be important here.

into the body first goes through the digestive tract and the small intestine, where it is broken down, digested, and absorbed so that beneficial, life-sustaining nutrients can enter the bloodstream and circulate through the body. Along with digestion, the digestive system prevents incompletely digested foods, toxins, and irritants from being absorbed into the blood. The barrier that prevents early absorption from the walls of the intestines into the bloodstream is the epithelial (inside) lining of the small intestine, which functions like cheesecloth: Only very small molecules are supposed to get through into the bloodstream.

The brain has its own protective cheeseclothlike lining that functions in much the same way as the epithelial lining in the small intestine, and, in fact, it's made of similar materials. It's referred to as the blood-brain barrier (BBB), and its main role is to block large molecules from entering into the brain from the bloodstream. The brain's cheesecloth is even finer than the one in the intestine because most molecules are too big to fit in the blood vessels that service the brain. Just as the intestinal lining can tear, resulting in a leaky gut, the cheesecloth of the brain can tear, resulting in a leaky brain. Scientists refer to these tears as a *breach of the blood-brain barrier*. I like to call it B4.

A leaky brain can occur for many reasons, especially when there is trauma to the head. When you have a concussion, you tear that cheesecloth a little bit. Even smaller, repeated traumas (think of head butts during soccer practice that can happen 20, 30, or 50 times a day, 3, 4, or even 5 days a week) can cause tears. You don't even have to hit your head to cause these tears: Shaken baby syndrome is one example; excessive exercise is another.[4] It makes me wonder about the long-term value of endurance events such as triathlons and marathons. I ran marathons earlier in life, and as I write this, I understand why runners refer to running at times as pounding the pavement. Now, the other side of the picture is that a modest amount of exercise is beneficial to brain function, tightens the BBB, and even prevents tumor cells that may be in the bloodstream from getting into the brain.[5] It's all about balance.

Inflammation from the immune system's antibody production protecting us from macromolecules of foods that get into the bloodstream causes tears in the blood-brain barrier; the most notorious are wheat and dairy.[6] In fact, inflammation stemming from many sources, including bacterial parasites, viral parasites, or autoimmune diseases, can tear the blood-brain barrier as well. Even proteins that are exposed to sugar and become overheated, crisping the tissue, such as the crust of bread or the surface of crème brûlée, produce a new molecule called advanced glycation end products (AGEs), which will also tear the cheesecloth in the gut and the brain, producing B4.[7] This is important to know, because every time you eat charred meats or barbecued chicken, the blackened coating you eat might be causing small tears in your brain.

Usually, the blood-brain barrier heals quickly, within 4 hours.[8] But if there is a recurring insult, B4 will remain, allowing macromolecules to penetrate the very sensitive brain. As a result, the glial cells of the usually calm immune system in the brain become overactivated to protect you and are continually firing their bazookas, which may create a whole lot of collateral damage. With the collateral damage, your immune system creates antibodies to eliminate the damaged cells, as well as antibodies to the macromolecules that got through the blood-brain barrier in the first place. Both of these types of antibodies are really big—much larger than what should be allowed to get through the blood-brain barrier. So just by definition, when you have elevated antibodies to the blood-brain barrier, you have a problem, and you're fueling the inflammatory cascade in the brain.

With a simple blood test, you'll be able to identify where you are on the B4 scale. Two of the biomarkers used in emergency rooms for severe trauma to the blood-brain barrier are called S100B[9] and neuron-specific enolase (NSE).[10] If they are elevated, it means that you're leaking S100B and NSE into your bloodstream. If you have high levels of S100B and/or NSE in your bloodstream long-term (for instance, as a result of playing soccer or football regularly), your body will make antibodies to them in order to get rid of the excess. When you have elevated antibodies to S100B and NSE, it strongly suggests that you have an ongoing tearing of your blood-brain barrier. These are extremely accurate biomarkers that show up with damage to the blood-brain barrier from any cause, not just physical trauma. They identify that the floodgates are open, allowing macromolecules into the brain, which then will activate the immune response, causing the inflammation that eventually manifests as brain fog, forgetfulness, ADHD, seizures, anxiety, depression, schizophrenia, bipolar disorder, and eventually dementia, Parkinson's, MS, and Alzheimer's.

Any tissue in the brain may be affected once you're suffering from B4. How you've lived your life, what toxins you have been exposed to and where they deposit, and your genetics determine your weak link, and that's the disease you will be vulnerable to eventually manifesting. The only difference is where the molecular mimicry is located. If the A-A-B-C-D from wheat looks similar to your cerebellum, you will have elevated antibodies to cerebellum, which will destroy cerebellar tissue and eventually cause signs of cerebellar degeneration (like elders who can no longer "two-step" up or down the stairs).[11] If the A-A-B-C-D from dairy looks similar to your myelin, you may make elevated antibodies to myelin, which will destroy myelin tissue and eventually cause signs of myelin degeneration (numbness and tingling) with a loss of motor function eventually manifesting as MS. If the molecular mimicry is to the toxic chemical bisphenol A (found in plastic water bottles, plastic wrap, storage containers, and to-go coffee lids, etc.), you may make elevated antibodies to a variety of different parts of your brain.[12] If the molecular mimicry is to corn, tomato, spinach, soy, or tobacco, you may make elevated antibodies to cells in the nerves of your brain and eyes called aquaporin-4, and here come vision problems along with brain dysfunction.[13]

The mechanism is very similar for most, if not all, chronic brain dysfunction. First you get B4. Then a toxin you are exposed to stimulates a response from the immune system to protect you (elevated antibodies to that substance), and those toxins look enough like your own tissue that the antibodies attack your tissue. When this goes on long enough, the attacked tissue cannot function normally anymore, and then here come your symptoms, usually mild at first, but getting progressively worse.

Whether you are worried about your child with attention-deficit disorder, your mother with memory loss, or your own constant brain fa-

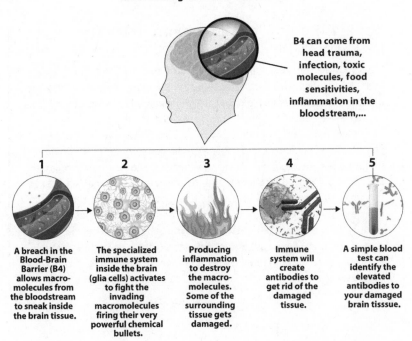

B4: Breaching the Blood-Brain Barrier

B4 can come from head trauma, infection, toxic molecules, food sensitivities, inflammation in the bloodstream,...

1 A breach in the Blood-Brain Barrier (B4) allows macro-molecules from the bloodstream to sneak inside the brain tissue.

2 The specialized immune system inside the brain (glia cells) activates to fight the invading macromolecules firing their very powerful chemical bullets.

3 Producing inflammation to destroy the macro-molecules. Some of the surrounding tissue gets damaged.

4 Immune system will create antibodies to get rid of the damaged tissue.

5 A simple blood test can identify the elevated antibodies to your damaged brain tisssue.

tigue, addressing this mechanism will lead to healing, regeneration, and improving function of the brain. Identifying what caused you to fall in the water and eventually go downstream and over the waterfall into the pool of symptoms below is the first step. What was the A-A-B-C-D? Was it mercury, wheat, dairy, toxic air? What has accumulated in your body that is causing the inflammation in your brain?

In order to stop the insanity of just taking drugs for symptoms, hoping your life jacket is going to keep you from drowning (i.e., symptoms getting worse), we must first identify if you are suffering from B4 and then follow the protocols in this book that will create the environment to restore the blood-brain barrier, stop the leakage of crud into the brain, and calm down the inflammatory cascade. This is the foundational tenet for reversing Alzheimer's and other brain-deteriorating conditions. Identifying the triggers, eliminating them, and creating the right environment for optimal neural regeneration is the path for restoring brain health.

> ### DR. TOM'S TIP
> ### SCREENING FOR THE TRIGGERS OF BRAIN INFLAMMATION
>
> Have your doctor order the Neural Zoomer blood test from Vibrant Wellness laboratories. This cutting-edge test is the most sensitive biomarker of brain antibodies available today. It includes all 6 of the most important categories to set a benchmark for: demyelination (the condition of your nerves in your brain, related to MS), the blood-brain barrier, peripheral neuropathies (numbness and tingling), brain autoimmunity (antibodies to brain tissue), herpes (there are more than 100 studies connecting herpes simplex 1 and Alzheimer's), and the genes for Alzheimer's. I believe this test is a game-changer. It can identify, years in advance, the ongoing mechanisms that can cause degenerative brain diseases. When you can identify the mechanism before there is so much tissue damage that symptoms appear, you have a window of opportunity to do something about it.
>
> If your doctor can't get the test, or is reluctant to order it, go to my Web site, theDr.com/neuralzoomer, where you can order the test yourself.

HYPOPERFUSION MEANS REDUCED BLOODFLOW

The effect of your heart function on your brain is profound. We know that the heart actually sends more signals to the brain than the brain sends to the heart. These signals regulate bloodflow to and away from the brain. Imagine that you have two garden hoses coming up from the neck into the brain: Those are your carotid arteries. Those hoses are connected to lawn sprinklers that distribute blood to the entire brain. Just as you need to soak your lawn in the summer to have lush, green grass, we need to soak our brains to have luscious brain function. In fact, the quantity and quality of the blood flowing to the brain determine how well your brain works.

Bloodflow is called *perfusion;* when you have a lack of bloodflow, it's called *hypo,* or low, perfusion. When *hypoperfusion* occurs in the brain, it creates B4.[14] When you have a lack of bloodflow into the brain, it creates inflammation all by itself, and you can start killing off the brain's nerve tissue. The messages sent from one neuron to another can get lost or dropped, causing brain dysfunction (as in "Where are my keys?"). If the back of the brain isn't getting enough blood, people may get seizures. If it occurs in the front of the brain, you are more prone to depression and anxiety.

In a 2009 study in *BMC Pediatrics*, researchers found a common link between a lack of cerebral bloodflow and children with autism, using a SPECT study that looks at bloodflow into the brain. In the study, 75 percent of the kids with autism had a lack of bloodflow into their brain. But what was even more interesting was that for each area of the brain where there was a lack of bloodflow, the symptom was different: The anatomical location of the lack of bloodflow significantly correlates with certain behaviors. For example, 30 of the children had hypoperfusion in the part of their brain called the thalamus, and those were the children exhibiting repetitive behavior patterns, a hallmark of autism. Twenty-three more

DR. TOM'S TIP
WHAT HYPOPERFUSION FEELS LIKE

Imagine this as an example of hypoperfusion. If you're sitting down, cross your legs. Leave them like that for 3 hours. Now stand up and run. You just can't. There's not enough blood getting to your legs.

If you feed your gluten-sensitive child toast for breakfast and then send her to school to learn, she just can't. There's not enough blood getting into her brain for it to function properly. That's why, within 6 months of going gluten-free, every celiac child who was also diagnosed with ADHD reported significant improvement (that's a geek's way of saying OMG) in all 12 markers of ADHD: fails to pay attention, interrupts frequently, blurts out answers, can't sit still, etc.[15]

Given that the primary symptom pattern for people with a sensitivity to wheat is brain dysfunction, now we understand that a primary trigger for this dysfunction is linked to the fact that 73 percent of all celiacs have hypoperfusion. The other ones are not exactly lucky: Their weak link in their chain (where their symptoms are going to manifest) is in other tissues of the body.

DR. TOM'S AT-HOME BIOMARKERS

Here's an example of how a dysfunction in the body can be a signal that there is also a dysfunction in your brain. Heart dysfunction and heart disease, as well as the medications necessary for treating them, are among the culprits that cause hypoperfusion in the brain. When you're walking up stairs and you're out of breath, this may be an early clue that there's a dysfunction not only with your cardiovascular system but also with your brain.

children had hypoperfusion of the right temporal lobes, which correlated with an obsessive desire for sameness: the need to wear the same shirt all the time, or to use only one particular bathroom, which is another hallmark of autism. Forty-five other children had hypoperfusion of the left temporal lobe, which associated with impairments in social interaction and communication, another hallmark of autism. These were the kids with the most severe autistic behavior.[16]

If you are wondering where the hypoperfusion came from, look at the same likely suspects we've been talking about. For example, food sensitivities can also cause hypoperfusion throughout the brain. Although this can occur in any gluten-sensitive person, 73 percent of celiacs have hypoperfusion. And the average number of locations is 4 out of 12 areas of the brain: That's one-third of your brain that can't work optimally because it's starving for all the good things it's supposed to get from blood, like oxygen, glucose, and amino acids (the building blocks of new cells), among others. However, in a study of patients with celiac disease, within 1 year of following a wheat-free diet, all but one person had their bloodflow return to normal, and symptoms of brain dysfunction went away.[17] This occurred because their immune systems were no longer making antibodies to wheat, the inflammation returned to normal levels, and bloodflow increased.

Hypoperfusion may also be caused by a variety of behaviors and illnesses,[18] including:

- Allergic reactions
- Anaphylactic shock

- Blood donation
- Dehydration
- Depression
- Diabetes
- Diarrhea
- Diuretics
- Emotional stress
- Fatigue
- Fear
- Head trauma
- Heart dysfunction
- Heart medications
- Hemorrhage
- Jaundice
- Prolonged bed rest
- Severe burns
- Snake bite
- Surgery
- Toxic shock syndrome
- Trauma
- Vomiting

NEO-EPITOPES: THE EARLIEST RECOGNITION OF BEING ON THE AUTOIMMUNE SPECTRUM

A very common trigger to the immune system fueling the autoimmune cascade in the brain is the production of *neo-epitopes*. These occur when an outside compound sticks to your tissue and forms a completely new compound. For example, imagine you've left a water bottle in your car on a hot day. When you get back in the car, you're as thirsty as can be. You grab the water bottle, take a few big gulps, and immediately know that the water tastes different, a little like plastic. The taste is likely the chemicals in the plastic itself that have leached into the water as a result of the heat. You likely just swallowed a little bisphenol A, more commonly known as BPA.

Now, BPA is a nasty accumulative toxin. It's a synthetic that's used widely in many forms, including plastic food containers, toys, baby pacifiers, medical products, the lining of tin cans, coffee cup lids, and even thermal receipts. It binds onto human protein throughout the body and forms a neo-epitope, a new (neo) poison to our body. BPA is an endocrine (hormone) disruptor and has the potential to impact fetal, child, and adult

Common Dietary Lectins and Agglutinins That Bind to Different Body Tissues and Cells

Human cells lectins can bind to (and form neo-epitopes)	WGA	SBA	PNA	LA	MA	TA	PA	POT.A	KBA+JBA
Skin	✓	✓	✓	✓				✓	✓
Lining of the nose and back of the throat	✓								
Inside lining of the mouth	✓	✓	✓	✓					
Stomach	✓								
Parietal cells (producers of hydrochloric acid)		✓	✓			✓			
Intestinal inside lining (brush border)	✓	✓				✓			✓
Inside lining of the large intestine	✓			✓					
Connective tissue	✓			✓			✓		✓
Thyroid	✓	✓		✓				✓	✓
Cartilage	✓	✓	✓						
Liver	✓	✓	✓						✓
Pancreas	✓				✓				✓
Kidney	✓		✓					✓	✓
Prostate	✓		✓	✓					
Skeletal muscle	✓	✓	✓				✓		
Cardiac muscle	✓	✓							
Breast	✓	✓	✓						
Pituitary			✓						
Eye	✓	✓	✓				✓		✓
Brain (myelin)	✓			✓					✓

Abbreviations: WGA, wheat germ agglutinin; SBA, soy bean agglutinin; PNA, peanut agglutinin; LA, lentil agglutinin; MA, mushroom agglutinin; TA, tomato agglutinin; PA, pea agglutinin; POT.A, potato agglutinin; KBA, kidney bean agglutinin; JBA, jack bean agglutinin.

DR. TOM'S TIP
A BIOMARKER FOR LECTINS

Lectins are peptides of partially digested wheat and other foods that are notorious for binding onto tissue and forming neo-epitopes. This is a major culprit when a wheat sensitivity causes the autoimmune mechanism to begin. Have your doctor check your lectin antibody levels by ordering a test from Cyrex Labs (Array 10). If your doctor can't get the test, or is reluctant to order it, go to my Web site, theDr.com/Cyrex10, where you can order the test yourself.

health. The BPA chemical has been found to bind to hormone receptors for estrogen and testosterone, creating a neo-epitope, which drastically interferes with the normal function of that receptor. What does that mean? Guys, low testosterone, erectile dysfunction, low sperm count, unable to impregnate. Ladies, low or high estrogen, low or high progesterone, osteoporosis, breast cancers, and other hormone-related cancers.

One of the neo-epitopes that have been studied a great deal is the gliadin-transglutaminase complex, or the gliadin-transglutaminase neo-epitope. When you have elevated antibodies to this complex, you are on the path to developing celiac disease. The research tells us that it is the earliest marker of non-celiac gluten sensitivity (NCGS), meaning that you may be on the celiac spectrum, and is often identifiable 7 years before you develop the disease.[19] This gliadin-transglutaminase neo-epitope is a primary mechanism in the development of gluten-related disorders.

This is how it works: Different kinds of peptides of poorly digested food stick to your tissue and form a new compound called a neo-epitope. For instance, the lectins (a type of sugar-binding protein that attaches to the outside of your cells) and the agglutinins (a substance that causes particles to stick together) in wheat, soy, peanuts, lentils, mushrooms, potatoes, kidney beans, and jack beans frequently form neo-epitopes in different tissues throughout the body.[20] The graph on page 47 shows how each of these types of food binds to different tissues and creates neo-epitopes. This neo-epitope is not part of our body, and our immune system sees it as a foreign threat and goes after it. The immune system thinks, "*This thing that is sticking onto my thyroid or onto areas of my brain, or to my testicles, is not part of me; this is not my own tissue,*" so it makes antibodies to attack this new compound. If the lectins of peanuts bind onto your prostate, your immune system may make antibodies to your prostate. If the lectins of peanuts bind onto your breast cells, your immune system may make antibodies to your breast cells. Or to your pituitary gland, eyes, muscles, liver . . . just look at the chart. These will be the locations where you might eventually experience symptoms due to the inflammation from the antibodies attacking your tissue. And, if you keep eating the food that sticks onto your tissue, forming neo-epitopes, you will continue to make antibodies to that tissue. Here comes the inflammatory cascade, with the eventual tissue dysfunction, then symptoms, and eventually disease.

A FEW WORDS ABOUT LPS

One mechanism that decreases bloodflow to and from the heart is called *arteriosclerosis,* the plugging up of your pipes. Here's another example of your immune system trying to protect you. Many people have heard that LDL is the "bad cholesterol." That's not true. Oxidized LDL cholesterol is the "bad" cholesterol. LDL cholesterol is the raw material that makes up your thyroid hormone, estrogen, progesterone, serotonin, cortisol, and stress hormones. That's a primary reason why your liver makes extra LDL

DR. TOM'S TIP
A BIOMARKER FOR LPS

Exhaust from bacteria called lipopolysaccharides (LPS), and viruses such as Epstein-Barr or herpes simplex, can also bind to tissue and form neo-epitopes. We can check for many of the most common LPS now with a simple blood test. This tells us where to focus our attention. For example, have your doctor check for LPS antibodies by ordering a blood test from Vibrant Wellness called the Wheat Zoomer. If your doctor can't get the test, or is reluctant to order it, go to my Web site, theDr.com/wheatzoomer, where you can order the test yourself.

cholesterol—to supply the raw material to accommodate your hormone needs. Most of the statin drugs prescribed to reduce your cholesterol do so by shutting down your liver's ability to make LDL cholesterol. Now, how smart is it to take that kind of drug if in fact you need more estrogen, or thyroid hormone, or stress hormones?

Here's one of the positive functions of LDL cholesterol. Lipopolysaccharides (LPS) are a by-product of bacteria that should never get into the bloodstream, yet they often do due to a leaky gut.[21] One of the critical functions of LDL cholesterol that is not recognized by most health-care practitioners is that LDL is an antibacterial compound that binds to LPS and makes the LPS less dangerous by forming an LDL/LPS neo-epitope. This is one of many reasons why your LDL cholesterol may be elevated: It increases in order to protect you from LPS.

When the LDL/LPS neo-epitope sticks to and penetrates the blood vessel wall, your immune system, trying to protect you, attacks this neo-epitope by making antibodies to it. Now you have what doctors call oxidized LDL; this is the bad guy in terms of cholesterol. The inflammation produced in this protective mechanism creates foam cells that then accumulate inside the blood vessel walls, and the blood vessel begins to swell.[22] As the blood vessels swell, your pipes plug up and bloodflow is constricted. As blockage in your blood vessels increases, the arteries become more rigid, and your heart has to work much harder to push the blood out. Here comes high blood pressure. This process slowly and silently builds

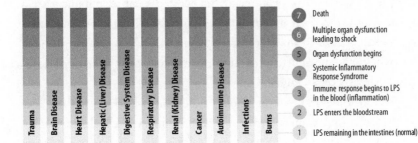

LPS in the intestines is a minimal threat to our health and is usually eliminated with the bowel movements. The greater the amount of LPS that gets through the intestines into the bloodstream, the greater the degree of responding inflammation, then tissue damage, then tissue dysfunction, then organ dysfunction leading to eventual death.

> ## DR. TOM'S TIP
> ### IDENTIFYING SEPSIS
>
> You can remember the symptoms of sepsis with the following mnemonic device:
>
> S—Shivering, fever, or very cold
> E—Extreme pain or general discomfort ("worst ever")
> P—Pale or discolored skin
> S—Sleepy, difficult to rouse, confused
> I—"I feel like I might die"
> S—Shortness of breath walking up stairs or uphill
>
> If you suspect sepsis (because you observe a combination of these symptoms), see your doctor immediately and say, "I am concerned about a systemic bacterial infection."

over time, until one day you have your blood pressure checked, and your doctor tells you that you've had a wake-up call and it's time to take blood pressure medication. Now you understand that LDL wasn't bad at all; it was just trying to protect you. The real culprit in this example was high levels of LPS in the bloodstream. Reducing LPS levels is how many functional medicine practitioners reduce and eventually eliminate the need for blood pressure medications for their patients.

LPS is particularly dangerous because when it gets into the bloodstream, having passed through the walls of the intestines, it's now categorized as an *endotoxin,* a toxin inside the body. The entire immune system reacts, causing systemic inflammation. And if there is a high enough concentration of LPS in the bloodstream, you can develop *sepsis,* the body's overwhelming and life-threatening response to a toxin that can lead to tissue damage, organ failure, or death.

The following information is going to be a little shocking, but I believe it's critically important: Sepsis from LPS infiltration killed my mother, and I do not want this to happen to you. LPS getting into the bloodstream strikes in unique and unexpected ways. The chart below demonstrates this. For instance, it is linked to periodontal disease: In one 2013 study, 100 percent of the participants who had a root canal tested positively for having LPS in the bloodstream.[23]

Even in otherwise healthy individuals, LPS moves fast. The damage will start at your weak link and spread throughout the body in what's known as multiple organ dysfunction syndrome (MODS).[24] Sepsis is the leading cause of death in US hospitals, killing 258,000 Americans every year, but not before it has negatively impacted brain health with conditions like hallucinations, delirium, and loss of cognitive function. This is a tragedy that almost always begins with and is fueled by LPS jetting through a leaky gut into a leaky brain.[25]

MEET THE MACAQUE MONKEYS

Scientists love to observe macaque monkeys, because they have a very similar intestinal tract to ours. They were used to develop the successful protocols that today allow people with HIV infections to live normal lives. But what's even more interesting about them is that within their species, there are different types of macaques, and each has a unique signature based on their digestion. Just like humans, some macaque monkeys are more likely to have diarrhea than others. In three laboratories across the globe, it was independently found that 51 percent of pigtail macaques have intestinal permeability, compared to 11 percent of rhesus macaque monkeys. To find

---

DR. TOM'S AT-HOME BIOMARKERS

Food sensitivities are a very common cause of systemic fluid retention. Have you ever noticed sock marks on your legs that weren't there earlier in the day? Or marks from your undergarments? It's certainly possible that you are wearing clothes that are too tight, but it's unlikely. It's more likely a sign that you're eating foods that are causing water retention, which, in an effort to protect you, is diluting the toxicity of those foods. The sock marks are a biomarker that something's in your system that is causing your body to react, and the most likely suspect is food sensitivities. The elimination diet we'll talk about in Chapter 9 will help you figure out which foods are causing this problem.

out why, researchers studied their epithelial borders, the inside lining of their intestines.[26] For an unknown reason, the pigtail macaque monkey has a leaky gut, while the rhesus macaque monkey does not. Because of the intestinal permeability, the pigtail macaques have loads of LPS traveling throughout their bodies, and consequently high levels of systemic inflammation, even in their brains, while rhesus macaques do not.

The pigtail macaques can't change their diet and heal their leaky gut, but we can. If we heal intestinal permeability, which you'll learn more about in the next chapter, you will reduce your LPS infiltration, which then lowers systemic inflammation throughout the body and the brain. This is another example of fix your body, fix your brain.

REDEFINING ALZHEIMER'S

Alzheimer's disease (AD) is a great example of the brain's relationship to autoimmunity, and one we'll use throughout the book because there is so much research available. According to the Alzheimer's Association, Alzheimer's disease is a specific type of dementia that causes problems with memory, thinking, and behavior serious enough to interfere with daily life. Symptoms usually develop slowly and get worse over time. The most common early symptom is difficulty remembering newly learned information, because the physical changes associated with the disease typically affect the hippocampus, the part of the brain that is responsible for short-term memory. As Alzheimer's advances through the brain, it leads to increasingly severe symptoms, including disorientation and confusion; mood and behavior changes; unfounded suspicions about family, friends, and professional caregivers; difficulty speaking, swallowing, and walking; and, ultimately, death. It is the third most common cause of death in the United States: For women the chance of developing AD is now greater than the chance of developing breast cancer.[27]

Alzheimer's is not a normal part of aging, although the majority of people with Alzheimer's are 65 or older, and we often think about it as a disease of old age. Yet approximately 200,000 Americans under the age of 65 have early-onset Alzheimer's. While there is no single known cause of Alzheimer's disease (and no known drug to arrest or cure it), there are hundreds of studies that point to antigens as a trigger, and these range from gluten to bacteria to the herpes virus. What unites all of them is a common presentation of B4.[28]

Alzheimer's disease can be positively diagnosed only on autopsy. There are two structures that are usually present in the brain of AD patients: *plaques* and *tangles*. Plaques are deposits of a protein fragment called *beta-amyloid* that build up in the spaces between neurons. Tangles are twisted fibers of another protein that build up inside neuronal cells. Scientists do not know exactly what role plaques and tangles play in Alzheimer's disease, but most experts believe they play a critical role in blocking communication among nerve cells.

Remember in the old movies when there's a building on fire, and 100 people stand in line, moving buckets from one person to the next? That's the way your neurons work. Each neuron passes on the chemical message it received from the one it's connected to. This happens again and again. If one person steps out of the line, it's difficult to move the bucket forward. At the beginning of brain dysfunction, you lose this ability to move the message from one neuron to the next. For you, it might look like something as benign as wondering, "Where are my keys?" If two people step out of line, it's almost impossible to move the bucket forward. In the brain, the message has stopped, and you might experience a blank moment or a slower reaction time, such as running a red light "accidentally" because you didn't respond to the yellow light fast enough. But when you kill off more neurons, or when there is a buildup of beta-amyloid plaques inside your brain, the neurons find it increasingly difficult to communicate with one another, and they can't pass the bucket along (now, for example, you might wonder, "What are keys for?"). That's being on the Alzheimer's spectrum, which eventually will develop into Alzheimer's disease.

We also know that the development of beta-amyloid is an immune function trying to protect you; it doesn't just "come out of nowhere." Beta-amyloid is the exhaust of an immune reaction, and we know this because beta-amyloid plaques are loaded with antibodies to various antigens (LPS, bacteria, toxic peptides of poorly digested food, viruses, etc.). For example, a very common antigen in beta-amyloid plaque is IgM antibodies to the herpes virus. What does this mean to you? If you get occasional cold sores, you are carrying the herpes virus, and your immune system is not always able to keep it in check. You see a cold sore on your lip when your internal immune system is unable to contain the virus and it starts to grow externally. It is likely that most of us have herpes virus in us: That's the price of living in our toxic world. However, if it grows unchecked because of a compromised immune system, here come the cold sores. Now you are at risk for B4 letting the herpes virus enter the brain, which would then activate the immune system and start creating those beta-amyloid plaques.[29]

Remember, there are more than 100 studies connecting herpes simplex 1 and Alzheimer's, and this is the mechanism: An activated immune system trying to protect you produces beta-amyloid plaques. That's quite an unintentional consequence, but one you need to know about. Now that you know, you can take action. By reading this book, you'll be able to identify if you currently have B4, and you can start taking the steps to heal the blood-brain barrier. Also, you'll need to stop those cold sores in their tracks by strengthening your immune system.

MEET DALE BREDESEN

My friend Dr. Dale Bredesen is internationally recognized as an expert in the mechanisms of neurodegenerative diseases such as Alzheimer's. He was a happy laboratory researcher for many years (a fellow geek) and told me that he never thought he'd be working with patients, but his work has become so impactful that he can no longer stand by and not help people reverse this deadly disease.

Since then, he has identified five separate categories of brain degeneration caused by more than 50 mechanisms (up from the original 37 he found in 2014) that contribute to the inflammation and the tissue destruction in Alzheimer's. He has also shown that the disease can be reversible if you address these causes. It took 5 years for his first set of dedicated patients to achieve great results reversing their cognitive decline, but what is more important to stay focused on than getting your brain back?

For example, a mold infestation in your house may cause B4. You breathe the air in your house, and the mold molecules get into your brain. If you have a gluten sensitivity, that may cause B4 and the gluten molecules get into your brain. Head traumas may cause B4, and the macromolecules in your bloodstream from a leaky gut get into your brain. If you have a bacterial infection or LPS in your bloodstream, that may cause B4, and the LPS gets into your brain. In all of these examples, your immune system inside the blood-brain barrier activates glial cells, which fire their bazookas in an effort to protect you. The beta-amyloid plaques are the exhaust of the glial cells attacking the mold, or gluten, or bacteria, or virus. Now here comes the collateral damage from this bazooka action, and the autoimmune response in your brain is initiated. This is why it is so important to check brain antibody levels. Do I have B4? Do I have antibodies to myelin? Do I have antibodies to my cerebellum? These types of biomarkers, which we'll talk about in Chapter 5, are critical to give you a "heads-up" if there is damage occurring in your brain right now. Because according to Dr. Bredesen, that damage will eventually lead to enough tissue dysfunction that you will have Alzheimer's. It's a step-by-step progression.

We have to take a functional medicine approach to uncovering how all of the potential causes are affecting you. When you walk into your house after returning from vacation, do you have to open your windows to air it out? That dank smell is likely a mold infestation. Do you have a gluten sensitivity? Do you have a dairy sensitivity? Do you sleep at least 7 to 8 hours a night? Do you exercise every day?

In his first study, Dr. Bredesen reversed Alzheimer's in 9 out of 10 people over the course of 5 years. These individuals are back to work, or back to living with their families. Now, 3 years later, he has more than 100 patients who have shown similar reversals.

All of Dr. Bredesen's work has been done with people who are already suffering with cognitive decline and Alzheimer's disease: They had cascaded far down the river and over the waterfall and into the pool of the autoimmune spectrum. The key to their successes has been reducing the inflammation in the brain and limiting the production of unnecessary antibodies. His work is a great example of how beneficial it is to calm down inflammation and allow the brain to heal itself. But you can do more. You don't have to wait until you have cognitive decline. Through proper testing, you can identify what is going on at a much earlier point on the spectrum and then initiate the proper protocols you'll learn about in this book. You'll be able to get out of the turbulent waters of brain dysfunction before you ever need a life jacket.

ACTION STEP WEEK 2: READ ABOUT DR. DALE BREDESEN'S RESULTS AND SHARE THEM WITH YOUR DOCTOR

Dr. Dale Bredesen's research and clinical practice with AD patients confirms the idea that there is no single cause of this terrible disease. In fact, in his 2014 landmark article, "Reversal of Cognitive Decline: A Novel Therapeutic Program," he identified 37 different mechanisms.[30] I consider this article so important that I'm providing here the link for you to download the article for free: www.theDr.com/bredesen. Read this so you can understand the results of his work, and take it to your doctor when you have your next physical.

3

A GREAT BRAIN
BEGINS IN YOUR GUT

WHILE THE BRAIN is involved in all bodily behaviors, surprisingly, it's the gastrointestinal tract, or the gut, that is in charge of the brain. We've known for almost 20 years that the gut has a role in modulating mood and thinking: It was in 1999 that Dr. Michael Gershon showed us in his book, *The Second Brain,* that the gut has its hands on the steering wheel of our brain. In this chapter, you'll learn the reasons why anytime you're dealing with a brain problem, the first place you most often have to look is the gut. A healthy gut is what makes it possible for us to have clear conscious thoughts. The reverse also applies: When you feel down in the dumps, you'll address your gut. When you want your brain to function better, pay attention to your gut.

Probably the most important lesson in this chapter is that the relationship between the gut and the brain is *bi-directional:* The gut sends messages to the brain, and the brain sends messages to the gut. This is one reason why when we feel stressed, we can have an upset stomach, or why digestive issues can cause us to feel stressed. You'll even learn the important connection between a poor attitude and poor health—what I call stinking thinking—and why it comes from the gut.[1]

THE ANATOMY OF THE GUT

The origin of a leaky brain is often a leaky gut. To understand the entire mechanism, you need a bit of gut knowledge, starting with how it works. The gut is an organ system that covers every aspect of digestion. Imagine your gut is one big, long tube—a 20- to 25-foot-long tube that starts at your mouth and goes to the other end. After you swallow food, the food starts its journey through the tube. The food has to be broken down into very small pieces (digestion) to fit through the lining inside the tube (absorption) in order to get into the bloodstream, where your body will use the smaller particles as the raw materials to make new cells. Some of the food we eat takes a long time to be broken down (prime rib is tougher to digest than a banana, for example) before it can be absorbed. That's a main reason why the digestive tract is 20 to 25 feet long.

The intestines are where the hard work of digestion takes place. They are lined with *microvilli*, microscopic cellular membrane bulges that increase the surface area of the intestines and function as the primary surface of nutrient absorption. The microvilli look like shag carpeting. If we could flatten out the microvilli, the surface of our intestines would be the size of a doubles tennis court. We need that much surface in the gut because there's so much activity going on.

This next part is a little geeky, but bear with me; it's critically important to understand this as we "digest" where your health and vitality come from. The intestines are covered by the *intestinal epithelium*, a single layer of cells that separates the contents of the intestines from the body. The epithelium serves a few crucial functions:

- It acts as a barrier, preventing the entry of harmful substances such as antigens, toxins, and microorganisms into the bloodstream.

Like the blood-brain barrier, it's a cheesecloth that allows only small molecules to pass through into the bloodstream.

- It acts as a selective filter that helps the distribution of nutrients and various other beneficial substances from the intestines to the rest of the body.
- It acts as a relay switch for the messages coming from the good bacteria in your gut to the rest of your body.

The microvilli are packed with *digestive enzymes* that act like scissors, aiding in the breakdown of complex nutrients into simpler compounds that can go through the cheesecloth and are then more easily absorbed. Every function of every organ depends on these enzymes to manufacture molecules, produce energy, and create cell structures. Snip, snip, snip—that's the process of digestion. If your scissors are dull and can't break down your food small enough (poor digestion), you don't get the nutrients you need out of the tube and into your body.

Sometimes, this intestinal cheesecloth gets torn, primarily due to inflammation. When this happens, larger molecules, called *macromolecules,* pass through the cheesecloth and into the bloodstream. This is referred to as intestinal permeability, or a leaky gut. Exactly which materials "sneak through" depends on how leaky someone's leaky gut happens to be.

THE IMMUNE SYSTEM OF THE GUT

Seventy percent of your entire immune system resides in the gut. The body is designed this way because the gut is where the greatest threat to our health comes through, every time you eat. You need the largest army in the right location so you can be protected.

When the gut is working well, and you feed it the right foods, digestion is efficient and effortless. Remember, some foods take longer to break down and digest than others; for example, it takes longer to digest a prime rib than it does a banana. If you have tears in your intestinal cheesecloth from other earlier exposures, big clumps of protein (macro-molecules) from the slowly digested prime rib will make it through the epithelial lining and get into your bloodstream before the proteins have been broken down in the intestines. The immune system recognizes these macromolecules as invaders and goes into instant defense mode, saying, "Whoa, what's this? I don't recognize it, so I better get rid of it." Now your body makes antibodies to beef. You develop a sensitivity to beef and any other macromolecule that penetrates the cheesecloth.

Even if you take an antacid and your stomach begins to feel better, you haven't addressed the tears in the cheesecloth. Further, antacids (also known as PPIs, or proton pump inhibitors) are the fourth most common medications prescribed today, yet they create havoc in the digestive tract.[2] Antacids dramatically reduce the production of hydrochloric acid (HCL). But HCL is good for you and necessary; too much HCL is not. The problem with PPIs is that they drastically reduce HCL, and the lack of HCL creates an environment that allows undesirable bacteria to flourish. When you have a gut overwhelmed with these undesirable bacteria, this is called *dysbiosis* (big Scrabble word). You might not notice it at all: It's as if you live in a moldy room but you don't notice the smell until the mold is overwhelming and your body can't compensate for it. The mold, however, is always there, affecting your lungs and your brain. A similar situation occurs in the gut with dysbiosis. You may not feel dysbiosis, but it's always there, affecting your gut and creating intestinal permeability. PPIs exacerbate dysbiosis, which causes intestinal permeability. A study from the Mayo Clinic tells us that even minor injuries to the intestinal mucosa can result in significant consequences, which may "seriously affect your health."[3]

If you take antacids for more than a few days, you're very likely creating a dysbiotic environment. However, you'll notice this problem only when there is so much damage to your gut that it becomes obvious: constipation, diarrhea, upset stomach, abdominal cramps, etc. And what do you do? Most people are told to take more antacids, which makes it worse. The vicious cycle begins:

"I feel bad" = take an antacid = create more dysbiosis = more tears in the cheesecloth = more macromolecules from other foods get through to the bloodstream = more activation of your immune system to protect you = more antibodies to different foods = more symptoms in or outside the gut = more antacids.

You never win in this very common scenario. Now, if you went to see a holistic, or integrative, or functional medicine doctor, she might order a 90-food blood test panel to see if your immune system identifies any foods as a problem. Lo and behold, the test results come back and show that you're "allergic" to 18 foods. You respond, "OMG, that's everything I eat."

Well, of course it is; your immune system is trying to protect you. However, the food you're eating is not necessarily the problem. You have tears in your cheesecloth, technically called pathogenic intestinal permeability. It's not the foods that are necessarily bad for you in the big picture (you do have to stop eating them for a while to calm down the immune protective mechanism); it's the leaky gut allowing macromolecules to get through that has to be fixed.

Here's the bottom line: When you eat something and feel anything less than perfect, your body's talking to you. It's telling you that some type of reaction is occurring and you need to pay attention. Are you feeling tired? Do you have a headache? The investigation of "why" begins with what you put in your mouth. Now that you understand this, I hope it's clear why what's on the end of your fork can be connected to any health complaint, and that every protocol you initiate must include making sure your gut is functioning adequately. Every system of your body improves when your gut functions more normally. And when you fix your body, you'll fix your brain. Your outlook on life improves, and so does your productivity. You'll have more energy (and sleep better), you'll be able to respond more quickly to life's challenges, your memory and attention will come back, and you will live a more vital life.

THE GUT'S MICROBIOME

Your state of mind is to a large degree controlled by your individualized output of brain hormones. But here's the big surprise: Your brain hormones are controlled by microbes—the bacteria, fungi, and viruses that live in your gut. The microvilli are covered in bacteria, packed in between each of the shags. There are millions and millions of bacteria in the gut, almost 10 times more than all the cells in the entire human body.

This community of microbes is called your gut's *microbiome* and is now thought to influence the entire body. We actually host many different microbiomes in and on our body. There is a microbiome of the skin and in each of our organs. In fact, if a woman has breast cancer, the breast with the cancer will have a different microbiome compared to the noncancerous breast.

The gut's microbiome can weigh up to 5 pounds—nearly twice as much as the brain—and each microbe within it is a living organism made up of cells and genes. There are about 23,000 genes in the human genome (our DNA). When genes turn on, they command the body to take an action, to do something. It doesn't matter if it's a human gene or a bacteria gene. If a bacteria gene turns on, it tells your gut to make a protein, to create an enzyme, to cause inflammation, to cause less inflammation—depending on the bacteria.

A primary function of the gut's microbiome is the development, regulation, and maintenance of the intestinal barrier. It is also linked to manufacturing vitamins, regulating metabolism and blood sugar, influencing genetic expression, and affecting brain chemical production. And because there are 100 to 150 times more bacterial genes in the microbiome than the human genome, they issue more orders than our own DNA, and therefore have a greater influence over our health.

We each host a completely unique microbiome that is influenced by our genetics, our antecedents (how we've lived our life), our environment, and our dietary selections. The vast majority of bacteria harbored in the gut's microbiome are thought to have beneficial effects, and while there are many different types of bacteria, they predominantly fall into two big groups. The

Bacteroidetes are the "good" bacteria and should be the dominant group that we host. The second group is the Firmicutes, and while they aren't dangerous, in high concentrations they can overwhelm the Bacteroidetes and take over. When the intestines contain the right balance of good and bad bacteria, our gut is in a state of *symbiosis*. An imbalance of the microbiome is referred to as *dysbiosis* and is a primary source of inflammation in the gut and throughout your body. A noticeable symptom of dysbiosis is fatigue.

Your immune cells in the gut sit on the same surface as your microbiome and are heavily influenced by it. In fact, the microbiome modulates, or controls, how immune cells operate much the same way the microbiome influences your brain hormone production. It takes many different parts to make your car move on down the road. The "primary control" is the part that has its hands on the steering wheel. Like it or not, feel the problem or not, your microbiome modulates (hands on the steering wheel) every body function.

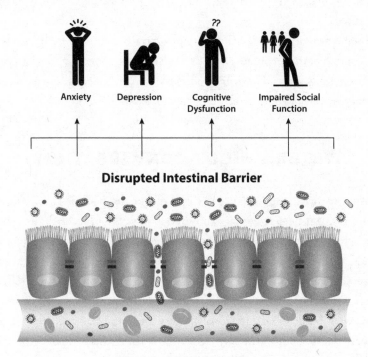

Where's the Weak Link in Your Brain?

The composition of the microbiome—based on the food you eat—can shape a healthy immune response or predispose you to disease.[4] An imbalanced microbiome creates an inflammatory environment that will create intestinal permeability, or a leaky gut. When it comes to the brain, a leaky gut can cause low-grade inflammation and affect brain hormone production, which leads to depression, anxiety, cognitive dysfunction, and impaired social function.[5] It increases inflammation throughout the brain and the body, which then increases our risk for Alzheimer's, anxiety, memory loss, brain fog, and mood swings. It also creates an environment for molecular mimicry, where antibodies attack the brain in areas that are molecularly similar to the offending foods.

If you take drugs to treat your depression, you may feel better because you are chemically overriding your brain hormone imbalance. These medications are great life jackets. If you need the drugs, take them. However, you'll still be sloshing against the inner turbulence of the waterfall. You haven't addressed the issue that caused the hormonal imbalance in the first place.

The microbiome also has a direct impact on B4: The intestinal and the blood-brain barriers contain some of the same components, and when you develop a leaky gut and have antibodies to your gut barrier, those antibodies can also attack your blood-brain barrier, leading to B4.

THE BRAIN-GUT CONVERSATION

In order to reach the ladder and climb out of the pool of autoimmune symptoms, you have to understand exactly how the brain and gut communicate. Think of the brain as a police chief who is in charge of all commands to the different precincts (your hormone production). The gut microbiota is the mayor of the city that contains the police precincts. The mayor modulates the police chief, telling him what to focus on, and explains what needs to be done to keep everyone in the city safe. This is true of every department in the city—the mayor always has his hands on the steering wheel.

For every message from the brain (the police chief) that goes down to the gut's microbiome (the mayor), there are nine messages from the gut going up to the brain: Remember, the brain and gut have a bi-directional relationship. These messages influence the brain's response to stressful situations, brain hormone production, the activation of the brain's immune system, the growth of new brain cells (neurogenesis), and the adaptability of these new cells to learn (neuroplasticity).

The foods you eat profoundly influence the microbiota, and its influence is evident in just 1 day. Thus, the messages from the microbiota to the brain can be changed just as quickly. The bacteria in the microbiome help your enzymes digest amino acids from the foods you eat and convert them into the different brain hormones, or neurotransmitters, our bodies need. These brain hormones control how the brain works, from brain speed (which is associated with attention) to mood to metabolism. If you get depressed or feel anxious, you are experiencing a neurotransmitter imbalance that started in your gut. In fact, 90 percent of all the serotonin (a critical hormone associated with mood and social behavior, appetite and digestion, sleep, memory, and sexual desire and function) you make is stored and produced in your gut, not in your brain.

STRESS IS A BI-DIRECTIONAL CHAT BETWEEN THE BRAIN AND THE GUT

Dysbiosis can also be caused by physical stress, which can range from environmental exposures like pollution, chemicals, and radiation, to the stresses of our everyday lives. And now the science is clearer than ever that the microbiota of the gut has its hands on the steering wheel and controls the entire relationship of how our bodies respond to the stress of life.[6] Here's how it works: The microbiota sends chemical messengers to the brain along the spinal cord and through the bloodstream. These messages instruct the hypothalamus how to respond to perceived stress. The hypothalamus tells the pituitary gland which stressors are the priorities, and the pituitary gland then sends messages telling the organs what hormones to produce.

For example, *Akkermansia* is a type of bacteria found in the intestines. It is considered one of the "good" bacteria, and if you are deficient in it, you're at much greater risk to develop type 1 diabetes and obesity. Stress hormones such as cortisol and the catecholamines epinephrine and norepinephrine will reduce your *Akkermansia* levels.

Suppose the first draft of your new book is due in 4 weeks (STRESS), and there is a tremendous amount that still needs to be done (STRESS). Your publisher has emphasized the critical nature of submitting it on time (STRESS), as there are a number of different departments that have blocked off the time to do their thing on the book and keep it moving through the process, making sure to have it out before the holidays (STRESS) (because it will make a great gift for someone you love:-)). You're up every day at 4:30 (STRESS); working all day until the brain starts blithering out what just doesn't make sense anymore (STRESS), and there's no time to shop for food (STRESS), thus you're living mostly on canned sardines with salad dressing and chopped fermented pickles on rice cakes (yum J). One of your staff who has been with you the longest just had a parent suddenly die in a traumatic fall (STRESS). You're supposed to be on stage tomorrow giving a talk on "Living a Healthy Lifestyle," and the presentation is not prepared yet (STRESS).

When you pause for a moment and reflect, you realize that all of these are First World problems. You have plenty of food and water; there's a nice roof over your head; everyone you love is happy and relatively healthy; and this book is the work you've always dreamt of doing. Suddenly a big smile comes across your face, visions of angels beaming down on you, the stress hormones calm down and are replaced by the feel-good endorphins produced in the brain from deep belly laughter or meditation, and all is well in the world.

If your microbiota is out of balance (low *Akkermansia*), the anxiety you woke up with won't go away and might even increase while you work all day. If you don't have the support in your gut needed to keep your brain calm (the right microbiota), the severity of the stress response is 2.8-fold higher, maintaining and reinforcing the stress hormones. But as you strengthen your microbiota by making better food choices, including eating the fermented foods listed in Chapter 9, your emotional resiliency increases. Base hit by base hit. Pickle by fermented pickle.

MEET MICHAEL MAES

Michael Maes, MD, PhD, is a psychiatrist who recognized 20 years ago that inflammation is a critical component in patients healing from emotional and cognitive problems. He was one of the first to connect inflammation in the brain, caused by intestinal permeability in the gut, with chronic fatigue syndrome, now called Systemic Exertion Intolerance Disease (SEID).[7]

Dr. Maes demonstrated that when you have a disrupted intestinal barrier, the undesirable bacteria from the gut's microbiome send chemical messages to the enteric nervous system in the intestines. This nervous system is connected to the spinal cord and sends those same messages up into the brain. This pathway is now referred to as the *brain-gut-microbiota axis*.

Now you've triggered the whole inflammatory cascade, first by activating the ancient immune system that produces cytokines, and then when you cross a line and that response is no longer enough, you get the adaptive immune system generating antibodies to the bad bacteria.

However, Dr. Maes realized that you can address a leaky gut and reverse brain dysfunction at the same time, following what he called a Leaky Gut Diet. His fix is much like the one you will be trying: eating gluten-free, dairy-free, and sugar-free, which we'll get to in Chapter 9.

FOODS OFTEN TRIGGER MOLECULAR MIMICRY

In the last chapter, we discussed molecular mimicry and how antibodies to wheat can also attack many different brain tissues that resemble the gliadin or other macromolecules of poorly digested wheat, A-A-B-C-D. These same antibodies can also attack the enzyme *glutamic acid decarboxylase (GAD),* which is necessary for converting glutamine, the most dominant amino acid in wheat and many other foods, into gamma-aminobutyric acid (GABA), a neurotransmitter known to calm the mind and reduce anxiety and depression.

If you have a sensitivity to wheat, you may create an antibody to the glutamic acid decarboxylase enzyme. These antibodies inhibit the enzyme from working. When you don't have enough GAD enzymes, you can't convert glutamic acid into GABA, so you'll have lower levels of GABA, which will make you feel more anxious. That's an example of molecular mimicry.

A groundbreaking 2013 study looked at people who reported no health concerns whatsoever. About half of the 400 participants had elevated antibodies to wheat that were also attacking the glutamic acid decarboxylase (GAD) enzyme. Another large percentage of the participants had elevated antibodies to casein (the protein in milk), and these people also had elevated antibodies to myelin basic protein and myelin oligoglycoproteins, which are the biomarkers of multiple sclerosis. Remember, having elevated enzymes means you are killing off more cells than you are making, whether you have symptoms or not. These participants were supposedly healthy (no symptoms yet). These were the "control group."[8] That's how prevalent wheat and dairy sensitivities affecting the brain can be, and how potentially devastating they are.

How many elders do you know whose brains are still active enough to want to learn more and explore new horizons? My guess is not many. Whether someone progresses to the point of MS or not, the brain function deterioration caused by elevated antibodies is happening to many of us silently, without symptoms. This is why if you want a healthy brain in your elder years, you must take the tests to see if you are already slowly killing off brain cells.

At the other end of the age spectrum, antibodies to gluten have been found in autistic children. Now, I know we talked about autism in the last chapter and how it relates to hypoperfusion (lack of bloodflow into the brain). Autism is very complicated, and we are just beginning to uncover the myriad of causes. Here's an example of how molecular mimicry plays a role in terms of food sensitivities affecting the brain. In one of my own published research studies in the journal *Nutritional Neuroscience*, we found that 87 percent of autistic children had antibodies against gluten, egg, and dairy, as compared to 1 percent of children without autism.[9] The damage the antibodies and associated inflammation cause may well be responsible for some of the neurological symptoms autistic children exhibit.

THE DESTRUCTIVE ROLL: THE PROBLEMS WITH WHEAT AND GLUTEN

Cereal grains, the world's most abundant food source, can affect human behavior and mental health. During digestion, wheat breaks down into different chemicals that have different reactions in the brain. First, it releases opiate-like molecules capable of causing mental derangement if they make it to the brain. These are called *exorphins,* and they trigger the same response as morphine. In the United States, we consume 132.5 pounds of wheat per person, per year. That is almost 165 grams a day. In Europe, the average is between 10 and 20 grams, although many people exceed 50 grams. Thus, Americans are eating more than three times as much gluten as other Western societies, and that's at their highest level. And every time you eat it, it may trigger your opioid receptors.

Remember the last time you laughed out loud during a movie or with your friends? Perhaps you even had belly laughter—when you laugh so hard your belly hurts. Remember how good you felt afterward? That's because your opiate receptors were stimulated, and you produced a little more endorphin, which was then circulating in your bloodstream. Chocolate stimulates your opiate receptors, too, and when you eat it, you just feel good. The same is true when you eat some wheat. It's satisfying, and it makes you feel good. At first.

But if you are eating lots of bread products every day—toast for breakfast, a sandwich for lunch, pasta for dinner—you're getting large amounts of these exorphins, and they are hitting your opium receptors constantly. Day after day, meal after meal, until eventually you dumb down those receptor sites and they become less efficient. They won't work very well anymore. You get opium receptor resistance. Over time, you need to eat more bread products to get the same good feeling. And that's addictive behavior. Now you can begin to understand why depression is so prevalent in our culture today. Some of these people have damaged their opiate receptors from a lifetime of eating bread. Today, the United States is ranked third in the world for depressive disorders, just after India and China. About one in five adults in the United States experiences some form of mental illness each year, according to the National Alliance on Mental Illness.[10]

Second, there is an entire family of chemicals found in wheat called *benzodiazepines*, which are the same chemicals used in drugs to treat mental health issues.[11] Take, for example, a study done shortly after World War II. One of the first hints that wheat and gluten could have implications for the brain was the observation that, in several countries, hospitalization rates for schizophrenia dropped in direct proportion to wheat shortages during the war. After the war was over, they went back up again within a couple of years. The number of schizophrenics rose dramatically from 1 out of 30,000 to 1 out of 100 when Western grains were reintroduced.

There are no enzymes in humans that can fully digest the gluten proteins found in wheat, rye, and barley. These grains will cause inflammation and intestinal permeability every time they are eaten. My friend and colleague Alessio Fasano, MD, conducted research at Harvard University and published a paper that showed that gluten in wheat causes intestinal permeability in every human.[12] As wheat and gluten macromolecules migrate to sites where they are not expected, including the brain, they prompt the immune system to attack both these particles and the substances that resemble them.

More than half of those with celiac disease (CD) have one or more psychiatric diagnoses or gluten ataxia, a loss of balance when walking, which occurs with antibodies to the cerebellum.[13] In a landmark study that covered 34 centers for gluten-related disorders in Italy, researchers found that in those patients without celiac, but with a non-celiac gluten sensitivity, the most frequent symptoms outside of the gut are tiredness and lack of well-being, reported by 64 percent and 68 percent, respectively. In addition, a high prevalence of neuropsychiatric symptoms, including headache (54 percent), anxiety (39 percent), "foggy mind" (38 percent), and arm/leg numbness (32 percent), was recorded.[14] That's how frequently a sensitivity to wheat affects your brain.

DR. TOM'S TIP
LOOK CLOSELY AT YOUR FACE

Wherever diets based on grain replaced the traditional diets of hunter-gatherers, life span and stature has been shown to have decreased, while infant mortality, infectious diseases, bone mineral disorders, and the frequency of dental disease increased. In fact, the human face, jaw, and teeth have become smaller in response to the requirements for chewing the soft texture of bread; they can be smaller because they're not working as hard.

We also know that celiacs often have a disproportionately large forehead. A 2005 study proved that 86 percent of celiac adults have an enlarged forehead; that doesn't mean that everyone with an enlarged forehead has celiac, but biomarkers do encourage further investigation.[16] Why investigate? Children identified with a sensitivity to wheat are at risk of developing enlarged foreheads, but if they get off of wheat completely before the age of 5, while their head is still growing, they have a better chance of developing a more symmetrical skull.

People with celiac disease also have a hard time digesting other foods and properly absorbing nutrients. When you can't absorb nutrients very well, you will have deficiencies of amino acids, and without the proper amount of amino acids, you cannot make a balanced amount of the brain hormones called neurotransmitters, which are essential for balanced brain function. In one study, it was shown that amino acid deficiencies contribute to psychiatric diagnoses in patients with celiac disease.[15] These lower levels of neurotransmitters are directly associated with Parkinson's, attention deficit disorder, schizophrenia, addictive personality disorder, fibromyalgia, and depression.

MEET KELLY

Kelly wasn't a patient of mine, but I know her story well.[17] When I read it in the literature, I realized that it is a perfect example of how devastating toxic foods can be.

Kelly was just 14 years old when she started to exhibit symptoms of brain dysfunction. She became increasingly irritable and had daily headaches and concentration difficulties. Four months later, her symptoms were worse. Her headaches became more severe, and she had sleep problems, behavior alterations, unmotivated crying spells, and lethargy. Her school performance deteriorated as well. Her mother noted that Kelly had severe bad breath, which she never had experienced before. Her behavior was so erratic that she was referred to a psychiatric outpatient clinic and was prescribed benzodiazepine, a pretty strong antipsychotic medication.

In June, at the end of the school year and during her final exams, Kelly experienced psychiatric symptoms, and although they were sporadic, they became more intense. She began to have complex hallucinations where she believed that people were coming out of the television to follow and scare her. She had weight loss, abdominal bloating, and severe constipation. None of the doctors she saw investigated these gut symptoms, but instead admitted her to a hospital psych ward.

In the hospital, they ran all sorts of tests, but all came back in the normal range. She did have gliadin antibodies checked, but they were not elevated. However, many labs test only gliadin, but there are 62 different peptides in poorly digested wheat that could trigger a reaction like what Kelly was experiencing. This lab checked only one, so the doctors never thought that she was sensitive to wheat because this one came back normal.

Her overall health was otherwise normal, including a CT scan. There was some sluggishness to her thyroid, and an EEG showed mild, nonspecific abnormalities in slow-wave activity. Had the doctors realized what they were seeing, this would have been a crucial clue: This type of brain rhythm (a sluggish brain-wave pattern) is a telltale sign of a sensitivity to wheat. Instead, because they didn't know what to do with the finding, they ignored it and focused on her abnormal autoimmune parameters, her thyroid, and the occurrence of psychotic symptoms. They suspected that she had a rare autoimmune encephalitis—a fire on the brain—so they put her on steroids and sent her home. The steroids reduced inflammation and led to partial temporary clinical improvement, but Kelly's mental symptoms persisted: She had emotional apathy, social withdrawal, and self-neglect.

By September, shortly after eating pasta, she started crying for no reason. She then experienced crying spells, confusion, difficulty walking, severe anxiety, and paranoid delirium. She was sent back to the psych ward, and over the next few months, she was hospitalized several more times. They did spinal cord MRIs, lumbar punctures, and more lab tests, which only showed a mild anemia and inflammation in the gut.

A year later, Kelly was doing worse. She exhibited paranoid thinking and suicidal ideation. Stronger antipsychotic drugs were prescribed, but the psychotic symptoms persisted. By this time, she had lost 15 percent of her weight over the course of the last year, and a nutritionist was consulted. The nutritionist was the first person to take her digestive issues into account and immediately put Kelly on a gluten-free diet. Unexpectedly, within a week, all of her symptoms dramatically improved.

Despite her best efforts, Kelly occasionally experienced inadvertent gluten exposures that triggered the recurrence of her psychotic symptoms within hours. Her symptoms would resolve in 2 to 3 days. She was repeatedly tested for celiac disease, but the tests repeatedly came back negative. This is a classic example of non-celiac gluten sensitivity severely affecting the brain. Finally, Kelly and her mother realized the necessity of being meticulous in avoiding all wheat. And she got better. Here's how the author of this study summarized the case:

> Until a few years ago, the spectrum of gluten-related disorders included only CD and wheat allergy, therefore our patient would be turned back home as a "psychotic patient" and receive lifelong treatment with antipsychotic drugs . . . It has been hypothesized that some neuro-psychiatric symptoms related to gluten may be the consequence of the excessive absorption of peptides with opioid activity that formed from incomplete breakdown of gluten. Increased intestinal permeability, also referred to as "leaky gut syndrome," may allow these peptides to cross the intestinal membrane, enter the bloodstream, and cross the blood-brain barrier, affecting the endogenous opiate system and neurotransmission within the nervous system.

This young girl was destined for a life spent in a psychiatric ward had it not been for an intrepid nutritionist. It pains me that even today, so many doctors do not know that a sensitivity to wheat can cause brain health problems without causing celiac disease. Unfortunately, this case study is not all that unusual. For many people, their weak link is their brain. That's why the information in this book is so important to understand—not only for you, but maybe for someone you know.

THERE ARE SO MANY PROBLEMS WITH COW'S MILK

Wheat isn't the only food that can cause leaky gut and leaky brain. Humans have a very difficult time digesting cow's milk. During digestion, the proteins of dairy are not fully digested into individual amino acids, and we are left with the clumps called peptides. These peptides create inflammation in the intestines, ripping the cheesecloth and allowing macromolecules to get into the bloodstream. Some of these macromolecules are exorphins that stimulate the opiate receptors in our bodies, just like those found in wheat. For instance, milk is broken down into the protein casein, which contains an exorphin called *casomorphin*. Just 1 gram of casein—found in 2 tablespoons of cow's milk—produces casomorphins in large enough amounts to have a negative impact on brain function. These casomorphins are 10 times stronger than those found in human milk.[18]

Even human breast milk contains exorphins that stimulate the opiate receptors. Why? We have been perfectly designed for survival, so it's no surprise that babies have to *want* to suckle, and breast milk stimulates opiate receptors (feel-good receptors), which is one sure way to get baby interested in suckling.

Not only are the opioids in cow's milk 10 times stronger than those in human milk, but the type of opioids concentrated in casomorphins have been shown to be 10 times more potent in the brain than morphine. Now we can start to make a connection between casomorphins and the many studies identifying an association between life-threatening brain impact and cow's milk. One particular type, bovine casomorphin-7 (BCM-7), is associated with disruptive brain function and neurological disorders, such

I JUST WANT MY PIZZA

Of course you do! Who could blame you: It's a perfect storm of wheat and dairy exorphins stimulating your opiate receptors, so it's literally addictive. I have never seen a study of a deficiency of pizza causing symptoms. But now you can decide if it's worth the risk. You can make the right food decisions for you once you understand a little more about how these foods can impact you.

as autism and schizophrenia. Another type is thought to bind to opiate receptors in the brain, and a number of studies are associating this type with sudden infant death syndrome (SIDS).[19, 20, 21]

Casomorphins also exaggerate the histamine release of food allergies, stimulate cravings for more high-fat foods, and diminish cognitive function ranging from ADHD to autism.[22] I know all of this sounds scary. And it is. When your immune system decides that your casomorphin level has crossed a threshold and is a threat, you will make antibodies to it. You have to know the impact of what you are eating.

IF YOU WANT TO THINK MORE CLEARLY, AVOID SUGAR

I cannot say this any more clearly: Eating processed sugar increases systemic inflammation. In fact, refined sugar is one of the most inflammatory foods in any quantity. There is no "little bit" of sugar that enhances your health. If you want to maintain or improve your brain function, you must stop eating the foods that are loaded with sugar so that your brain and body can have a chance to recalibrate. Without sugar, you may find that many of your emotional problems, including anxiousness, depression, and irritability, may dissipate. It's that simple.

But if that is not enough information, here's another, and probably the biggest, reason why you should transition out of a sugar habit. We've all heard that eating too much sugar is a trigger in developing diabetes, and you probably know that there are two types of diabetes. Type 1 diabetes has always been known to be an autoimmune disease, and it occurs when antibodies have destroyed enough cells of the pancreas so that it is unable to produce enough insulin. Type 2 diabetes is related to years of excessive intake of sugar, wearing out our sugar-regulating system. People with type 2 diabetes do not need extra insulin; they need medications that help get the insulin from the bloodstream into their cells. This is called insulin resistance, which is another autoimmune mechanism.

Every cell in the body uses glucose (blood sugar) for fuel. Glucose piggybacks onto the hormone insulin, produced in the pancreas, which then escorts glucose into insulin receptor sites in each and every cell. This mechanism literally turns the doorknob, opening the door to the cell, allowing the glucose molecules to enter and fuel the cell. It's a beautiful system. The problem is that table sugar (sucrose) will stimulate insulin production just like glucose will. How many sugar-laden foods have you eaten just this week? Each of those foods requires the production of more insulin than the body is meant to produce. That excess insulin goes ahead and opens cell doors, flooding cells with excess sugar. Now multiply your week of sugar by 20 or 30 years of day-in and day-out eating sugar-laden foods. All this consumption wears out the insulin receptor sites; now the doors to the cells won't open, sugar stays in the blood at dangerous levels,

DR. TOM'S BIOMARKERS

A very simple way of measuring your insulin sensitivity or your insulin resistance is called your HOMA score: Homeostasis Model Assessment. It's a simple calculation based on a fasting insulin and glucose blood test. You can use your HOMA score, checked every 8 weeks, to confirm that your protocols are improving your insulin receptor function and lowering your diabetes risk. To check your HOMA score, first have your doctor order a fasting insulin and glucose blood test. Get the results, go to theDr.com/HOMA, enter your results, and you'll see what your score is. As you follow the suggestions in this book, your score should be improving toward normal every 2 months.

and the cells are left craving glucose. This is called insulin-resistant diabetes.[23]

Researchers believe that insulin-resistant diabetes initiates a strong inflammatory response in the brain, resulting in the same plaques that are linked to dementia and Alzheimer's disease. In fact, Dr. Dale Bredesen believes that it is a primary cause of Alzheimer's. No one wants to end up living their golden years with Alzheimer's, so wouldn't you do everything in your power to avoid it? Stabilizing blood sugar function is a primary component of Dr. Bredesen's and every other brain enhancement protocol I've ever read about.

THE GUT'S ROLE IN ALZHEIMER'S AND PARKINSON'S

A number of studies suggest that both Alzheimer's and Parkinson's[24] diseases begin in the gut, though each condition manifests in the brain. As we've discussed, the gut-brain communication is primarily controlled by the microbiome. There are two separate mechanisms that are associated with misfolded proteins that eventually produce both Parkinson's and Alzheimer's. The proteins associated with Parkinson's are called *alpha synuclein proteins*. These become twisted in the gut years before there are any symptoms. A large percentage of Parkinson's patients suffer for years with constipation—usually because the microbiota in their gut is out of balance. It's a telltale sign. The ensuing inflammation from constipation can affect any tissue in the body, including the brain. Scientists are now identifying that the imbalance of good bacteria in the gut (dysbiosis) may be twisting proteins in the gut (misfolded proteins), which then can creep up your spine over the years, deposit in your brain, and then 10 years, 20 years later, you develop Parkinson's.

The microbiota also plays a role in affecting the proteins that cause Alzheimer's—the beta-amyloid. Researchers are now identifying that the gut's microbiome controls the brain's metabolism, the brain's immune response, and the brain's function.[25]

Remember, no one gets Alzheimer's or Parkinson's disease in their sixties or seventies. It begins much earlier. Usually it doesn't manifest in your twenties or thirties, though the process of killing off cells begins then. It continues for decades until you hit a threshold where the symptoms begin to manifest. What people don't realize is that when you say, "Oh, I'm getting old—I don't remember stuff like I used to," at age 42, that's a problem. It means that the brain's not working right and something is out of balance. Once you cross the line of critical damage decades after the process began, the symptoms appear. And where did this all begin? In the gut. Later, you'll learn exactly what foods you should eat, and the ones to avoid, in order to maintain the healthiest microbiome that will optimize brain function. The dozens of incredibly delicious recipes in this book will help you start off a whole new way of thinking about your diet.

ACTION STEP WEEK 3: KEEP TRACK OF WHAT YOU'RE EATING

Let's do a reality check and see how much of the three problematic foods we discussed in this chapter you are actually eating. Every day for 1 week, write down or enter into your smartphone when you've had wheat, dairy, or sugar. Start by reading labels more carefully. You'll be surprised where these three lurk (there are full instructions for finding these culprits in Chapter 9).

Later, you'll find lots of great suggestions for healthier options that can serve as replacements.

GARBAGE IN, GARBAGE OUT: HOW OUR TOXIC ENVIRONMENT AFFECTS THE BRAIN

MOM ALWAYS SAID we learn from our mistakes. Well, if that's the case, we all have a lot to learn when it comes to how we treat our bodies, our brains, and how we've been treating our world.

Let's start this chapter with a case study, but I have to warn you that this one doesn't have a good outcome. However, the message here is so helpful for all of us.

Sabina's family reached out to me through my Facebook page. The e-mail header just read "Please help," and attached was a photo of a 28-year-old woman and her 4-year-old son. The message said that Sabina had been diagnosed with *necrotizing autoimmune myofasciitis,* an autoimmune disease. Necrotizing fasciitis is an aggressive infection affecting the skin and soft tissue; this is the "flesh-eating bacteria" you may have heard about. This particular disease has a rapid rate of progression and a very high acute mortality rate.[1] Necrotizing autoimmune myofasciitis occurs when doctors can't find the source of the infection destroying the muscle. Sabina was being treated at the very famous Karolinska Institute in Sweden, one of the largest and most prestigious medical universities in the world. She was seeing world experts in muscle diseases, but every day she was getting worse, even though the doctors there had put her on steroids and chemotherapy to shut down the immune reaction that was killing her muscles.

My wife, Marzi, read the message and forwarded it to me with her own header, "Honey, please help." So I wrote to Sabina's family and said, "You know, I learned that one of the secrets of life is to always say 'yes, dear' to my wife. You caught her attention, so I am happy to help if I can." I told them to fill out our standard intake forms, and in the meantime, I studied the photo they attached to the original message to see if there were any clues.

Sabina was a lovely looking young woman, and the photo was adorable. She was wearing a three-quarter-length-sleeved white blouse with black polka dots and black pants, and her son was wearing a black shirt and white pants with black polka dots. Then I looked more closely at the parts of her arms, hands, and feet that were visible and realized that she had tattoos from her forearms down to her fingertips. There were tattoos on her lower legs going to her ankles and on her feet. There were also tattoos on her neck, coming up just below her face. I could only imagine that a large part of her torso was also covered in tattoos, but even if I was wrong, I had a pretty good clue as to the line of questioning I needed to begin with.

What's the potential problem with tattoos? There are a few, and not all of them are well known.

First, 10 percent of unopened bottles of tattoo ink and 17 percent of open bottles are contaminated with bacteria known to create infections.[2] In research from Denmark, these types of bacterial infections appear shortly after getting a tattoo, and they cause both chronic and mild complaints for 4 out of 10 of all the tattooed. These infections also create a localized sun sensitivity for 2 out of 10 people who have been tattooed.[3]

Second, the inks, and whatever bacteria is growing in them, don't just stay at the site of the tattoo. They are absorbed and travel throughout the body,[4] and can cause disease away from the initial site of the tattoo. For instance, sarcoidosis, a collection of tiny inflammatory cells called granulomas that usually develop in the lungs, skin, and lymph nodes, is known to affect people after they have been tattooed.[5]

Third, we know that having just one tattoo nearly triples the risk of getting other immune diseases, such as a hepatitis C infection, and increases the risk of developing a hepatitis B infection by 48 percent.[6] In Sabina's case, her tattoos could have triggered an immune response creating a necrotizing reaction.[7] Standard tattoo ink is also full of toxic heavy metals, as well as the family of endocrine-disrupting chemicals called phthalates.[8] Every tattoo could be exposing your body to high concentrations of these toxic chemicals, which your immune system will try to protect you from.

I had a very clear idea what was likely contributing to Sabina's autoimmune disease. Was it possible that the inks in the tattoos were slowly leaching into the surrounding tissue, forming neo-epitopes that her immune system was attacking? Was it possible that toxic bacteria were introduced to her tissue? Of course it was possible. Was it possible the toxic chemicals in the inks triggered an immune response? Of course it was possible. And none of her doctors had investigated *why* her immune system was attacking her muscles. She had not been tested for an immune reaction to either bacteria or toxic chemicals. Instead, they valiantly gave her the best life jacket possible by suppressing her immune system with steroids and chemotherapy. But it wasn't working. Her immune system kept attacking, and she was still drowning.

Few people think about the toxic effect of tattoos. And certainly not the world experts in necrotizing autoimmune myofasciitis. I couldn't wait for the family to get back to me, so I wrote them a note and told them that Sabina must be checked for bacteria as well as heavy metals and phthalate toxicity immediately.

Unfortunately, I heard from the family only one more time. They told me that Sabina was very sick and having such a difficult time that she couldn't make it to the doctor's office at all. I'm afraid that this woman has passed, and I believe in my heart and soul that this toxicity was a contributor, and perhaps the primary contributor, to her problem.

DR. TOM'S TIP
IF YOU MUST GET A TATTOO

I personally do not recommend tattoos, as they are a pocket of toxicity in your body that can leach into your circulatory system and activate an immune response. But if you must:

✓ Make sure the artist uses a brand-new needle, or buy one yourself.
✓ Ensure that the artist never dips a tattoo needle into bottles of ink that have already been used. Better still, buy your own ink.
✓ It is possible to get vegetable-based tattoo ink, but it's not very common.

Now I know that many people have full-body (or close to it) tattoos and don't get sick to this degree. In this chapter, you'll learn about the concept of the body burden, and how the immune system can become hyperactivated from environmental exposures that are seemingly innocuous to most others. I'm not going to judge anyone on their desire to get a tattoo or two. However, toxins are real, and when the immune system is overburdened, it can result in devastating outcomes. Sabina's weak link in her chain was likely her muscles, but the same mechanism that protects us from toxic exposures can affect any area of the body, especially the brain. What's more, the same few mechanisms that I'll describe in this chapter occur for a wide variety of toxins.

The biggest health problem we face—an activated immune system trying to protect you—cannot be resolved with detoxification. Don't get me wrong, detoxication is essential; you must clean up all of the accumulated crud and debris in the body. But detoxification is only a Band-Aid. Detoxification by itself is not going to create vibrant health if you keep exposing yourself to tattoo ink, or toxic chemicals, or toxic foods.

In the triad of factors that must be present to trigger autoimmunity, we've discussed your genetics and a dysfunctional gut. Now you'll learn about the third component—how environmental exposures are the trigger that initiates the immune response. This chapter is meant to provide the facts you need to know about the toxic world we live in, how these toxins accumulate in the body, and how they affect our thinking and our health.

WHAT HAVE WE DONE?

I was flying home from giving a lecture in Austin, Texas, a few months ago and read an article that deeply disturbed me. The World Wildlife Fund, in conjunction with two major universities, had just published a report showing there has been on average a 52 percent reduction of all wildlife on the planet from 1970 to 2010.[9] I thought, "Oh, that's too bad," and turned the page. But when I arrived back in San Diego, I was driving home on the freeway when I almost hit the brakes—I was so startled. "Wait a minute. Did I just read that there has been a 58 percent loss of wildlife on the planet in just 42 years? Fifty-eight percent of every mammal on the planet? Is that possible?"

I was startled by two things. First, I was incredulous at my initial reaction, which was blasé at best, numb at worst. We're so overwhelmed by the bombardment of statistics in our world today that it's easy, and even tempting, to go numb. Then I thought about the science, the facts themselves. In 42 years, we've lost more than half of every living thing.

When I got home, I pulled up the study. And of course, the numbers don't lie. The world wildlife study monitored 14,152 different animal populations within 3,706 species. The numbers are worse for animal populations that live near fresh water—an 81 percent decimation. This higher number is due to animals drinking water from rivers and streams that are filled with horrendous concentrations of toxic chemicals. Farmers spray their fields with pesticides, and when the rains come, it washes off and goes down into the streams and into the rivers. The bees die off and can't fertilize the orchards. The fruit doesn't grow and a whole cascade effect occurs.

But it's not just the animals—pollution is affecting our health and well-being. The same pollutants that are causing the loss of the wildlife affect humans. If we drank the same unfiltered water, we'd be so constantly inflamed from the toxic chemicals that we'd die younger and be unable to reproduce, just like the animals. We're only mildly luckier, because when we filter our drinking water, the toxic exposures are reduced but not eliminated. The truth is, they have been accumulating in our bodies and have contributed to the unbelievable rise in all autoimmune diseases over the last 30 years. When researchers reviewed 185 studies on male fertility in 2017, they found that between 1973 and 2011, there had been a 59 percent reduction in male sperm counts. The researchers referred to this in their paper as "the canary in the coal mine for male health across the life span," as low sperm count is associated with "overall morbidity and mortality," a.k.a. getting sick and dying earlier.[10]

According to the *Journal of Pediatrics*, 250 pounds of toxic chemicals per person per day are being dumped in the United States. That is every single day, 7 days per week. In China, 70 percent of the entire country's lakes and rivers are contaminated. In three-quarters of all countries, industrial waste is simply released into their water systems. America's not that much better—40 percent of our own waterways are deemed unsafe for swimming or fishing. Pretty scary. If we gloss over this, stay numb to this, our immediate future is at grave risk.

Our polluting habits can be directly linked to climate change. If you are a believer, as I am, I know that I'm preaching to the choir. But if you aren't, I hope you stay here with me for these next few bullets. This information can be so overwhelming that the tendency is to become numb (like I did on the plane) and start thinking about something else. Please stay.

- The medical journal *Lancet* tells us climate change is "the greatest threat to human health of the 21st century."[11] Our polluting habits affect our lungs, our cardiovascular system, and, as you'll see shortly, our brain.
- The Intergovernmental Panel on Climate Change's latest report links climate change to increased scarcity of food and fresh water; extreme weather events; rise in sea level; loss of biodiversity; and

areas around the globe becoming uninhabitable, leading to mass human migration, conflict, and violence.[12] For instance, a scarcity of food on the planet, especially fresh fruits and vegetables, will cause a scarcity of antioxidants in our diet. Given that antioxidants and polyphenols are the fire extinguishers for inflammation, without them, inflammation will go unchecked, like a forest fire that's very difficult to put out, ultimately creating B4 and diminished brain function.

- The American Association for the Advancement of Science states that climate change has caused a "real chance of abrupt, unpredictable, and potentially irreversible changes with highly damaging impacts on people around the globe."[13] The study points out that "lingering consequences [of storms and floods] may range from mold growth in flooded buildings, to contaminated drinking water supplies, to post-traumatic stress and other mental health disorders." You'll learn more about mold and its direct effect on the brain later in this chapter.

- The *British Medical Journal* tells us that "this [climate change] is an emergency. Immediate and transformative action is needed at every level: individual, local, and national; personal, political, and financial."[14]

The stakes are higher than they have ever been. The *New England Journal of Medicine* published a report stating that for the first time in history, our children are likely to die at an earlier age than their parents.[15] The impact of our lifestyle, including what we are exposed to, is affecting our children right now: They are getting sick at an earlier age, getting diagnosed with disease at earlier ages, and dying earlier than the age their parents will die at.

Technology is improving exponentially, and we really don't know what the world will look like in 10 years. Our environment is changing just as rapidly, causing our bodies and brains to change. Many of my doctor friends talk about the therapies we gave to patients 10 years ago, and how they no longer work as well because we have so much more internal toxicity today than we did even 10 years ago. The environmental toxins that we are exposed to are increasing exponentially (250 pounds per person per day), causing more neo-epitopes, triggering a greater immune response, more collateral damage, and a more severe autoimmune response.

The Environmental Working Group (EWG) once ran separate tests from different laboratories and demonstrated there was an average of 200 industrial toxic chemicals and pollutants in umbilical cord blood from babies born in US hospitals. The umbilical cord blood contained pesticides, consumer product ingredients, and wastes from burning coal, gasoline, and garbage.[16] This is an overwhelming amount of toxins that the human body, especially at infancy, is not designed to deal with. These chemicals would then enter the infant's bloodstream and could interfere with both brain development and endocrine/hormone development.

This EWG study was conducted more than 10 years ago, but if anything, things have gotten worse. Today, every child in Mexico City who is checked has beta-amyloid plaque in the brain, the mechanism of Alzheimer's we learned about in Chapter 2. While the study looked at children, we can only imagine that all 40 million people in this one city are being contaminated by what they breathe. In a 2016 study, Dr. Dale Bredesen refers to the impact of toxic air on the brain as "Inhalational Alzheimer's."[17] Air pollution goes into the lungs, right into the bloodstream, and straight to the brain. In an effort to protect you, the body triggers an immune response, and here comes the inflammation, collateral damage, antibody damage, and tissue destruction that can eventually lead to Alzheimer's or Parkinson's or dementia.

Overwhelmed? Me too. Feeling guilty? That's totally understandable. But once you understand how the body processes and stores toxins, you can begin to make sense of what the best next steps should be. Read on. Just remember, base hits win the ball game. There are no "home runs" to stop the effects of pollution. The world we live in is not going to get less toxic in the immediate future. Thus, day in and day out, you and your children will all be exposed to overwhelming levels of accumulative toxic debris from this world we have created. This is why you must stop throwing gasoline on the fire by avoiding toxins whenever possible and detoxifying your system as necessary.

THE CONCEPT OF BODY BURDEN

The human body is confronted with toxic exposures every day: Toxins are in the air we breathe and the foods we eat, and they get absorbed into our skin. We deal with these toxic exposures like a glass that is being continuously filled with water. Think of a glass that is already half full. If you continue pouring water into it, eventually the water will overflow. When toxic exposures are limited and the body can process them through its own mechanisms of detoxification and elimination before the glass is full, the toxins aren't likely to trigger an immune response and cause eventual health problems.

But when the glass is completely full and water is spilling over the sides, it means the body's detoxification mechanisms are overwhelmed and we have crossed a threshold: the total toxic body burden. When our natural detoxification mechanisms are overwhelmed, we do not get rid of the toxins, so they begin to accumulate in the body. When this happens, these external environmental toxins have now become internal endotoxins. And just like LPS and the neo-epitopes we learned about in Chapter 2, once endotoxins are in the body, they are circulating in your bloodstream and very difficult to remove.

Your body has a natural defense mechanism toward toxins: If you cannot break the toxins down and eliminate them, you must get them out of circulation to keep them away from the brain. Usually, these toxins become stored. Most often, they are stored in your fat cells. Here comes your spare tire around your midsection. Other toxins, like heavy metals, can get stored in your bones.

When toxins do make their way up to the brain, the effects can be devastating. The Centers for Disease Control and Prevention's Autism and Developmental Disabilities Monitoring Network reported in 2014 that approximately 1 in 68 children in the United States has an autism spectrum disorder.[18] When I started my practice in 1980, autism prevalence was reported as about 1 in 10,000. Stephanie Seneff, PhD, from MIT, who researches the connection between autism and glyphosate exposure from this widely used insecticide, has publicly said, "At today's rate, by 2025, one in two children will be autistic."[19] Might chemical exposures and toxic foods that overtax the body's detoxification systems be reasons why the incidence of autism today is so incredibly high? Yes, they might be. There are no new tests that identify autism better that make diagnosis more prevalent; rather, it's that more kids are being correctly diagnosed, and their exposure to toxins may be a cause.

Adult brains can be affected by chemicals as well. No longer does an apple a day keep the doctor away. Apples contain more pesticides than any other fruit or vegetable. For starters, Joseph Pizzorno, ND, states in his book *The Toxin Solution* that 80 percent of apples grown in the United States have a chemical called diphenylamine sprayed on them (a known neurotoxin), which breaks down into cancer-causing nitrosamines. Increased levels of nitrosamines are linked to increased incidence of both Alzheimer's and Parkinson's disease.

This does not mean that all apples will affect all of us in the exact same way. Just as each of us is a unique and distinct individual, we each have our own threshold or body burden. Our genetics make some of us better than others at detoxifying. It is possible to deal with toxic chemicals without overwhelming the detoxification capabilities of our bodies. But nowadays, we're all exposed to a constant onslaught of toxic chemicals, plus daily exposure to foods that our bodies are sensitive to. As a result, we are more likely to fill the glass to overflowing and cross the line.

We need to lower our body burden. There are two ways of doing this: The first is to reduce exposures. The second way is to enhance our liver's ability to break down toxic chemicals. That detoxification pathway is referred to as Phase II detoxification. One of the best ways to enhance Phase II detoxification is to include cruciferous vegetables in your diet every day. Modifying your diet by eliminating toxic foods that can trigger

Cruciferous Vegetables Enhance Phase II Liver Detoxification		
Arugula	Bok Choi	Broccoli
Broccoli Rabe	Broccoli Romanesco	Brussels Sprouts
Cabbage	Cauliflower	Chinese Broccoli
Chinese Cabbage	Collard Greens	Daikon
Garden Cress	Horseradish	Kale
Kohlrabi	Komatsuna	Land Cress
Mizuna	Mustard – seeds and leaves	Pak Choi
Radish	Rutabaga	Tatsoi
Turnips – root and greens	Wasabi	Watercress

an immune response will give your body a chance to flush out the deposits of toxins it's storing. At least one daily serving of cruciferous vegetables will enhance your liver's ability to breakdown and flush out these toxic chemicals.

What's more, lowering the body burden means that when we are next faced with an exposure, we'll be better equipped to deal with it. Then minor toxins such as most food sensitivities won't become major issues. If your threshold is eliminating 20 toxins per day, but you are bombarded with 100, your body becomes a metabolically toxic pool. Here comes whatever autoimmune disease you are vulnerable to (the weak link in your chain). However, if you can reduce 80 of the toxic exposures, then your body can handle the other 20 much more easily. The goal is to avoid being in a deficit where the level of toxins you are being exposed to is greater than your body's ability to detoxify. This is a primary benefit of detoxification programs—to clean out the accumulated, not-yet-broken-down toxins like lead, mercury, polychlorinated biphenyls (PCBs), and more.

Here's a scenario I come across all the time: A patient gets excited about the ideas behind detoxification. He wants more information, so he watches the videos on the Internet that detox experts have posted. He finds out what his likely exposures could be by checking his biomarkers. Then he follows a 3-week detox program to get rid of toxins in his body,

> ## DR. TOM'S TIP
> ### A SECRET BENEFIT OF VITAMIN C
>
> Nitrites and nitrates convert into dangerous nitrosamines in the absence of vitamin C. Back in the late '80s when my son was small, a big treat was a meatball sandwich at the Subway on the corner. When he wanted to go, we always made sure to give him a chewable vitamin C before he walked out the door. Putting vitamin C in the stomach within 15 to 20 minutes of eating these meats will greatly reduce or eliminate any conversion into the carcinogenic nitrosamines. We all eat hot dogs, hamburgers, or cured meats on occasion at picnics or ball games, etc. Just make sure to take some vitamin C beforehand.[20]
>
> The detrimental effects of nitrosamines and many other environmental toxin exposures can also be reduced by including certain foods in our diet, such as garlic,[21] curcumin (the active anti-inflammatory in the spice turmeric[22]), purple sweet potatoes,[23] cruciferous vegetables, and berries.[24]

and he feels like a million bucks. But 6 months later, he starts to feel sick again. He comes back to my office and asks, "What happened?" The answer is that despite his best efforts, he was still exposed to more toxins every day than his body could handle. Whatever detox program he did, he now has to do it again. Because of the body burden, in this toxic world, we have to constantly fight back.

HOW THE IMMUNE SYSTEM DEALS WITH ENVIRONMENTAL INSULTS

My friend Mark Houston, MD, at Vanderbilt University helped frame the discussion about our immune system's capabilities when he said, "The body has a limited number of options for an unlimited number of insults." In other words, there is only so much that the body can do to respond to the monstrous number of insults that we confront every day.

The immune system that we have to protect us is the exact same immune system our ancestors had thousands of years ago. What did our ancestors have to fight a thousand years ago? Bugs, parasites, viruses, molds, and fungus. That was it. There wasn't a high concentration of mercury in the air or in the fish they ate. There weren't high levels of lead in the water like in Flint, Michigan. There was no DDT sprayed on crops, no bisphenol A in water bottles. No nitrosamines in the meats. If our ancestors ate bad meat or got some bug or ingested too much of the wrong bacteria, the immune system kicked into action. If a dead carcass polluted a water pond and our ancestors drank the water, their immune systems were up to the task to protect them.

The problem is that our immune system has to fight all of these toxins with the same ammunition it uses for viruses, parasites, bugs, mold, and fungi. It starts fighting with everything at its disposal—inflammation and antibodies. But if the body burden is too high, and we cross the threshold of exposures (more toxins than the immune system can handle), our immune system becomes overwhelmed, and we accumulate excess inflammation, elevated antibodies, collateral damage, tissue destruction, and eventual autoimmune symptoms. We are ill-equipped to fight bisphenol A binding to our estrogen or testosterone receptor sites, or mercury binding to our BBB, or gluten getting through the intestines and into the bloodstream. We are exposed every day to thousands of different chemicals (I'm not exaggerating), and all our immune system can do is respond as if it's defending against a bug, parasite, virus, mold, or fungus.

Eventually your immune system can't keep up anymore. This can happen in utero (if Mom had an excessive amount of toxin storage or exposures during pregnancy), or at any age after birth. It just depends on your genetics and what you've been exposed to. But eventually we cross the line. And when we do, minor toxins like wheat get treated just like a bug, parasite, virus, mold, or fungus.

Now I'm going to "geek out" on you for a moment, but I hope the point comes across. Here are a few graphs from a research paper we published back in 2008, demonstrating how the immune system was tolerant to a minor irritant (wheat), and when we cross the line and lose oral tolerance. Notice that Box J of the following graph is a controlled response to the minor toxin wheat. This is our immune system saying, "Relax, it's a minor bug, parasite, virus, mold, or fungus; it's no big deal." But when we cross

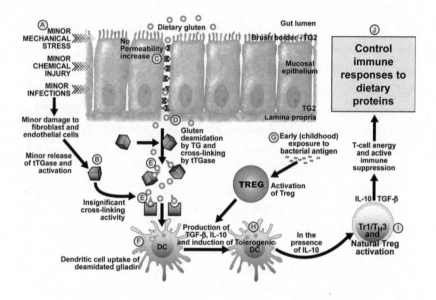

the line and our immune system becomes "trigger happy" because we are fighting toxins so often that any irritant is now more than a minor annoyance, the end result is the development of an autoimmune response wherever the weak link in our chain is (M, on the next page, Multi-Organ System Disorder). That's oral intolerance in action.[25]

Add to this the fact that you also get some bisphenol A (BPA) in your system. Your body believes that it's a bug, parasite, virus, mold, or fungus. All your body can do is go after the toxin in the same way—first with the pistols (innate immune system), and then, if necessary, with the bazookas (antibodies). If this occurs rarely, not a problem. But when it's a repetitive exposure and there's constant antibody formation, now we start getting collateral damage. Now, because the bisphenol A molecules have bound to your tissue, forming a neo-epitope, and your immune system attacks this neo-epitope, the collateral damage occurs to the cells on your thyroid, or your adrenals, or ovaries, or testes, or the brain. Your body then makes antibodies to get rid of the damaged cells. Because of the constant exposure to toxins, you continue to kill off cells until this mechanism of getting rid of the old organ cells becomes self-perpetuating. That's why every small bit you do to reduce your toxic load, every base hit, will make

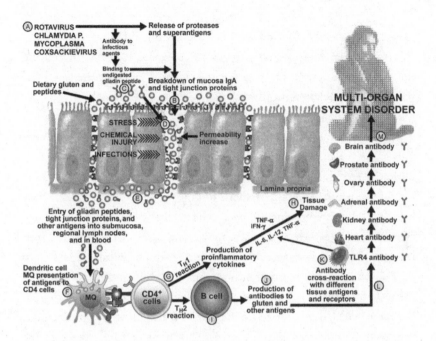

a difference. The goal is to get your body burden below threshold levels so your immune system no longer has to be activated.

Remember, antibodies are not neutral. If they're elevated, you lose more cells than you make. When that happens, you eventually get dysfunction of the affected area—any area, every area, including your brain. Depending on the type of toxin and the area of the brain it attacks, your symptoms can range from mild to severe and can affect all aspects of brain health.

THE PROBLEM WITH ENDOCRINE DISRUPTORS

Every cell in your body has many receptor sites sitting on its outer surface facing the bloodstream. Each receptor site acts as a catcher's mitt. For example, if a receptor site is for thyroid hormone, then when that hormone approaches as it travels through the bloodstream, a magnetic charge grabs it right into the receptor, like a pitcher throwing a fastball into the catcher's mitt. Only thyroid hormones will go into a thyroid receptor site. When estrogen goes into an estrogen receptor site, it opens the cell and the estrogen goes right in. Then the cell closes. A receptor site is a doorway, which is locked until the hormone comes in. It unlocks the lock so that the cell opens and the hormone goes in.

However, some of the chemicals we are exposed to are called *endocrine disruptors*. These chemicals look just like your hormones, creep into your hormone receptor sites, and disrupt your hormone balance by blocking the catcher's mitt. Sometimes, they don't open the door into the cell; they just sit in the receptor site, filling up the catcher's mitt. When the body cannot eliminate these chemicals, they accumulate in the catcher's mitt receptor sites. For instance, chlorine, fluoride, and bromine are known to fill thyroid hormone receptor sites. When these chemicals are sitting in the receptor sites, the hormones can't get in, causing a functional thyroid hormone deficiency. Your hormone levels in the blood are normal, but your cells are functioning as if there is a hormone deficiency because the hormone can't get into the receptor sites, unlock the doors, and go into the cells. This might look like the signs of a sluggish thyroid—cold hands and feet (perhaps wearing socks to bed), constant fatigue, inability to lose weight, brain fog—but when you go to a doctor who runs a blood test because it sounds like thyroid symptoms, your thyroid blood levels will be normal. The problem isn't your thyroid; it's your thyroid receptors.

Autoimmune diseases are nine times more common in women than they are in men. Endocrine disruptors affect women much more than they affect men because these chemicals are mostly attracted to estrogen receptor sites, which are located in brain, uterine, ovarian, and breast tissue. If the estrogen catcher's mitt is full, whenever estrogen travels by these sites, the hormone can't enter because the receptor site is full of the toxic chemicals. The estrogen then bounces out of the cell site, causing an estrogen deficiency to those tissues.

In men, endocrine disruptors can manifest health issues like low testosterone, testicular cancer, extremely small testicle development, or low sperm count concentrations causing male infertility. Guys who are diagnosed with infertility must check their toxicity levels of these endocrine-disrupting chemicals.[26] The average male today has one-third the level of testosterone that his grandfather had. As I mentioned earlier, a 2017 study shows sperm counts around the world have declined by more than 50 percent in the past 40 years. A second paper, published the same month, links this decline in fertility to endocrine disruptors.[27] And as reported by my good friend Joe Mercola, DO, Danish researcher and pediatrician Niels Skakkebæk, MD, DMSc, commented on the findings, saying:

> These two new papers add significantly to existing literature on adverse trends in male reproductive health problems.... Here in Denmark, there is an epidemic of infertility. More than 20 percent of Danish men do not father children. Most worryingly is that semen quality is in general so poor that an average young Danish man has much fewer sperm than men had a couple of generations ago, and more than 90 percent of their sperm are abnormal.

If a man's testosterone is below 550 nanograms per deciliter (which is still in the normal range), he is edging toward the cutoff point at which a man will have trouble fertilizing an egg. Plus, he will not have the 30 percent benefit of a reduction in risks of heart attacks that those above 550 have. Why? Testosterone is necessary to assist the "good" HDL cholesterol that cleans the blood vessels in your heart.[28]

Women face ovarian cysts, uterine fibroids, breast and other hormone-related cancers, and brain dysfunction. This may be why some women with autoimmune disease feel so much better when they're pregnant. Women make higher concentrations of hormones when they are pregnant, and higher levels of hormones have a better chance of getting into the cells.

PCBs, for example, are an entire family of toxic chemicals that are also endocrine disruptors. Originally used industrially, PCBs have found their way into the food chain. They are known to bind with estrogen receptors. There is a high concentration of estrogen-loving cells in breast tissue, where endocrine-disrupting chemicals can accumulate. When a pregnant woman delivers a baby, the mammary cells in the breasts become activated to produce first colostrum and then breast milk. For most women today, especially in their first pregnancy, that colostrum and breast milk is loaded—not just laced, but loaded—with PCBs. A nursing baby will immediately become exposed to huge amounts of PCBs, which are toxic to the brain, affecting both brain development and brain function. Could this be one of the contributing factors to the ridiculously high increased level of autism we're seeing today? The answer is yes, it could be. Although researchers have identified that these toxic chemicals have an effect on brain development and thyroid, estrogen, and immune function, the consensus among pediatricians is that the benefits of breastfeeding still far outweigh the risks of exposure.[29] From that perspective, whenever a mom can lower her risk of exposures to these toxic chemicals, there will be less of a toxic load in her breast milk. I also strongly believe every woman of child-bearing age needs to detoxify her body before she becomes pregnant. By doing so, you are ensuring a higher likelihood that your future baby will have every opportunity to have a well-developed brain.

EIGHT WAYS TOXINS AFFECT OUR BRAINS

Toxins can cause inflammation, oxidative stress, infection, and allergy. Dr. Joe Pizzorno, a founding godfather of functional medicine, shares in his book *The Toxin Solution* that there are eight basic mechanisms by which environmental toxins affect our brain health:

1. Enzymes are molecules that speed up the rate of all chemical reactions inside our cells. Toxins poison enzymes, leaving them less effective.
2. Toxins displace structural minerals, resulting in weaker bones. When toxins displace the calcium in your bones, there is a twofold effect: weaker skeletal structures and risk of increased toxin release when you start losing bone cells (for women, in menopause). The

toxins being released by the loss of bone now circulate throughout the body and ultimately can affect the brain, increasing inflammation and brain cell loss in our elder years.

3. Toxins damage organs like the brain through B4, molecular mimicry, and collateral damage from neo-epitope formation. For instance, when chlorine binds onto thyroid receptor sites, it forms a neo-epitope. Then your immune system will make antibodies to that chlorine thyroid neo-epitope.

4. Toxins damage DNA, which increases the rate of aging and cellular degeneration. Many commonly used pesticides, phthalates, improperly detoxified estrogens, and products containing benzene damage DNA.

5. Toxins modify gene expression. Our genes switch on and off to adapt to changes in our bodies and the outer environment. Many toxins activate or suppress our genes in undesirable ways. This not only results in individual brain health problems (such as depression and dementia) but also causes effects that can span generations.

6. Toxins directly affect the function of our cell receptor sites (by filling up the catcher's mitts so our hormones can't get in). Damage to these cells prevents them from getting important messages, which may result in anxiety.[30]

7. Toxins interfere with hormones and cause imbalances, as in the case of endocrine disruptors. Toxins such as BPA can also induce, inhibit, and mimic hormones.

8. Toxins actually impair your body's ability to detoxify—again, the body burden—and this is the worst problem of all.

THE TOXINS YOU NEED TO AVOID

There are thousands of toxins we're exposed to every day, but in this next section, I'm going to highlight the worst offenders. The same toxins that are detrimental to the brain can also affect the body. A tool used by scientists to measure how long a substance will stick around in your body is referred to as its half-life. The half-life of a drug or a chemical is the amount of time it takes before half of the active elements are either eliminated or broken down by the body. The half-life of benzene is 1 day (breathe the fumes when filling your gas tank, and for an entire day there is an inflammatory cascade in your lungs and bloodstream). The half-life of mercury is 2 months (eat a tuna fish sandwich and risk having 2 months of inflammation in your gut). The half-life of PCBs is 2 to 30 years, depending on which type comes your way.[31] This means that eating just one nonorganic apple may lead you to carry those endocrine-disrupting chemicals in your body, activating an immune response and causing more inflammation, for up to 30 years.

Do you see how overwhelming all of these exposures are to your immune system? As far as I can tell, our only hope right now to get a handle on this is to reduce the added exposures, help our bodies eliminate the accumulated loads in our body (detox), and enhance our detoxification capabilities by our food selections and the nutrients we take.

Half-Lives of Typical Toxins in the Blood

TOXIN	HALF-LIFE
Arsenic	2-4 days (CDC)
Benzene	0.5-1 day
Cadmium	16 years
Chlordane	3-4 days
DDT	6-10 years
Dieldrin	2-12 months
Ethanol	15 percent/hour
Lead	1-1.5 months (2-30 years in bone)
Mercury	2 months (CDC)
Production of antibodies to toxins	As long as toxin is in the tissue over threshold levels
Antibodies to toxins	3-8 weeks

BPA: IS YOUR COFFEE CUP KILLING YOU?

Bisphenol A, the chemical that allows plastics to be molded and then hardened so that they can be used to make food and beverage containers, the resin lining of cans, adhesives, building materials, optical lenses, plastic dental sealants, baby bottles, water bottles, soft lids on coffee cups, and a thousand other products, is one of the top offenders in the family of endocrine disruptors. Molecule for molecule, BPA is as potent as the strongest estrogen, estradiol.[33]

When you get bisphenol A in your body, it can bind on estrogen receptor sites. The body immediately responds when you cross a threshold, and your immune system starts making antibodies to bisphenol A. The antibodies attack bisphenol A that may be sitting in the receptor site on a breast cell, or on an ovarian cell, or on a brain cell, causing damage to the cell itself. The inflammation from the antibodies, trying to protect you, also causes collateral damage on the cell. Now your body has to make antibodies to that damaged cell. Let's say it is a brain cell. Your immune system attacks it. It breaks up the bisphenol A to get rid of it, and in the process, it causes collateral damage. When you have elevated antibodies to your brain, that means you are killing off more brain cells than you're making. Or, if Mom had elevated BPA levels during pregnancy (nowadays that's almost a given), a boy's testes may not develop properly in utero, and years later that boy has problems making enough sperm, leading to infertility. Or if the baby was a girl, her breast cells do not develop properly, and years later she has a much higher risk of breast cancer. This is the horrible reality today of what we are doing to our newborns, our next generation.

Remember that if you pull on a chain, it always breaks at the weakest link—your heart, your brain, your liver, your kidneys, your skin, your hormones, wherever you have a genetically weak link. One person gets Hashimoto's thyroid disease from exposure to endocrine disruptors like bisphenol A. The next person is a child whose mom had high levels of bisphenol A and breast-fed, and the child is born with brain dysfunction.

DR. TOM'S TIP
GET A NEW SHOWERHEAD

If you are in an elevator in a hotel, and the elevator door opens, can you tell right away that the swimming pool is on that floor? If you can smell the chlorine, it may suggest you have a sensitivity to chlorine and it's been accumulating in your system. It would be wise to see if you have a sensitivity to chlorine by testing for antibodies.

Chlorine is an endocrine disruptor we are all exposed to because it's used to treat our water supply. Chlorine binds on thyroid receptor sites and blocks thyroid hormone from getting into the cell.[32]

It would be helpful to reduce your chlorine exposure, but we shouldn't drink less water. But we can get a chlorine shower filter, which is much more effective because we get the most exposure to chlorine in the shower. You breathe the steam, and the steam goes through the permeable membranes of the lungs, into the bloodstream, and right up to the brain. Chlorine filters remove the chlorine before it touches your body.

Chlorine filters are inexpensive and easy to install; you don't even need to hire a plumber. Just remember to change them out every 6 months. You'll know it's working because within a few days, your skin and hair will feel softer. Your skin, your hair, and especially your thyroid receptor sites will love you.

This may be why it is now so common to have hormone-related symptoms. Millions of women are prescribed hormones every year for birth control, menopause, or conditions like low thyroid or low bone density, among others. Unfortunately, it's rare that their doctors checked their hormone levels to identify a deficiency before prescribing hormone replacement therapies. Functional medicine doctors like me frequently see hormone-related symptoms with normal hormone levels. This is when we must consider if there is a toxic overload of endocrine disruptors affecting hormone function.

It is also very likely that their doctor never checked to see if they are carrying a toxic load. Instead, the doctor is handing out life jackets. Remember, if you need a good life jacket, take the hormones; just take the safest hormones you can (choose natural over synthetic). Now that you have a life jacket, you can start going upstream. Think about your body burden. Ask your doctor to check for accumulated levels of endocrine-disrupting chemicals.

Ten years ago, many forward-thinking doctors were saying that we have to check people for their BPA levels because it's a prevalent toxin in our environment and it can cause a lot of damage. Today, scientists say, "That's a waste of time and money because everyone has BPA in their bodies." Both are correct. When checked, practically every newborn child today has BPA in their urine. It came from Mom's exposure during pregnancy. And then babies start accumulating their own exposures with plastic baby bottles and sucking on plastic pacifiers. Now scientists tell us that what we have to check for is not *if* we have BPA in our bodies, but rather is our immune system activated from the exposures to BPA that took us over the threshold?

So what's the big deal about BPA if our immune system is actively fighting it? It's a losing battle. The exposures we get to BPA are so high that if you do not become conscious of reducing your exposure when you can, you are at a higher risk of developing what can be gently called a world of trouble.

In random human blood tests of healthy donors, IgG antibodies (the army) to BPA were found in 13 percent of participants, and IgM antibodies (the navy) to BPA in 15 percent. Adding these two groups together means that 28 percent—more than one out of four—of "healthy people" are fighting this one toxin, with all of the collateral damage this fight will incur.[34]

The primary category of detoxification for many endocrine-disrupting chemicals, including BPA, is *methylation*. The better a person can methylate, the more toxic chemicals get broken down. Green tea (any amount is helpful, but target at least 3 cups per day), vitamin B_{12}, folic acid (another B vitamin), choline, and betaine are the best methylating substances.

FIGHTING BACK AGAINST BPA EXPOSURES

The lid on your coffee cup, the water bottle you drink out of, the plastic wrap you use to store your food—are all loaded with BPA. We use these products on a daily basis, and we don't always realize when we're making a mistake when it comes to our health. For instance, when reading, I often take off my glasses to think about something, and the arms of my glasses end up in my mouth. I am unconsciously chewing on the frame or just like the feel of the plastic in my mouth (probably some oral familiarity from my smoking days in my early twenties). But as I chew on the plastic, my saliva, which is a little bit acidic, pulls out a little bit of the bisphenol A. When I realize what I'm doing, I take them out of my mouth.

There are small changes we can adopt that will make a big difference in getting our toxic levels down. For example, when you go to the local coffee shop to get your coffee, and they give you a lid, immediately throw away the lid, or ask not to be given one. Why? The steam from the hot coffee comes up to the underside of the lid, which is made of BPA (unless it's marked BPA-free, and then the manufacturer has substituted BPF, which is worse). The steam rises, condenses, and drips back down into the coffee, full of bisphenol A. It's best to arrive at the coffee shop with your own stainless-steel mug and say, "Fill 'er up, please." By the way, it may also save you money, as many coffee shops will charge you less if you don't need a cup.

Next, get rid of all brands of plastic wrap. Every time you wrap leftovers in plastic wrap and put them in the refrigerator, the next day your

Estimated Daily Intake of PCB and Dioxin Toxic Equivalents (TEQ) from Birth Until 25 Years of Age for Males and Females

Age Group	Males		Females	
	Total daily TEQ intake (pg)	Daily TEQ intake (pg/kg bw)	Total daily TEQ intake (pg)	Daily TEQ intake (pg/kg bw)
Birth–6 months	852	112	852	118
1–5 years	110	6.5	102	6.3
6–10 years	109	3.9	97	3.5
10–15 years	144	3.0	129	2.7
16–20 years	172	2.5	125	2.1
20–25 years	171	2.4	126	2.2

Modified (shortened) from *Dietary Exposure to Polychlorinated Biphenyls and Dioxins from Infancy until Adulthood: A Comparison between Breast-feeding, Toddler, and Long-term Exposure* Environ Health Perspect. Jan;107(1):45-51 food is loaded with measurable levels of BPA. Not only does heat allow BPA to transfer, but even when cold, the acidity of the food will pull it out. Instead, use waxed paper or parchment paper, and secure the wrappings with rubber bands. Alternatively, try glass storage containers with glass lids to avoid the plastic. Miles Kimball, an online retailer (www .mileskimball.com), sells all kinds of glass storage containers, and they're available in different sizes and shapes with glass lids.

Plastic baby bottles pose another problem. Parents often heat baby bottles in a microwave, leaching plasticizer chemicals into the milk and, at the same time, killing most of the nutrients. This is why it's always better to use glass bottles. Mothers who choose to breast-feed (a smart idea because it's critically important for baby's health) have to recognize that they likely have accumulative levels of BPA, PCBs, and dioxins that have been building up in their bloodstream for years, which can transfer to the baby while nursing. Look at the graph below of the amount of these toxic chemicals children get in the first 5 years of life. The shocking numbers in the first 6 months of life are due to breast milk secreting the toxins that have been accumulating in Mom's breasts over her lifetime.

When a woman has measurable levels of BPA in her blood during pregnancy, the developing area of the baby's brain that controls hormones and the stress response throughout life does not mature properly. In 2015, researchers identified a deficiency of the myelin protective coating around the hypothalamus connected to BPA exposure:[35] For the baby in utero, this means that a crucial area of the brain that controls hormones and emotions will not work as well as it's genetically designed to. This can manifest as anxiety, depression, hyperactivity, or Attention-Deficit/Hyperactivity Disorder (ADHD). And what happens to children and young adults diagnosed with anxiety, depression, hyperactivity, or ADHD? They're prescribed medications.

While I'm not suggesting that *all* children and teens who take ADHD medications will become violent adults, the fact is that these medications are the single largest common factor in all suicides and mass shootings in the United States in the last 25 years. These offenders all were on medications for anxiety, depression, hyperactivity, or ADHD. Multiple credible scientific studies going back more than a decade, as well as internal documents from pharmaceutical companies, show that the class of antidepressant drugs called selective serotonin reuptake inhibitors (SSRIs) have well-known but unreported side effects, including but not limited to suicide and other violent behavior. Think I'm exaggerating? Listen to this summary statement from a review published by the Royal Society of Medicine of 137 different studies on the topic:

> There can be little doubt that we underestimated the harms of antidepressants. Antidepressants double the occurrence of events in adult healthy volunteers that can lead to suicide and violence.[36]

These are uncomfortable issues to talk about, but we must because they are not going away. They're getting worse. So what can we do? The first thing we must do is to become educated in the chain reaction of toxic chemical exposure. Second, all women of child-bearing age should make detoxing a priority *before* they get pregnant. Moms and dads, it's time to model making less harmful choices in front of your children.

If you love drinking sparkling water or soda out of metal cans, think again. The metal cans are lined with BPA. Carbonated beverages are more

DR. TOM'S TIP
PURCHASING BABY BOTTLES

✓ Avoid clear plastic baby bottles and containers with the recycling number 7 and the letters "PC" imprinted on them. Many contain BPA.
✓ Choose bottles made of opaque plastic. These bottles (made of polyethylene or polypropylene) do not contain BPA. You can also look for the recycle symbols with the number 2 or 5 in them.
✓ Glass bottles can be an alternative, but be aware of the risk of injury to you or your baby if the bottle is dropped or broken.
✓ Because heat may cause the release of BPA from plastic:
 » Do not boil polycarbonate bottles.
 » Do not heat polycarbonate bottles in the microwave.
 » Do not wash polycarbonate bottles in the dishwasher.[38]

acidic and cause more of the BPA to leach out of the can. Switch to a Soda Stream, where you can make your own carbonated beverages out of your own filtered water. This way, you will know that you get the purest beverages possible.

Credit card receipts are covered in bisphenol A.[37] We fold them up, and the BPA goes onto our hands, and from there it can get into the bloodstream. Instead, use your phone to take a picture of the credit card receipt for your files and do not handle or carry that receipt—leave it on the table.

HEAVY METALS

Heavy metals are physically dense natural elements including lead, cadmium, arsenic, chromium, and mercury. They are known to be toxic to the brain and are implicated in brain health issues ranging from headaches to fatigue to neurodegeneration. Both cadmium and lead have been linked to learning disabilities and decreased IQ. Lead exposure can also cause impulsivity and violent behavior. Mercury has been linked to attention-deficit disorder, learning disabilities, and memory impairment as well as motor dysfunction.

Many studies support the correlation between a large, single exposure to any of the heavy metals and damage to the brain.[39] However, continued exposures over many decades to even minute quantities may have a cumulative detrimental effect. Worse, the exposure to several different heavy metals in combination can affect our health, even in minuscule doses.

For instance, lead is known to cause major permanent brain dysfunction in both children and adults. This is one of the reasons why the water crisis in Flint, Michigan, was so devastating. These children will never be able to think clearly again (unless they completely get the lead out of their bodies and rebuild healthier brain tissue—more on that in Chapter 5). Lead pipes tainted the water supply for more than a year before the US government took action. Worldwide, it is estimated that about 800,000 children are affected by exposure to lead each year.[40] According to the World Health Organization, loss of IQ points can be traced to lead exposure in early childhood.

When the body cannot detoxify lead naturally, it accumulates in the brain and bones. When women go through the hormonal changes of menopause, they often have an estrogen deficiency and are at risk for osteoporosis because estrogen is necessary to keep the bones strong. When you have osteoporosis, the bones will start breaking down. If they were storing lead, those molecules will recirculate throughout the blood and deposit in the body and the brain, accelerating brain deterioration. Here comes dementia.

Any house built before 1978 may still contain lead paint and lead plumbing, exposing you daily to particles in the air or in your tap water. Small quantities of lead can also be found in places you would never suspect, including personal cosmetics, toys, earthenware pottery, lead crystal, and the soil around your home. It can also be found in foods grown in soil treated with fertilizers containing lead, and in bone broth: Although it's no guarantee of being free of heavy metals, choosing organic whenever possible is the safest alternative.

Mercury is present in some dental fillings, cosmetics, fungicides and pesticides, medicines, some vaccines, and large fatty fish. As far as I know, all tuna now has mercury at close to or actually toxic levels. All of it. You'll learn in Chapter 9 which fish are safe to eat, and why it makes a difference where they come from.

Dental amalgam is the largest contributor of neurotoxic mercury exposure and affects more than 120 million Americans. Mercury has been the most studied and most closely linked heavy metal that affects brain health. The World Health Organization tells us that children can suffer from the entire spectrum of brain dysfunction with mild to moderate levels of mercury toxicity (from mild Attention-Deficit/Hyperactivity Disorder to mental retardation).[41]

Remember the Mad Hatter in *Alice in Wonderland*? Hat makers (or milliners) used to dip their creations in a vat of mercury to stiffen them up. The absorption of the mercury over time through their skin, and probably from being inhaled, would affect the milliners' brains and they would become unpredictable, volatile, and "mad"—thus the term *mad hatter* or *mad as a hatter*.

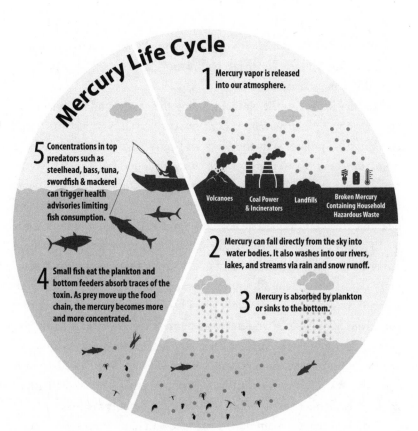

Mercury Life Cycle

1 Mercury vapor is released into our atmosphere.

Volcanoes | Coal Power & Incinerators | Landfills | Broken Mercury Containing Household Hazardous Waste

5 Concentrations in top predators such as steelhead, bass, tuna, swordfish & mackerel can trigger health advisories limiting fish consumption.

2 Mercury can fall directly from the sky into water bodies. It also washes into our rivers, lakes, and streams via rain and snow runoff.

3 Mercury is absorbed by plankton or sinks to the bottom.

4 Small fish eat the plankton and bottom feeders absorb traces of the toxin. As prey move up the food chain, the mercury becomes more and more concentrated.

Boston Corbett, a hat industry worker who killed John Wilkes Booth, President Abraham Lincoln's assassin, might have suffered from poor mental health due to mercury poisoning. Corbett, who'd been employed as a hat maker since he was a young man, became a religious zealot and in 1858, at the age of 26, castrated himself with a pair of scissors as a way to curb his libido—I'd say that qualifies as insane. He went on to serve in the Union Army during the Civil War, and after Lincoln was shot by Booth on April 14, 1865, at Ford's Theatre in Washington, DC, Corbett and his regiment, the 16th New York Cavalry, were sent to track down the gunman, who was on the lam. On April 26, the soldiers surrounded Booth in a Virginia barn; however, Corbett disobeyed orders to capture the fugitive alive and instead shot and killed him. Corbett was cleared of blame by the military and lauded by many in the public as a hero for his role in avenging the president's death. Eventually, he resumed working in the hat industry in the Northeast before moving to Kansas, and in 1887, he landed in a mental asylum.

Mercury is toxic to the brain, including the central and peripheral nervous systems: When you have high mercury levels, you just can't think straight, can't process your thoughts, and can't send the correct messages from your brain to your muscles. Neurological and behavioral disorders have been observed after inhalation, ingestion, or skin exposure to different mercury compounds. Symptoms include tremors, insomnia, memory loss, neuromuscular effects, headaches, and cognitive and motor dysfunction.

The most protected tissue in the human body is the fetus as it is developing inside the mother. Nothing gets to baby that hasn't gone through every detoxification and filtering pathway a mom has. Thus it gives you a sense of the scope of the problem when I tell you a fetus will absorb mercury from Mom's blood and have concentrations 40 percent higher than Mom, especially in the brain—a disaster for a developing neurological system. Most of that mercury comes from Mom's fillings. This is another reason why I consider it so critically important that women detoxify, including removing mercury fillings, before they become pregnant.[42]

Cadmium depresses immune system function, interferes with kidney function, and is associated with high blood pressure and cancer. It can be found in electronic cigarettes,[43] traditional cigarettes,[44] old water pipes,[45] white bread,[46] and white rice.[47] I have found in my clinical practice that when my patient's blood pressure medications weren't working, he or she often had high levels of cadmium.

Avoidance is the best way to decrease your exposure, but if you think you have high levels of heavy metals, talk to your doctor, do the tests listed in Chapter 5, and think about therapies like chelation, which is meant to pull these heavy metals out of your system.

MOLD

The toxins from mold, called *mycotoxins,* may have developed as a chemical defense against insects, microorganisms, nematodes, grazing animals, and humans. These mycotoxins have been used in many beneficial ways, including antibiotics (penicillin) and immunosuppressants (cyclosporine). However, they're also capable of producing illness and causing allergic reactions and, in some cases, death.[48, 49]

Mold can cause both infections and brain irritation, although it is easily overlooked as a source of the problem. The chemicals and spores released by mold disrupt the immune system and increase inflammation. Mold can cause infections anywhere in the body. For example, one study showed that 100 percent of children with high eosinophils (a type of white blood cell) or ear infections with effusions (runny ears) were found to have mold infections in their ears.[50] For these children and others who have recurrent ear infections, antibiotics won't work, because they will not destroy a mold infection. It can grow inside of your gut, in your nostrils, and on practically any body tissue, although it doesn't show up on standard blood tests.[51]

Have you ever returned home from vacation and needed to air out the house? Mold can live under carpets, in ventilation shafts, or behind walls, so you might never see the signs of mold growth that would make you suspicious of its presence. Do you have any "dark spots" in the corners of the shower, or along the track for the shower door, or on curtains? Whether you see it or not, it's estimated that as much as 50 percent of commercial and residential buildings contain toxic mold, according to the CDC's National Institute for Occupational Safety and Health analysis. Fifty percent! I'd suggest you stop the thought "Oh, that's not in *my* house." Although this occurs mostly in bathrooms and kitchens, where there is water, you should carefully check the outside of your house as well for leaks that may allow water into the insulation in the walls—a perfect incubating place where you'll breathe it for years. Most every city now has mold inspectors.

Mold exposure can be a problem both indoors and outdoors in wet and dry climates, but levels can be especially toxic in high-humidity environments, including places like indoor pools, fitness centers, and aquariums.

Food spoilage results in mold and mycotoxin contamination, which can then be either ingested or inhaled. It's always been a frustration of mine that I'll spend a few dollars for some beautiful-looking raspberries, and in

2 days, they're already growing white fuzz. Don't think for a second that they are okay to eat if there's "only a little." Throw them out. Mold is also commonly found in small quantities in wheat and corn: It grows on these grains during storage.[52] The problem here is that you can't see the mold growing on the wheat or corn, but it makes its way into the end products.

Mold exposure from food is another example of a frequent exposure that poses little immediate damage, yet contributes to your total body burden. The beneficial bacteria in your gut will break down small exposures until you've crossed the threshold of tolerance for toxins. When your immune system can no longer protect you completely, excess inflammation begins causing tissue damage that eventually leads to symptoms. These can include headaches or even sudden unexplained "rage" or anger. There are actually 37 different neurological and physiological complaints associated with mold exposure to be aware of:

- Abdominal pain
- Aches
- Appetite swings
- Blurred vision
- Confusion
- Cough
- Decreased learning of new knowledge
- Diarrhea
- Disorientation
- Excessive thirst
- Fatigue
- Focus/concentration issues
- Headache
- Ice pick pain
- Increased urination
- Joint pain
- Light sensitivity
- Memory issues
- Metallic taste
- Mood swings
- Morning stiffness
- Muscle cramps
- Numbness
- Red eyes
- Shortness of breath
- Sinus problems
- Skin sensitivity
- Static shocks
- Sweats (especially night sweats)
- Tearing
- Temperature regulation or dysregulation problems
- Tingling
- Tremors

- Unusual pain
- Vertigo

- Weakness
- Word recollection issues

MEET STEVE

Steve is a senior executive of an oil company. He reached out and asked if I'd take a look at his medical file. With complaints of brain fog that was so severe it was affecting his performance at work, he didn't have word recollection. He couldn't put sophisticated thoughts together. He couldn't hold on to multiple projects at one time.

Steve had already been to the Mayo Clinic twice, as well as other famous clinics around the world, and I asked him to send me his test results before we met. I love these types of cases. When someone says, "I've been to Mayo and they don't know what's wrong," my response is always the same. "That's great! That means you do not have a disease, because if you had a disease, Mayo would find it. You've got dysfunction. Let's see what is not functioning right." And sure enough, none of his test results gave us a clue—there were no disease markers, which intrigued me, so we set up an appointment for him to come to my office.

Within the first 2 minutes of Steve walking in the door, I knew the answer to his problem. Steve was a handsome man, but there was something off with his complexion. I noticed that he was beyond pale, and actually looking pasty. He did not have the look of a CEO of a major company.

DR. TOM'S TIP
ENSURING YOUR HOME IS SAFE TO BREATHE IN

It's a good idea to have your house inspected for mold. The National Organization of Remediators and Mold Inspectors (normi.org) has trained thousands of construction professionals throughout the United States, Canada, Europe, and South America. NORMI provides more than 14 certifications to meet licensing laws now established in the states of Texas, Louisiana, New York, and Washington, DC.

I made Steve a cup of coffee and asked him, "So, when did your basement flood?"

Steve was so startled he almost spilled his coffee. He said, "What? How did you know?"

A pasty complexion can be one of the biomarkers of a chronic mold infection in the body. For Steve, it turned out that his basement had flooded a couple of years ago, and as he was telling me this, he realized that within 6 months of this, his symptoms began. He told me, "The basement flooded; we had a couple inches of water. I had a team come out and clean it up. They put some dehumidifiers down there, some big machines sucking out water, and then everything seemed fine. But 6 months later, I started feeling anxious and confused, and over time, things have only gotten worse."

I ran just one test on Steve: a urine test for mold. His results came back sky-high. The mold endotoxin had accumulated in his body, causing a recurring mold infection that was constantly being retriggered because he was living in the house, still breathing in the air that had mold in it. The weak link in his chain was his brain, which is notoriously vulnerable to mold.

I sent Steve home to clean out his house again. This time he had to hire an expert who dealt specifically with mold. It could be harboring in drywall, the air filtration system, or in the heating and cooling system.

Steve reported back a few months later that he was making huge progress. He completely remediated his home and then followed the instructions in this book to get rid of the toxic mold in his body. When he did, his mental capacity returned and he regained his confidence at work.

GETTING RID OF MOLD ENDOTOXINS

In order to get rid of mold growing in your body, you have to first stop throwing gasoline on the fire, so to speak, and get your house and work environment checked to find the source and remediate it. Next, increase your immune system's ability to fight the mold that may have accumulated in your body. This means checking to see how strong, or burnt out, or anywhere in between your immune system's ability is right now. Have your doctor check your immune system function through the bloodwork we'll discuss in Chapter 5.

Next, have your doctor check your glutathione levels via a urine or blood test. Glutathione is the master antioxidant that works inside your cells to break down and eliminate heavy metals and environmental toxins like mold. Some people carry the gene that makes utilizing the body's natural glutathione very difficult, so taking more will not benefit you much. You have to check to see what the deck of cards is you were dealt in this lifetime with regard to the genes for glutathione production and utilization. Have your doctor check your genetic detoxification panel listed in Chapter 5.

There are many different supplements that support glutathione and methylation, including:

- Alpha-lipoic acid
- Betaine
- Choline
- Folic acid
- Milk thistle (herbal supplement)
- N-acetyl cysteine (NAC)
- Selenium
- Vitamin B_6
- Vitamin B_{12}
- Vitamins C and E (taken together)

Foods that support detoxification, including mold:

- Asparagus
- Avocado
- Beets
- Black-eyed peas
- Broccoli

- Cruciferous vegetables
- Garbanzo beans (chickpeas)
- Garlic
- Lentils
- Liver
- Onions
- Pinto beans
- Spinach

Foods that are high in vitamin C and vitamin E are important to include in a healthy diet, because they promote a stronger immune system. Foods high in vitamin C include:

- Broccoli
- Brussels sprouts
- Grapefruit
- Green peppers
- Guava
- Kale
- Kiwifruit
- Oranges
- Red peppers
- Strawberries

Foods high in vitamin E include:

- Almonds
- Avocado
- Butternut squash
- Olive oil
- Spinach
- Sunflower seeds
- Sweet potato
- Trout

ANTIBIOTICS ARE TOXIC TO THE MICROBIOME

While antibiotics have saved millions of lives, the way they do so is actually toxic to the microbiome. They wipe out the bacteria in your gut in a nonselective manner. With each exposure, the good bacteria actually get wiped out first, along with small amounts of the bad bacteria. Some people start feeling better after a few days and stop a 10-day prescription early. Well, the bad bacteria that are still there become resistant to the antibiotics, and instead of dying off, they will prosper and create colonies of antibiotic-resistant bacteria, leading to dysbiosis that leads to long-term inflammation.[53] In one meta-analysis of 4,373 papers, researchers concluded that individuals prescribed an antibiotic for a respiratory or urinary infection develop bacterial resistance to that antibiotic.[54] The effect is greatest in the month immediately after treatment but may persist for up to 12 months.

If you are prescribed antibiotics but stop taking them because you feel a little better, you will not wipe out all of the bad guys. These remaining undesirable bacteria produce an outer defense wall called a *biofilm*, which acts as a protective shield against further antibiotic attacks. The CDC tells us it can take up to 100 times the usual dose of antibiotics to kill the bad bacteria if they've developed a biofilm.[55] This is the primary mechanism behind what we call antibiotic-resistant bacteria. So if you have to take an antibiotic, take it for the full course—do not stop early.

When you wipe out your immune system's army, you have to rebuild it. Yet studies show that even 2 years after a single dose of antibiotics, our microbiome is not back to normal. What's more, we know that when you take antibiotics, the incidence of developing a different disease later on increases.[56] In children, the number of antibiotics taken before the age of 5 has a direct effect on their IQ.[57]

The excess-antibiotic problem isn't just with prescription antibiotics: These drugs have worked their way deep into our food chain. The vast majority of antibiotics are given not to people, but to animals—cattle, chicken, pork, and farm-raised fish—and its residue remains in the meats we eat. They are also sprayed on vegetables just before harvest to keep the bugs away. When we eat these foods, we get minute dosages that in isolation are not necessarily a big problem, but there is a cumulative effect.

ALTERNATIVES FOR ANTIBIOTIC USE

One way to lower your exposure to antibiotics is to try the more natural antibiotics first. These include phage therapy and herbs, both of which do not have the same type of scattershot effect throughout the entire intestine. The challenge is that the natural antibiotics usually are not as strong. However, they can still play a critical part of a more effective strategy—the "base hits" approach again.

Remember the old adage "All roads lead to Rome"? I believe in taking a pleiotropic approach to medicine: Greek *pleio*, meaning "many," and *trepein*, meaning "to turn, to convert"; thus, many that convert. With an approach that uses many safe, natural substances that provide multiple weaker benefits, you not only reduce excess inflammation, you also activate the genes to begin the healing process.

Phage therapy utilizes *bacteriophages*, which are viruses that live inside bacteria. These supplements can invade bacteria cells, disrupt bacterial metabolism, and cause the bad bacteria to die. For example, *Bacillus subtilis* is a bacterium that has phage capabilities. Phage therapy is more specific than antibiotics: They will not harm the good bacteria in their efforts to attack the bad. The product I recommend is called Mega-Spore. If your doctor cannot order it for you, find it on my Web site at theDr .com/megaspore. It works very well as a component of a "big picture," all-roads-lead-to-Rome approach.

Biocidin (also available on my Web site at theDr.com/biocidin) is a combination of herbs that targets the gut and supports microbiome balance. It can address many different viruses and bacteria. I've used Biocidin for 25 years in my clinical practice, and it is my go-to product whenever I feel my immune system needs a reset. Over the years, I have found that it is helpful for addressing inflammation, whether it's on my gums, or muscles, or if I'm battling a cold. If my patients required long-term antibiotics, if there was ever a safe window to pause using them, we would try Biocidin to see if there was a beneficial effect. It comes in drops, capsules, and as a spray, which is helpful for treating recurrent sinus infections. While it's true that natural antibiotics may not work as fast as prescription medication, for many infections, treating them is not a race, but a journey to wellness.

It's always safer to take a natural approach, which will also have fewer side effects. However, if the natural approach isn't working, take the medications: You need the life jacket.

FOODS TO EAT WHILE TAKING ANTIBIOTICS

- Homemade applesauce: Dr. Michael Ash and Antony Haynes recommend eating stewed apples or applesauce while taking antibiotics. Applesauce is highly effective at healing your gut after damage from antibiotics and helps to repopulate the gut with good bacteria. For best results, make it yourself. Just take four apples (organic if possible) and dice them up to about a half inch in size, with the skins on. Throw them in a pot about a third of the way full with water. Add a handful of raisins and some cinnamon. Bring it to a boil and let it cook for 8 to 10 minutes. When the skin starts to get a little shine, it's a signal that you've released the pectin, the fiber from inside the skin. The pectin helps to heal and seal the lining of your gut quickly.
- Chicken bone broth. The collagen in chicken bone broth acts as a natural probiotic, meaning that it feeds the good bacteria and helps to seal a leaky gut. Store-bought is fine, and organic is best (remember the lead?).
- Pomegranate juice. When you drink pomegranate juice, you rebuild the good bacteria in your gut.

PAY ATTENTION TO YOUR BEDROOM

There are families of chemicals in your bedroom furniture called isocyanates, as well as flame retardants that are found on our sheets if they are not made of pure cotton. If the wood of your bed is pressboard, it may be loaded with formaldehyde. All of these chemicals feed the Firmicutes, the bad bacteria in your gut, and suppress the preferential Bacteroidetes, resulting in dysbiosis, the bacterial imbalance that causes leaky gut and leads to leaky brain.

Stop the cycle by swapping out your blended sheets for organic cotton sheets and blankets. If you change your bedroom, within 3 months, you'll start seeing better digestive and brain function. And, of course, the air we are breathing is often very toxic for us. Get the best air filtration system you can afford in your bedroom. That's where you spend 6 to 8 hours per day, so that's where you should be breathing the purest air you can.

DETOX VIA INTERMITTENT FASTING: EVERYTHING OLD IS NEW AGAIN

I clearly remember the man I met years ago who first got me interested in health care and, specifically, in chiropractic. As a young man of 22, I had to carry my girlfriend into Dr. Harold Swanson's office because she had immobilizing back pain. I didn't know what a chiropractor was, but when she walked out without pain, I was intrigued to learn more about his healing protocol. The compassion this man emanated was compelling. I hadn't met many men yet in my life whom I would want to emulate, but this kind, gentle giant of a man "caught" me. He must have "seen" with deep eyes, because he said to me that day, "You come back, Tom, and watch me work."

I used to visit Dr. Swanson on occasion when I was in my undergraduate years in Ann Arbor, Michigan. He would ask his patients if I could watch, and then he would explain to me about chiropractic, and the patient's situation. Every patient would come out of the visit feeling better. Every patient.

At the time, Dr. Swanson was 78 years old. One of the things he always told me was, "One day a week, Tom, the body needs to rest." On that day, all he would eat was vegetable juice. Just think, this guy had graduated from chiropractic college in 1924, and he was already onto detoxing!

Dr. Swanson's instinct was correct, although the science wasn't there at the time to back up his ideas. Now, of course, we know that what he did was brilliant. I'm not saying you have to fast 1 day a week. But, if you elevate your consciousness a little bit more about "when" you eat, you can change how you think about health. It's about the choices we make every day.

For example, we have a genetic "backup" system to burn excess fat, and now we know how to activate it. In fact, we can activate these genes without having to starve ourselves: It's called intermittent fasting. This is an eating program where you make sure to eat within a specific window of time. The result in test animals was a 20 percent increase in life span.[58]

In a 2016 study, where the participants ate within a 12-hour range and then fasted for the remaining 12 hours, they were able to burn stored fat cells, which then released stored toxins that were easily eliminated. Over the course of 3 weeks, the weight loss was obvious, but when the liver enzymes were tested, the results were pretty impressive.[59] The liver is your primary organ for detoxification, and once the participants were able to get rid of a lot of persistent organic pollutants, their liver enzyme numbers went down. This meant that the liver had to work less on detoxification.

Some of its other benefits include:[60]

- Gene repair
- Improved cardiovascular health
- Increased insulin sensitivity, reducing your risk of developing obesity and/or diabetes
- Less accumulation of damaged cells and less damaging of cells (reduced oxidative stress)
- Lowered triglyceride levels if they were too high
- Normalized levels of the "hunger hormone" ghrelin
- Normalized insulin and leptin levels
- Reduced cancer risk

DR. TOM'S TIP
TRY INTERMITTENT FASTING

Intermittent fasting turns on your "survival genes" so that you use stored body fat as fuel.[61] When you turn on survival genes, genes always win.

Try this for a week while following the gluten-free, dairy-free, sugar-free eating plan described in Part 2: Skip breakfast and eat lunch and dinner within a 6- to 8-hour time frame, and stop eating 3 hours before you go to bed. This schedule is thought to put the body in a state to burn more fat. Make sure to drink water all day long, and that you have good bowel activity before you start.

After a week, see if it's right for you. If you like the results, keep going, every day. After you've achieved the result you would like, you'll find you don't have to focus 7 days a week on intermittent fasting.

However, people who should think twice before trying this regimen are those living with chronic stress, anyone taking steroid medications, and women who are pregnant or nursing.

TOXIC EXPOSURES OCCUR IN THE MOST UNLIKELY PLACES: PERSONAL CARE PRODUCTS

While we are doing our absolute best to keep our bodies clean from the inside out, we also have to examine how we take care of our outer selves. For instance, sunscreen—which is crucial for preventing sunburn, early skin aging, and skin cancer—contains more than 20 chemicals that are not approved for use by the US Food and Drug Administration. The benzophenones and dibenzoyl methanes are the most commonly implicated chemicals.[62]

The Environmental Working Group puts their stamp of approval on zinc-based sunscreens. In their words, "Sunscreens using zinc oxide and titanium dioxide tend to rate well in our analysis: They are stable in sunlight, offer a good balance between protection from the two types of ultraviolet radiation—UVA and UVB—and don't often contain potentially harmful additives."[63]

Some soaps, nail polish, hairspray, and dryer sheets contain phthalate plasticizers such as BPA. In one recent study, children whose mothers were exposed to higher levels of phthalates in late pregnancy tended to score lower than other kids on intelligence tests by the age of 7.[64]

There are also hidden sources of gluten that we can come in contact with just by using everyday commercial products, including those you use on your body. The science behind the effect of gluten in commercial products is real and well documented.[65] That said, some researchers argue that gluten molecules cannot penetrate the skin. They say that gluten-filled products such as shampoos, lipsticks, and even eye makeup cannot penetrate the skin or scalp and should not pose a problem. However, for some people, they do. It is possible that these molecules enter our bodies through our respiratory system when we smell them. The respiratory route of delivery of a food toxin is well referenced in the literature. When you are using any of these gluten-containing products, you're breathing in the tiniest particles, and they can activate an immune response.[66] Even if you don't experience symptoms, you could be doing damage to your internal tissue.

Gluten proteins found in cosmetics can be a problem for some highly sensitive individuals. At the annual meeting of the American College of Gastroenterology in 2013, researchers presented a case study of a 28-year-old woman who successfully managed her celiac disease through diet. After trying a new body lotion, however, she developed an itchy, blistering rash on her arms, along with stomach bloating and diarrhea. Once she stopped using the lotion, her symptoms disappeared. Further, in a 2014 scientific article titled "Food Allergen in Cosmetics," the authors reported a meta-analysis of eight different studies on more than 1,900 patients who suffered with symptoms from severe wheat allergies, yet these patients were not eating wheat. The authors found it was a facial soap containing wheat protein that caused this reaction. Once the patients stopped using the soap, their symptoms disappeared.[67]

The most common symptom of a wheat-sensitive reaction to body-care products is hives. Other reported symptoms include asthma and atopic dermatitis, a chronic inflammatory skin condition marked by severe itching, dry skin, and visible lesions. The estimated prevalence of atopic dermatitis has dramatically increased over the past 30 years, especially in urban areas, emphasizing both the loss of oral tolerance and the prevalence of environmental exposures like cosmetics in triggering the disease.[68] For a complete list of ingredients in cosmetics and body-care products that may contain gluten, go to my Web site at www.theDr.com/productswithgluten.

Luckily, specialty manufacturers have created entire lines of organic, gluten-free, dairy-free, and sugar-free beauty products. Annmarie Skin Care (theDr.com/annmariegianni) is one company my patients rave about, and to learn more about these products, go to theDr.com/skincare. The Environmental Working Group's Web site (www.ewg.org) keeps a running list of chemicals in products to avoid.

HOUSEHOLD CLEANING PRODUCTS

Household cleaners may trigger intestinal permeability and cause inflammation due to a direct inflammatory response or indirectly from one of the hidden ingredients (such as gluten). Symptoms may or may not be obvious. For some people, it's obvious. If they're exposed to a particular product or chemical, they have a reaction. Yet for most, it's not so clear-cut. The symptom might be low energy or joint pains that come and go.

One difficulty in isolating a product that may cause symptoms is that for most products, there is no government oversight. For example, the Environmental Protection Agency (EPA) governs the labeling of laundry detergents, and it does not adhere to the labeling requirements set forth by the FDA. The EPA's concern is whether a laundry detergent is "environmentally friendly," not whether the detergent contains gluten as a filler, and so it does not require labels on household products to list all ingredients.

For those of us who need to avoid gluten or have other chemical sensitivities, it's buyer beware. The following chart lists some of the biggest offenders that we are often exposed to, and what you can use as a better replacement.

PRODUCT	REASON TO AVOID	SOLUTION
Charcoal briquettes	May contain wheat as a binding agent.	Replace with natural wood charcoal.
Charcoal lighter fluid	Releases toxic chemicals into the air.	Old newspapers or twigs
Dish soap/washing-up liquid	May contain proteins from gluten grains.	Look for organic, gluten-free options.
Disinfectant	May contain alcohol from a gluten-containing grain.	See "All-Purpose Disinfectant" recipe on page 123.
Drywall/plasterboard	Starch from gluten-containing grain may be used in the manufacture of drywall.	If you feel better when you're away from home for a few days, it might be your home that is the toxin. You'll have to hire a remediator, who will locate the source of the problem and then remove and replace the affected drywall.
Envelopes	Envelope glue is primarily derived from cornstarch or gum arabic. However, it can also be produced from other starches, including dextrin (from wheat).	Use a wet sponge to seal envelopes instead of licking them.
Glue	Some household glues may contain wheat starch.	Wear cotton gloves when applying glue.
Hair care	**Avoid:** Dark permanent hair dyes, chemical hair straighteners that may contain toxins, including formaldehyde, p-Phenylenediamine (PPD), DMDM hydantoin, ammonia, coal tar, or resorcinol	Look for organic, semipermanent options.
Hand soap	May contain ingredients derived from gluten grains. **Avoid:** triclosan and triclocarban.	Look for organic, gluten-free options.

Product	Reason to Avoid	Solution
Household cleaning products	May contain proteins or starches from gluten grains.	See recipes for "All-Purpose Cleaner" and "All-Purpose Scouring Powder" on page 123.
Laundry detergent/washing powder/washing liquid/fabric softeners/stain removers	May contain proteins from gluten grains.	Look for organic, gluten-free options.
Nail polish/remover	**Avoid:** formaldehyde or formalin in polish, hardeners, or other nail products; toluene and dibutyl phthalate (DBP) in polish.	Look for an organic, gluten-free brand.
Paste for craft purposes	Wheat paste may be used for papier-mâché, decoupage, book binding, and collage. Wheat paste may also be used to glue posters or flyers.	Wear cotton gloves when applying pastes.
Pet food	May contain gluten grains.	Look for an organic, gluten-free brand.
Pet litter	May contain wheat.	Look for an organic, gluten-free brand.
Plywood glue	May be made from wheat flour.	Wear cotton gloves when applying glue.
Skin moisturizer and lip products	**Avoid:** retinyl palmitate, retinyl acetate, and retinoic acid and retinol in daytime products.	Look for organic, gluten-free options.
Sunscreen	**Avoid:** retinyl palmitate, aerosol spray and powder sunscreen, oxybenzone, products with added insect repellent	Look for products with zinc oxide or titanium dioxide as active ingredients, otherwise avobenzone (at 3%)
Toothpaste	**Avoid:** triclosan	Look for organic, gluten-free options.
Wallpaper paste	May contain wheat starch: In Poland, wheat plus water is used as wallpaper paste.	Remove wallpaper from your home.

DIY CLEANERS

Some manufacturers produce nontoxic cleaners by using natural ingredients that do not release harmful fumes or contain gluten. Their formulas are based on the same tried-and-true ingredients used for generations, and I've found that it's easy enough just to make your own. The formulas are easy to mix, and the ingredients are inexpensive. The only downside is they often require a little more elbow grease.

The following formulas are some of my favorites:

ALL-PURPOSE CLEANER

1 cup water
¼ teaspoon organic, gluten-free liquid dishwashing soap
1 tablespoon baking soda
½ teaspoon borax

In a spray bottle, mix together the water, dishwashing soap, baking soda, and borax.

ALL-PURPOSE SCOURING POWDER

1 cup baking soda
10 drops rosemary essential oil

In a can with a perforated lid, mix together the baking soda and rosemary essential oil.

ALL-PURPOSE DISINFECTANT

1 cup water
2 tablespoons Castile soap
1 teaspoon tea tree oil
8 drops eucalyptus essential oil

In a spray bottle, mix together the water, Castile soap, tea tree oil, and eucalyptus essential oil.

GLASS CLEANER

1 cup water
1 cup vinegar
10 drops lemon essential oil

In a spray bottle, mix together the water, vinegar, and lemon essential oil.

PORCELAIN POLISH

2 tablespoons cream of tartar
½ cup hydrogen peroxide

In a small bowl, mix together the cream of tartar and hydrogen peroxide.

WOOD FLOOR CLEANER

3 tablespoons Castile soap
½ cup vinegar
½ cup black tea
2 gallons water

In a large bucket, mix together the Castile soap, vinegar, tea, and water.

WOOD CABINET CLEANER

2 cups water
2 tablespoons vinegar
1 tablespoon lemon oil

In a squirt bottle, mix together the water, vinegar, and lemon oil.

WHAT'S NEXT?

In the next chapter, we are going to talk about a variety of tests that show where the problem in your brain is located, and what's causing it. You can also undergo testing to identify the kind of toxins that are in your system. Knowing these answers is the key for going upstream and identifying the reason why you fell over the waterfall.

Then you can start to implement simple lifestyle changes—the base hits—that will enhance every aspect of your health, particularly your brain. Each suggestion builds on the next, creating that pleiotropic approach we discussed in this chapter. When you implement all of these suggestions together, you'll begin to see real improvements in the way you think and feel. Looking for a better life jacket isn't the answer.

ACTION STEP WEEK 4: REVIEW THE EWG'S WEB SITE

Once a month, allocate your "1 hour a week" to reviewing the Environmental Working Group's Web site—ewg.org—and learning more about healthy consumer products, so you can avoid the toxic ones.

PART II

THE LADDER: CREATING BETTER BRAIN HEALTH

5

KNOW YOUR BIOMARKERS

A FUNCTIONAL MEDICINE checkup includes every detail about your health, starting with your mother's health history during her pregnancy with you; your birth history; your health in infancy, childhood, and young adulthood; vaccinations; fevers; antibiotic use; and more. It includes everything and anything that has happened that may have contributed to the "you" of today. I work together with every patient I treat to create a timeline so we can easily visualize the development of the imbalance that eventually caused the symptoms he or she now has. Many times, adults will come into my office with the symptoms of autoimmune disease, and we can trace the first symptoms back to when they were very young. Understanding your timeline allows you to grasp how far along you are on the autoimmune spectrum, because you will see how the earliest symptoms have progressed over time. It's usually a jaw-dropping experience when patients realize how it is all connected. Their current health symptoms began many years earlier.

You can use the following chart to create your timeline. First, plug in the symptoms you are currently dealing with. They can be related directly to your brain or not. See if you can determine when the symptoms started and how they have changed over time. Then dial down to the details of any chronic or recurring symptoms, or the minor pains that are more of an annoyance. Think back to your youth and record on your timeline each major or minor physical or emotional health upset. Include what you did at the time to address each event. You can ask your parents or relatives if they have any information about your mother's pregnancy and delivery. The major events will quickly come to mind, like ear infections, repeated bouts of strep throat, or having your tonsils removed.

MY TIMELINE

Copy this chart into a journal if you need more space. Then transfer this information onto a linear graph. Use the following sample as a guide.

Age	Key Event	Treatment and Outcome

MEET PENNY

Penny is a lovely 42-year-old woman who came to see me complaining of short-term memory loss. She would occasionally get in the car and forget where she was supposed to be headed, or would walk into a room at home without remembering what she needed to pick up. She was highly concerned because her aunt recently had been diagnosed with Alzheimer's disease (AD), and Penny worried that the same fate was her future. She told me that she was healthy but occasionally had menstrual cramps and constipation. Her previous standardized blood tests were always in the normal range. Her family doctor told Penny that her forgetfulness was nothing more than anxiety, a stress response to her busy life, and if she just slowed down, her thinking would bounce back to normal.

I asked Penny to fill out the Living Matrix timeline before our first visit, starting with her parents' health history. I asked her to pay attention to any known toxins she or her parents might have been exposed to. She interviewed both her mother and her father and found out that the old Victorian house her mother grew up in, and that her aunt was still living in, had at one time been covered in lead paint. Penny's mother also told her that when Penny was a baby, she had multiple ear infections. Penny filled in the rest. She wrote down when she was first diagnosed with ADHD (8 years old) and when she started seeing a dermatologist for troublesome acne (13 years) and when her menstrual problems became an issue.

With this information, I could see a clear pattern of chronic infections and chronic inflammation. Penny's graph below is an example of a visual health history (the timeline) that allows both a doctor and the patient to see where health complaints may be coming from. Given Penny's presenting concerns of brain dysfunction and memory loss, the possibility of lead accumulation was one that needed to be explored.

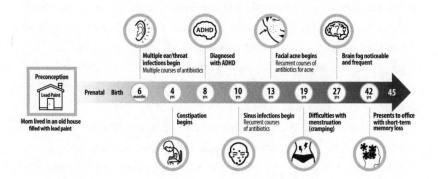

GENETIC TESTING

We get our genes from our mother and father. There's nothing you can do about that—it's the owner's manual you have been given in this lifetime. If you look at the owner's manual for your car, it tells you exactly how to operate the different buttons and switches. When it comes to your genes, epigenetics teaches us that you can turn on and off your genes based on the lifestyle you're leading. That's why your genes show the weak link in your chain but they are not your destiny.

The genes that are strongly associated with a risk of developing cognitive decline and Alzheimer's disease are within the ApoE family. There are three versions (ApoE2, ApoE3, and ApoE4). You get one from your mother and one from your father. You can be carrying an ApoE2/2 (a 2 from both your mother and father), 2/3 (a 2 from one parent and a 3 from the other), 2/4, 3/3, 3/4, or 4/4. ApoE3/3 is the most common—that's what I have. When I opened my test results and saw that I was a 3/3, I noticed I breathed a sigh of relief, as it's the ApoE4 gene that puts you at a much higher risk for developing Alzheimer's.

The ApoE4 variant is the largest known genetic risk factor for late-onset Alzheimer's disease in a variety of ethnic groups. Caucasian and Japanese individuals who carry two ApoE4 genes have a ten- and thirtyfold increased risk, respectively, of developing AD by 75 years of age, as compared to those not carrying an ApoE4 gene. Although 40 to 65 percent of AD patients have at least one copy of this ApoE4 gene, ApoE4 is not a determinant of the disease, but it is a risk factor for the disease— at least a third of patients with AD are ApoE4 negative, and some with ApoE4 never develop the disease.[1] Yet in another study, those with two ApoE4 genes have up to 20 times the risk of developing AD. Nigerian blacks have the highest observed frequency of the ApoE4 gene in the world, yet AD is rare among them.[2] There is growing evidence that suggests this may be because they do not eat a Western diet.

If you have an ApoE4 gene (one or two of them), it's not good. But here's the reality: The thousands of people in these studies, every single one of them, did not have the information you now have just from reading this book. They did not know there are biomarkers that identify the mechanisms causing the inflammation that sets this disease in motion. When you identify the biomarker, it gives you the window of opportunity to go back upstream and fix the problem.

I am strongly of the opinion that if you don't know you have a "weak link in your chain," you are very likely to keep doing what you've always done. And your lifestyle, unknown to you, could be producing B4 (a breach of the blood-brain barrier), allowing macromolecules to get inside your brain, creating inflammation in your brain, causing collateral damage to surrounding tissue, stimulating your immune system to produce elevated antibodies to the damaged tissue, leaving white matter lesions and beta-amyloid plaque deposits, diminishing brain function as a result, and eventually leading to a diagnosis of Alzheimer's disease. So get the tests, apply the principles in this book, check your results every 6 months to a year to confirm you've calmed down the inflammatory cascade, and pay it forward. Go out in the world and tell everyone you know about going upstream and learning to identify brain inflammation before it becomes brain degeneration. You'll be doing your part to make this world a better place.

THE SCIENCE OF PREDICTIVE AUTOIMMUNITY

What if you could find out if your brain was being affected by autoimmunity *before* there was enough tissue damage to produce a single symptom? That's the science of predictive autoimmunity. It is now possible to test for many of the different factors that influence the immune system's production of antibodies to your own tissue.

I'm a firm believer in identifying "what's brewing" in your body as early as possible. Knowledge is power, especially if you couple that knowledge with action. When we can pinpoint which imbalances are occurring in our brains, whether or not we currently experience symptoms, it gives us a window of opportunity to make informed decisions: "What do I do?"

"Can I stop this from progressing?" "Can it be reversed?" This is why the world of predictive autoimmunity is of such value.

According to Professor Yehuda Shoenfeld, MD, one of the world's leading medical experts in autoimmunity, autoimmune diseases have incubation periods that range from as little as a few years to as long as 40 years. That's how long it may take before a person has enough tissue damage that would generate strong enough symptoms that warrant a trip to the doctor, and usually it takes multiple doctor visits before receiving an accurate diagnosis. This is particularly true if you have issues with your brain function. Without a baseline, only you can tell if your memory is slipping, if your attention is waning, or if you are having trouble sleeping.

Sometimes, these symptoms are subtle. Other times, they are pronounced, but you might connect them to something else that's going on in your body or your life: a stressful time at work or at home, an infection, or even a thought like "My brain doesn't seem to be working as well as it used to." Often, even if you're unaware, these issues can be traced to your immune system, which, in its efforts to try to protect you, is creating inflammation in your brain.

Autoimmune diseases can be identified by testing properly for elevated levels of autoantibodies—the antibodies to your own tissue—that can tell doctors when a certain disease is "brewing," sometimes years before there is enough tissue damage to produce symptoms. I like to think of these autoantibody levels as messengers from the future. Furthermore, when these autoantibodies appear, they tend to follow a predictable course, with a progressive accumulation of specific autoantibodies before the onset of the disease, even while patients are still asymptomatic.

Antibody levels of any type are referred to as *biomarkers* because they measure body function. Doctors already use biomarkers to predict a host of illnesses; for instance, a biomarker of inflammation (hs-CRP) is a more accurate predictor of heart disease than having high cholesterol. These biomarker tests confirm why we know that you don't wake up with Alzheimer's—the biomarkers are there years before the disease shows up.

Biomarker testing gives us a positive predictive value (PPV) when we are looking for the earliest stages of autoimmune disease. The biomarkers of predictive autoimmunity are the temperature gauges on the dashboard of your immune system. Some cars have only a "hot light" that turns on when the engine is overheating. If you have only a hot light on the dashboard, you don't get advance warning, and you don't know there's a problem until smoke is coming out of your engine. When that happens, you have no choice but to pull over—your engine is about to blow up. That's what a diagnosis of a disease is: You get symptoms, have to "pull over" right away (go to a doctor), and then receive a diagnosis of a disease. That's the "hot light" approach to your health. Other cars have a temperature gauge that inches up toward the red zone. When you see the needle climbing toward the red zone, it gives you an opportunity to get your engine checked before it overheats. That's my approach to health care, and the reason I feel so strongly about predictive autoimmunity.

Predictive autoimmunity may seem almost magical, but it's not fortune-telling. It doesn't actually predict what the future will be. It identifies the direction your health is heading. What you will learn is that the lifestyle choices you make interact with your genetic vulnerabilities and determine if your immune system is called into action. For example, one study showed that if you have elevated autoantibodies to the Purkinje cells in your brain, there is a 52 percent PPV you are killing off brain tissue years before there is so much damage it becomes obvious and you receive a diagnosis of brain atrophy (shrinkage). Now, you may not currently have symptoms of brain dysfunction, but if you test positively for elevated autoantibodies to Purkinje cells, the mechanism is occurring that is killing off your tissue; those symptoms are coming.[3]

The blood tests described in this chapter are not always included in the battery of testing most doctors will offer during an annual physical. However, I believe they are an essential tool in identifying the early indicators of where the weak link in your chain is pulling at your health. Because of the terrifying increase in brain diseases, everyone should have a baseline set of biomarker tests for their brain health, even if you are not currently experiencing symptoms. This is a revolutionary, groundbreaking testing protocol that can wipe away years or even decades of mystery, confusion, and loss of hope.

As you begin to follow the recommendations in the rest of this book, you can use these tests to track your progress by continuing to monitor your autoantibodies. Many people believe that once their thinking or mood returns to normal, their brain health problems are gone. Nothing is further from the truth in the world of autoimmunity. Although eliminating the symptoms is a primary goal, even when there is symptom relief, we are still on the spectrum. The only way to know if you have silenced the autoimmune cascade is to retest. Otherwise, we may think that since our symptoms are controlled, we do not have to be as vigilant in following the recommendations outlined in this book. I have seen this happen many times over the years, where "surprise" flare-ups reappear seemingly out of nowhere. The problem was that the brain hadn't fully healed, and when an irritant like gluten was reintroduced, the inflammatory cascade began again.

A classic example of this is with celiac disease (CD), where only 8 percent of people heal completely on a gluten-free diet, although many more will remark that they feel significantly better. According to a 2009 study published in the journal *Alimentary Pharmacology and Therapeutics*, 65 percent of celiac patients feel better but still have underlying, excessive inflammation in their intestines,[4] causing intestinal permeability that opens a gateway to the development of other autoimmune diseases, even when they are following a gluten-free diet. The remaining patients did not heal at all, even on a gluten-free diet (they have other compounding triggers that need to be addressed). The advice for all celiac patients, then, is to get retested for the biomarkers of intestinal permeability. Without retesting, you will never know if you have completely healed. If your intestinal permeability has not completely healed, the damage will continue at your weakest link, which often is the brain. Unfortunately, even if your gut completely heals, your body remembers that you once crossed the line and wheat became a problem. Now you've produced a Memory B cell to wheat (like the one you produce after having a vaccination for measles that keeps you protected for life), and a sensitivity to wheat is now permanent. You'll always need to be vigilant and avoid gluten. Just as you can't be a little pregnant, you can't have a little wheat.

WHEN IT COMES TO THE BRAIN, BIOMARKERS HAVE THE POTENTIAL TO . . .

✓ Confirm if and where the immune system is attacking your own tissue

✓ Enable diagnosis before the onset of symptoms

✓ Predict disease flares

✓ Predict and monitor response to therapy

✓ Describe organ or tissue damage

COMMON BRAIN SYMPTOMS OF CELIAC DISEASE AND NON-CELIAC WHEAT SENSITIVITY

Given that gluten is such a common contributor to brain dysfunction, comprehensive testing for a gluten-related disorder is essential. Talk with your doctor about the Wheat Zoomer test we discussed in Chapter 2, which is the most cutting-edge test for a wheat sensitivity. If you have, or had during your lifetime, any of the following symptoms (and add them to your timeline), you'll need that test as well as the brain-related antibody tests listed in this chapter.

When you look at the list, you might not see the connection between these symptoms and your brain health, but there often is a direct correlation. Symptoms that develop in the body may in fact be the only red light on the dashboard that shows you have a problem with your brain. For instance, when your doctor checks your reflexes by tapping your elbow or knee, she's actually testing for an abnormal communication pathway from your brain to your muscles.

Most patients who present with neurological manifestations of gluten sensitivity have no gastrointestinal symptoms. Patients with celiac disease might not have gastrointestinal symptoms either.[5] For every celiac patient with gut symptoms, there are eight more that present with symptoms elsewhere in the body,[6] and most commonly in the brain. These symptoms might include:

- Anxiety[7]
- Ataxia[8] (loss of balance)
- Attention-Deficit Disorder (ADD/ADHD)[9]
- Brain fog[10]
- Chronic fatigue[11]
- Cognitive impairment[12]
- Delayed puberty[13]
- Dementia/Alzheimer's disease[14]
- Depression[15]
- Down Syndrome[16]
- Epilepsy[17] (seizures)
- Failure to thrive or short stature[18]
- Headache[19]
- Hypotonia[20] (Low muscle tone)
- Learning disorders[21]
- Peripheral neuropathy[22] (numbness and tingling)
- Psychosis[23]
- Recurring pain[24] anywhere in the body
- Short-term memory loss[25] (forgetfulness)
- Sleep disturbances[26]

BRAIN-RELATED BLOOD TESTS

There are simple blood tests available that can tell you if the mechanism that causes blood-brain barrier permeability, or leaky brain, is active in you. You can identify increased inflammation. You can determine sensitivities to certain foods. You can find out if you have environmental sensitivities to the air you're breathing. You can trace mercury levels from eating too much tuna fish. You have to go upstream to see what set off the mechanism that is causing the damage.

For example, any patient who has the ApoE4 gene is at a higher risk of having excessive inflammation. The end result of an unchecked, exaggerated inflammatory response due to a genetic overreaction is a much higher risk of Alzheimer's disease. If you know you have one or two ApoE4 genes, then you need to make sure your biomarkers of inflammation in the brain do not elevate. If you check and they are elevated, then you know that something in your lifestyle, food choices, or environment is triggering an immune response. Then the question is "what is it?" And now you'll work with a functional medicine practitioner and you'll find out what it is. You will take the steps necessary to identify the inflammatory trigger, get the inflammation down, and recheck the biomarkers 6 months later. This is the best way that I know of to prevent the development of Alzheimer's.

Now more than ever, we have the ability to identify the vulnerability of any human being to developing degenerative brain disease. We can identify what is going on upstream before someone tumbles over the waterfall and falls in the whirlpool of brain symptoms, frantically looking for the best life jacket to keep them afloat. This is true "health care," as opposed to the "disease care" that is most prevalent today. We need to listen to our body, test with biomarkers, and figure out where we are, what we're currently doing, and, more important, what we can do to prevent these conditions based on whatever situation is going on. First we'll talk about how to identify the biomarkers. Then we'll talk about how to address this.

If there is one area of the body where we want the earliest indicators possible—the "temperature gauges" that will tell us our engine is overheating—it's the brain. There are a few categories we'll address here. The first is elevated antibodies, the biomarker that tells us when your immune system says, "We've got a problem here." Having measurable levels of antibodies to your brain tissue is not a bad thing; that's how we regenerate new brain cells. The immune system gets rid of the old and damaged cells to make room for the new cells. But when you have *elevated* levels of antibodies to your brain tissue, you are killing off more cells than you're making. When we can identify the elevated levels of antibodies to your brain, we now have something to focus on to get the antibody load down to normal levels.

WHY LOOK FOR ANTIBODY BIOMARKERS?

There is an increased interest in predictive autoimmunity antibody biomarkers for several reasons.

- Autoantibodies can be correlated to disease activity and severity.
- Antibodies are shown to be related to a particular clinical manifestation or tissue injury presenting years before disease onset, and they may constitute potential biomarkers of the disease.
- Antibodies act as a predictive marker of disease occurrence.
- Antibodies are valuable indicators for therapeutic response to biologics (drugs) as well as to side effects.
- These autoantibodies can be a useful tool for diagnosis and management relevant to organ-specific or non-organ-specific disorders.[27]

By using a panel of several biomarkers of brain injury, the predictive capabilities toward long-term outcome have been shown to increase. No one elevated marker by itself gives a certain diagnosis of a disease or a risk of a disease. All a single elevated marker tells you is that something is out of balance. But when you have a number of biomarkers out of balance that have been shown to affect the brain, you now know with more certainty that you have a problem you should address right away. By monitoring several biomarkers that are out of balance, you can see if the protocols being applied are working to calm down the inflammation (and to what degree).[28]

ANTIBODY TESTING FOR B4 (theDr.com/B4)

If there is one group of biomarkers that are of the greatest value in identifying if the brain is under duress, it is the biomarkers that identify if there is a breach of the blood-brain barrier (B4). As far as I know, practically every brain disease and every brain dysfunction (anxiety, depression, schizophrenia, psychosis, etc.) is associated with B4. Listen to how researchers refer to the importance of the BBB: "The complex nature of blood-brain barrier dysfunction in psychosis might be relevant to many aspects of disrupted neuronal and synaptic function, increased permeability to inflammatory molecules, disrupted glutamate homoeostasis, impaired action of antipsychotics, and development of antipsychotic resistance."[29] The inflammation in the brain is creating a resistance to the drugs that are meant to treat these serious conditions.

I recommend the following biomarkers to identify B4. Interestingly, the antibodies that identify leaky gut (zonulin, actin, LPS) may also identify a leaky brain.

1. Antibodies to zonulin: Zonulin is a tight junction modulator (hands on the steering wheel) that is released by the small intestine mucosa upon gluten stimulation. Interestingly, the zonulin receptor has been found in the human BBB. Overexpression of zonulin and zonulin antibodies could be involved in the blood-brain barrier disruption in a role similar to the one that zonulin plays in increasing intestinal permeability.[30]

2. Antibodies to actin: BBB surface cells contain actin, a smooth muscle protein forming a cable network within the endothelial cell. Elevated antibodies to actin have been used as a measure of intestinal permeability and are now recognized as a biomarker of B4.

3. Antibodies to LPS: LPS are families of by-products from gram-negative bacteria. Their molecular size is much too big to be in the bloodstream, but it happens all the time. LPS binds on brain tissues, forming neo-epitopes. LPS has been identified in the brains of those with Alzheimer's, Parkinson's, or schizophrenia, and many other people with brain diseases. Thus, antibodies to LPS may be creating a bonfire in your brain.

4. Antibodies to S100B: S100B is the most studied biomarker of brain injury. First identified more than 50 years ago, it is now recognized as a biomarker of B4.[31] The detection of S100B antibodies actually indicates if the BBB has been damaged and if autoimmunity has

been activated against the damaged brain cells. It can even be used to indicate the degree of recovery and when a patient can return to normal activity.[32] When you have elevated levels of S100B antibodies, it validates that there's damage occurring in your BBB that will eventually cause the scar tissue called white matter abnormalities, which is what causes the loss of cognition (the loss of thinking capability).

5. Antibodies to neuron-specific enolase (NSE): Neuron-specific enolase is the most studied biomarker of predicted outcomes after head trauma. In one study it was found elevated in 34 of 35 head trauma cases. It's also a marker of damage to the BBB. Elevated antibodies to NSE tell us there is an ongoing leakage of this enzyme from certain damaged tissue.[33] That's one reason why it's so important to check a panel of markers, and not just one. This is a good biomarker, but it's not a "slam dunk" by itself for B4.

CHECK THESE ANTIBODIES TO BRAIN TISSUE

1. Antibodies to transglutaminase 2 (TG2): This marker is the "go-to" blood test for celiac disease. Interestingly, antibodies to TG2 can cross-react with TG3 (in your skin) and TG6 (a primary component of the brain). This means antibodies to TG2 (produced with a sensitivity to eating wheat) may trigger production of antibodies to TG6 and begin an inflammatory response in the brain. This is the most common identified mechanism behind a sensitivity to wheat creating brain symptoms.

2. Antibodies to transglutaminase 6 (TG6): As discussed, TG6 is a primary component of the brain. Elevated levels of antibodies mean the immune system is attacking your brain. These antibodies found in the bloodstream have to get through the BBB to attack the brain tissue. Thus, there likely is B4 occurring if these antibodies are being produced in the brain.[34]

3. Antibodies to gangliosides: Antibodies to gangliosides are thought to be involved in the development of some muscle diseases (motor neuropathies) due to relatively high levels detected prior to therapeutic intervention, and a subsequent decrease of antibodies that occurs with clinical improvement.[35] The most common neurological symptom in celiac disease is *peripheral neuropathies,* numbness and tingling that can occur anywhere in the body. Twenty-two percent of CD patients manifest peripheral neuropathies. Every one (100 percent) of these patients had elevated anti-ganglioside antibodies. Ganglioside antibodies can be produced as a cross-reactivity reaction with the bacterium *Campylobacter jejuni* or with *Haemophilus influenza.* This is thought to be a primary mechanism in Guillain-Barré syndrome.

4. Antibodies to herpes simplex: Between 20 and 40 percent of the population suffer from *herpes labialis* (cold sores), a disorder of the peripheral nervous system (PNS) caused by the virus herpes simplex 1 (HSV1). There are more than 100 studies on the association of HSV1 in elderly people and the development of Alzheimer's disease. In younger people, the virus is almost always absent in the brain.[36] If the viral load gets higher than your immune system can keep in check, it creates an infection. With a viral infection, your immune system brings out the big guns, antibodies, to deal with it. In this case, the immune system produces IgM antibodies to HSV1. The risk of an HSV1 infection causing the development of amyloid plaque in the aged brain is magnified dramatically if the person also carries the gene for ApoE4.

5. Antibodies to *Chlamydia pneumoniae:* Another organism that has been linked to Alzheimer's disease is *C. pneumoniae.* In this case, the bacterial DNA has been found to be present in the brains of a very high proportion of AD patients, but in very few age-matched controls (those without AD), indicating a greater susceptibility to entry and infection of the brain by the bacterium in AD patients rather than, as with HSV1, a greater susceptibility to damage of the nervous system.

WHAT YOU SEE IN AN MRI

The x-ray test to see if you have a problem with your brain is called an MRI. If it identifies *white matter lesions,* you know that there is something going on in the brain, that there's some type of pathology. Radiologists may tell you that it's normal to see white matter lesions. It is not. Remember, there's a big difference between "normal" and common. Normal means what we're designed to have, or do. Common just means it happens to a lot of us. It is not normal to have white matter lesions in the brain, but it sure is common.

6. Antibodies to gliofibrillar acid protein (GFAP): GFAP is a major component of the brain. Its levels elevate with inflammation of the brain from strokes, head injuries, and other trauma. Traumatic brain injury patients (such as those who have been in car accidents or had concussions) showed an average 3.77-fold increase in anti-GFAP autoantibody levels from early (0 to 1 days) to late (7 to 10 days) postinjury. The presence of these autoantibodies tells us just how bad the injury is. The higher the level, the worse the outcome. In cases of aging and senile dementia conditions, the brain is characterized by cell loss and neuron damage sustained over long periods and is associated with high levels of GFAP. When you have high levels of GFAP, your immune system will make antibodies to them. This data suggests that anti-GFAP autoantibodies represent excellent markers that can be used to monitor and assess brain injury in traumatic brain injury (TBI).

7. Antibodies to myelin basic protein (MBP): Myelin is the "plastic wrap" or protective sheath around all of your nerves and your brain. Every nerve and all bran tissue is wrapped with this covering. A primary mechanism in the development of multiple sclerosis (MS) is the antibody attack on the myelin coating of your nerves. When you develop an elevation of myelin antibodies, you destroy this coating, and the messages that are being sent across them will flicker. This is what causes the symptoms of MS.

Myelin basic protein antibodies are detected in various neuroimmune disorders including multiple sclerosis. Consequently, antibodies to MBP are accepted markers of inflammation in various neuroimmune disorders. In possible cases of multiple sclerosis, the measurement of antibodies against MBP may predict early conversion to clinically definite multiple sclerosis; in one study, patients who were positive for both antibodies to MBP and myelin oligodendrocyte glycoprotein had clinically definite multiple sclerosis within an average of 7.5 months.[37] Autism Spectrum Disorder (ASD) patients possess significantly higher levels of anti-brain antibodies, such as MBP antibodies, and brain endothelial cells or B4[38] antibodies. MBP antibodies may develop as a cross-reaction after a streptococcal (strep) infection. This autoimmune response triggers inflammation that compromises the blood-brain barrier.[39, 40, 41]

8. Antibodies to glutamic acid decarboxylase: These are antibodies to your brain and are also related to celiac disease, non-celiac gluten sensitivity, type 1 diabetes, stiff person syndrome, and cerebellar ataxia, which is a disorder affecting balance and muscle movement. These antibodies, when elevated, are also associated with insomnia and anxiety. This is one reason why following a gluten-free diet has been shown to be an effective remedy for these two conditions.

9. Antibodies to alpha + beta tubulin: Tubulin is a building-block protein and a major component of a cell's internal structure, called *microtubules*. These structures play key roles in many nerve functions. Elevated antibodies to tubulin appear in alcoholic liver disease, demyelinating diseases, recent-onset type 1 diabetes, Graves' disease, Hashimoto's, PANDAS, rheumatoid arthritis, and toxin exposures (including mercury and other heavy metals). This is another example of how an environmental trigger (like excessive heavy metal exposure) can trigger a neurological autoimmune disease.

10. Cerebellar antibodies: The cerebellum is the part of the brain controlling movement and balance. Inside the cerebellar cortex there are large neurons called Purkinje cells. The cerebellar antibodies

test measures antibodies against Purkinje cells. These antibodies are associated with autism, celiac disease, gluten ataxia, and paraneoplastic cerebellar degeneration syndrome.

Elevated levels of this antibody are often why people, as they begin aging, feel unsteady walking up and down stairs. Their cerebellum is shrinking due to years of elevated antibodies to the cerebellum, slowly killing off the Purkinje cells. In my office, if a patient had elevated antibodies to gluten, 26 percent of them also had elevated antibodies to their cerebellum. That's one out of four people whose brains were shrinking from years of eating a food that may not have given them stomach pains, yet their immune response was going after their cerebellum.

For example, my patient Sam came in one day and was feeling unsteady on his feet. We investigated and found that he had a gluten sensitivity manifesting as inflammation in his brain that was picked up with an MRI, yet there were no gut symptoms. His cerebellum looked normal on the MRI—just some inflammation. He refused to follow the recommendation to get off gluten. Seven years later, Sam came back, but this time he could hardly walk. The increased level of antibodies to the weak link in his chain (his cerebellum) kept killing his cerebellar cells, and his cerebellum had shrunk to the point where he now had a diagnosis of gluten ataxia. Unfortunately, his inability to walk became permanent.

11. Antibodies to synapsin: Synapsin is a major immunoreactive protein found in most neurons of the central and peripheral nervous systems. It is a brain protein involved in the regulation of brain hormones. When you have elevated antibodies to synapsin, you are very vulnerable to having imbalances in your brain hormones. This imbalance is a primary cause of anxiety, depression, bipolar disorder, and schizophrenia. These antibodies to your brain cause demyelinating diseases (like MS) and peripheral neuropathies, numbness and tingling, anywhere in your body. Antibodies to synapsin also will inhibit the release of the brain hormones and can contribute to the development of lupus.

TESTING FOR ENVIRONMENTAL EXPOSURES

There are many ways to test for toxic chemical accumulation in our bodies. We currently know that the clinical usefulness of identifying toxin levels in the body is not as important as it used to be. That's because practically everyone has some measurable levels of these toxins in their body. That they are there is almost a "given" in our society today. What is critically important is if your immune system is activated and producing antibodies to a toxin. This means that you have crossed the line of tolerance and your immune system has to allocate its precious energy to fighting this specific toxin.

Your doctor can order any of these tests, or you can get them from my Web site at theDr.com:

1. Cyrex Chemical Immune Reactivity Screen (Array 11): This excellent panel looks for 24 different toxins that can accumulate in your tissue. Remember, there are thousands of chemicals that we are exposed to, but these 24 are the top offenders (including PCBs, phthalates, BPA, dioxin, and more). (theDr.com/Cyrex11)

2. Cyrex Pathogen-Associated Immune Reactivity Screen (Array 12): This panel looks at 29 different pathogens (bacteria, viruses like herpes, and molds). There are hundreds of different bacteria and viruses that may be a problem, but these 29 are the primary pathogens associated with chronic fatigue, digestive upset, brain dysfunction, and compromised immune systems. (theDr.com/Cyrex12)

3. Real Time Labs Urinary Mold Panel: The most sensitive test I've found for mold is this urine test. It identifies if there is mold accumulation in your body. The three types of by-products for mold it looks for are ochratoxin, aflatoxin, and trichothecene. (theDr.com/realtimemold)

4. Provocative Challenge Urine Test for Heavy Metals: There are three methodologies for testing for heavy metals: blood, hair, and urine. Blood tests are what most doctors and schools recommend

when you are looking for lead, mercury, etc. However, the body does everything it can to keep heavy metals out of the blood and away from the brain. Thus, a blood test is accurate for testing an acute heavy metal exposure within 2 weeks. However, if you believe you have an accumulative or long-term exposure, a blood test will not accurately identify it. A hair analysis can identify an exposure for a longer period of time, up to 2 months. However, it is also of limited value, because only the first inch of hair from the nape of the neck can be used. The third and most accurate method for determining heavy metal accumulation is a special urine analysis. The standard analysis can identify only what the kidneys have filtered

DR. TOM'S AT-HOME BIOMARKER FOR LIVER FUNCTION

The liver is your primary organ for detoxification. It has more than 360 functions, but one of the primary ones is that it is your body's oil filter for the blood. If you drop an apple on the ground, wipe it off, and eat it, it's the job of the liver to catch any leftover dirt and prevent it from entering your bloodstream. The liver is built with thousands of honeycombs, each of which is lined with a different kind of cheesecloth than your intestines and brain have. All three are designed to stop large molecules from getting through.

Here's a simple indicator that suggests you have a dirty oil filter (liver congestion). Have someone press a finger on your back between your shoulder blades, close to your spine. When they take their finger away, they will see a blemish or fingerprint where they had pressed. Count how many seconds it takes before the blemish disappears. It should take 1 to 2 seconds for the blemish to disappear as the blood flows back to your skin. Four seconds or more suggests liver congestion. If you need detoxing soon, you might have blemishes that last as long as 7 or 8 seconds.

Why does this work? When the blood comes out of the liver, it travels right past this area on your back. If you have a congested liver, the blood pools and can't get through fast enough to keep traveling through the body without a bit of a damming effect. Increased liver blemish time suggests sluggish bloodflow coming out of the liver. Intermittent fasting, and many of the specific foods we discussed in Chapter 4, will help to detox the liver.

from the blood over the last 2 weeks. However, if you take a chelating substance, which pulls the metals out of storage in your fat cells and bones, and then collect a 24-hour urine sample, you'll get a much more accurate result. The chelating substances most often used are EDTA and DMSA. Have your doctor do a provocative challenge urine test to identify accumulative heavy metals (lead, mercury, arsenic, cadmium, aluminum). (theDr.com/heavymetals)

5. DetoxiGenomic Profile: The genes that you've inherited make you more or less susceptible to having problems breaking down environmental toxins, including prescription medications. This is a major reason why some people have side effects when taking medications, and others do not. This genetic test is an excellent way to identify if you have the genes that inhibit your ability to break down toxins that can directly make you vulnerable to a host of brain dysfunction, including chronic fatigue, anxiety, depression, ADHD, alcoholism, bipolar disorders, schizophrenia, as well as an increased risk of lung, colon, bladder, head, and neck cancers. (theDr.com/geneticdetoxification)

SHOW THIS BOOK TO YOUR DOCTOR

If you would like to order these tests from your doctor, you might be met with some resistance. He or she may say, "It's not possible to check all of these antibodies." Explain that it is, and show your doctor this book. If your doctor still doesn't believe you, it might be time to include another doctor on your health-care team. If your doctor refuses to do the tests you request, you can learn more about ordering these tests on my Web site (theDr.com).

I am on the teaching faculty of the Institute for Functional Medicine (functionalmedicine.org). To find a certified functional medicine practitioner like me in your area, visit that Web site. Most health insurance plans will cover services provided by a functional medicine practitioner. The type of practitioner (MD, DO, DC, acupuncturist) is not as important as the certified training in functional medicine that they have received.

The world of autoimmune disease is the best example of the limitations of conventional medicine. Just as a farm has individual silos to hold different grains, the silos of traditional medicine are referred to as specialties. And the vast majority of medical specialists have very little training in autoimmunity. They all have their own silo, and few practitioners look for clues to solve a medical problem outside their training and expertise. In fact, 46 percent of internists and general practitioners surveyed acknowledge they only received 1 or 2 lectures, not courses, in autoimmunity during medical school.

For instance, your family doctor may refer you to an endocrinologist to examine hormonal output, or to a rheumatologist for musculoskeletal diseases like arthritis. All know how to respond to autoimmune issues within their specialty, but few are trained to see the big picture. A traditional dermatologist focuses on the skin and treats the skin, whereas a functional medicine practitioner looks at the skin but treats the whole body. The functional medicine doctor knows, for example, that many times skin issues from acne to psoriasis resolve completely when diet is addressed.

Traditional medical doctors usually treat only the symptoms (and usually through drugs and/or surgery) and rarely offer diet or an examination of environmental toxins as a solution (or the initial problem) of autoimmunity. Here's an example of how this can be a problem: Imagine that your child is suffering from seizures. You've been to three different doctors, and still the drugs are not controlling the seizures. This is called drug-resistant epilepsy. Fifty percent of children with drug-resistant epilepsy are found to go into complete remission on a gluten-free diet.[42] Why don't our neurologists know this and test for it? The reason was that this research was not published in a neurology journal; it was published in a general medicine journal.

The bottom line is that these tests exist, and the results are accurate. In today's modern era, new science is coming out exponentially quicker. Your doctor needs to get on board. It's not that these antibody tests are new. It's that we're now measuring a large variety of antibodies to see where the inflammation is occurring.

By initiating the appropriate lifestyle interventions (diet, limiting envi-

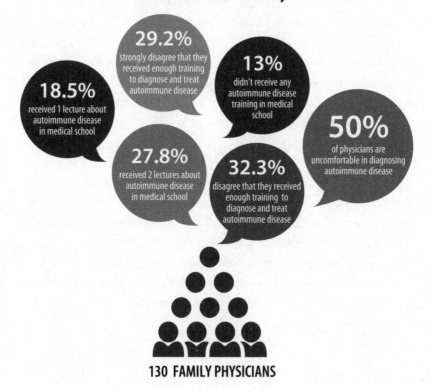

The Limited Training Our Medical Doctors Receive on Autoimmunity

29.2% strongly disagree that they received enough training to diagnose and treat autoimmune disease

13% didn't receive any autoimmune disease training in medical school

18.5% received 1 lecture about autoimmune disease in medical school

27.8% received 2 lectures about autoimmune disease in medical school

32.3% disagree that they received enough training to diagnose and treat autoimmune disease

50% of physicians are uncomfortable in diagnosing autoimmune disease

130 FAMILY PHYSICIANS

ronmental exposures, stress reduction, exercise), you should be able to not only feel the difference but also demonstrate a reduction of antibody levels. It will take a minimum of 6 months before the antibody load reduces enough to show up in bloodwork. That's why you have to retest 6 months or a year after initiating a program.

Like peeling away the layers of an onion, it can take time to find the bottom-line trigger. Meanwhile, any life jacket might help, but it's unlikely that your symptoms will go away completely. You might be able to mask the symptoms with a powerful drug, but the underlying pathology continues. Please don't get me wrong: I think that drugs for symptom relief can be very useful at times—get the safest life jacket you can when you're drowning in symptoms. However, the exclusive emphasis on symptom relief has produced the results that our current health-care system suffers from: shorter life spans for our children, terrible rankings by the World Health Organization for the quality of health care in the United States, and much more. Yet by identifying the underlying cause of your symptoms, you can arrest the development of brain dysfunction and have the brainpower to learn a new language in your eighties. In the next few chapters, you'll learn exactly what you can do to light up your brain.

ACTION STEP WEEK 5: WORK ON YOUR TIMELINE

I cannot overemphasize the importance of taking the time to get your timeline to be as accurate as possible. My friends at Living Matrix have created a way to assist functional medicine doctors to guide their patients in creating their own health timeline. Using this free resource, you can create a completely comprehensive timeline and then find a functional medicine practitioner in your area who understands how to work with you and your timeline. Visit theDr.com/livingmatrix for more information.

6

THE PYRAMID
OF HEALTH

*The problems we have created today cannot be solved with the same
level of thinking that created the problem.*
—ALBERT EINSTEIN

YOU ARE NOW on the journey, making your way farther upstream, where you'll be introduced to new foods, new habits, and new ideas that will have a profound and lasting effect on your brain health. The most essential of the three are the new ideas. A major goal of this book has been to change how you think about your health, to stop looking for the better life jacket. You've learned how your brain function has been affected by a toxic environment, whether it's the foods you've been eating or the world around you. The research we've been discovering together has hopefully shaped your understanding and provided real, scientific reasons why we have to take this journey: We must restore our health, and our world.

Now it's time to grab onto the ladder and get yourself out of the pool. This second part of the book provides the tools you'll need. You will determine exactly how the foods you eat and the lifestyle choices you make are affecting how you think. And then you'll see how much better you can feel by removing the offending foods and chemical exposures that may have been holding you back. These changes are the base hits, and you'll see improvements in increments—building one small success on top of another.

The latest brain science focuses on the process of neurogenesis, where the brain continues to create new cells and grow throughout our lives. This mechanism teaches us that it is rarely too late to change our habits or our health. First, we have to stop the wear and tear on the leaky brain and the leaky gut (in other words, stop throwing gasoline on the fire). Then we can train the body so that it is in a constant "heal, seal, and repair" state that affects every cell. Every cell in your body regenerates; the entire body regenerates every 7 years. This is how I know it's entirely possible to create a healthier, stronger brain by creating the right internal environment. But in order to bring balance to an overactive or underperforming immune system and address the leaky gut/leaky brain, we cannot just take a pill. We must also address the lifestyle habits that caused this imbalance in the first place.

The ultimate goal is to reduce inflammation throughout the body and the brain, especially in the intestinal tract, which will set the stage to heal intestinal permeability. By healing a leaky gut, you are minimizing the passage of toxic bacteria and large food molecules into the body and the brain, which is what's causing the immune protective response that creates systemic inflammation.

You might have read in other books or on the Internet that we are supposed to "boost" the immune system with nutrients, such as antioxidants. That's not entirely correct. The truth is, immune *balancing* is more important than immune boosting. You don't want to boost the immune system if you already have an autoimmune disease. You don't want to suppress the immune system either. You want to balance immune function so it can protect us, but not overreact. Our goal in creating a balanced immune system is to allow it to function as it was intended so that you can stay healthy.

Now, are you ready and willing to put in 1 hour a week for 6 months to have a higher-functioning brain? I hope so, because once you balance your immune system by continually hitting base hits, your brain health symptoms begin diminishing—less brain fog, better attention, better mood, better sleep, better resiliency. You'll find that your vitality comes back, and you'll be better equipped to handle the challenges and stresses of everyday life. Let's get started.

THE PYRAMID OF HEALTH

The model we'll be using for addressing our concerns and making improvements is based on an establishing principle of chiropractic care: the Triangle of Health. One of my first mentors was George Goodheart, DC, the founder of applied kinesiology, a system of testing muscles as biomarkers of function for what's happening inside the body. Dr. Goodheart discovered that there were many associations between the organs in the body and the muscles that shared the same bloodflow. He created a method for addressing the muscles and the bone structure that led to a beneficial effect on the associated organs. Since then, tens of thousands of doctors and hundreds of thousands of patients have been helped through his muscle function and evaluation protocol.

In addressing any long-term or chronic health problem, Dr. Goodheart always talked about the Triangle of Health as a way to look at the three different underlying platforms from which our therapeutic protocols would have to come. First, we always evaluated and addressed the structure: the foundation that holds us together, including bones, muscles, ligaments, and posture. Next, we investigated the mind-set: our emotional or spiritual side, including our overall outlook on life. Finally, we had to look at the biochemistry: everything we put in our mouth, from medication to food. No one "platform" was more important than another. We had to determine which platform to begin with for each patient's complaint. In some cases, mind-set was the most important to begin with, and counseling in deep meditation techniques, or taking daily quiet walks, or seeing a therapist was the right prescription. In other cases, what was needed was addressing the structure, and chiropractic care, or massage therapy, or Feldenkrais Method sessions, or other approaches emphasizing the bones, muscles, and ligaments were what was needed. And sometimes it was biochemistry, and pharmaceuticals, dietary changes, or nutritional therapy, that was exactly "what the doctor ordered."

I had hundreds of hours of study with Dr. Goodheart. I am forever grateful that his teachings molded a large portion of how I think about health care, the paradigm that I come from, and my insatiable curiosity.

I loved going to his weekend seminars, where every Sunday morning he would begin with the exact same prayer. He would bow his head and say:

"One of the things that I like to do on a Saturday or a Sunday, or any day, is to ask for help from where it all comes from. I'm sure that there's someone who can do this better than I can, but if you will bear with me ... Dear Lord, Thou Great Physician, from whom every good and perfect gift must come, give kindness to our hearts, intelligence to our minds, and strength and skill to our hands so we may help our suffering fellow man through our chosen profession. We ask it in thy name, Amen." Then he would say, "If anyone doesn't like this, it's too bad; it's my football." And then he would talk for an hour or more about the philosophy of being a doctor and what our obligation was. His bottom line was always the same: We must continue to ask "why" the patient has what they have.

A few years before Dr. Goodheart passed away, I think it was 2004 or 2005, we got to talking about the Triangle of Health. I remember the conversation well. I said, "Dr. Goodheart, I don't think it's a Triangle of Health anymore. I think there are now four critical components, not three."

"And what do you think is the fourth component, Tom?"

"Well, sir, we certainly have the structure, the biochemistry, and the mind-set, but I think we have to consider a fourth category, and that is the electromagnetic field."

Dr. Goodheart smiled, nodded his head, and agreed with the logic. We all experience electromagnetic radiation from many sources. Each source produces its own electromagnetic field, or EMF—a wave of energy radiating outward, getting weaker with increasing distance. It disrupts the electrical frequencies in the brain and throughout the nervous system.

During my first week of my medical education, my very first week, I saw a notice in the hall saying that Sheldon Deal, DC, Mr. Arizona, would be speaking on campus the next weekend and the talk was open to all. It was that weekend talk with Dr. Deal back in 1978 that introduced me to the topic of electromagnetic pollution. Dr. Deal was not just a chiropractor, he was Mr. Arizona, a professional bodybuilder. I went to a

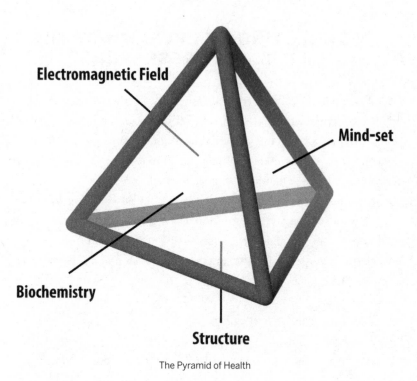

Electromagnetic Field

Mind-set

Biochemistry

Structure

The Pyramid of Health

seminar of his that first week and was completely floored. He had a color television on a stand in the lecture hall, and he had it turned on, but the volume was off. When we all were seated, he walked over to the podium, opened his briefcase, and took out a magnet about the size of an iPhone 7. When he walked toward the television holding the magnet in front of him, the picture turned upside down. When he walked away, the picture returned to normal. He did it twice, and both times walking toward the television with the magnet in hand turned the picture upside down. He said, "That's what electromagnetic pollution does to your brain." At the time, cell phones were not a "thing" yet, and the big concern was the batteries in watches.

Thus, my new Triangle of Health has four sides, so it's really more of a Pyramid of Health, and in the remainder of the book, we will explore each aspect, beginning with the structure, which I put at the base of the pyramid because that is the foundation.

CONNECTING THE PYRAMID WITH THE LATEST RESEARCH

Dale Bredesen, MD, has identified more than 100 factors that may contribute to the development of Alzheimer's disease. He believes, as I do, that Alzheimer's is not one disease process, but a name given to a cluster of symptoms. And as there are many symptoms, there are many mechanisms out of balance that need to be addressed.

Of the hundreds of factors that may impact our brain health, many are the result of the way we lead our lives. Throughout the rest of this book, we're going to review the base hits you can put into practice right now that can address your own brain health issues and are proven to be effective. These include:

- Increasing exercise (structure)
- Addressing diet by eliminating "The Big Three"—wheat, dairy, and sugar—and increasing vegetables, fruits, and non-farmed fish (biochemistry)
- Supplementing with the following detoxifying nutrients (biochemistry):
  - » Folate (vitamin B_9): This vitamin's name is derived from the Latin word *folium*, which means leaf. In fact, leafy vegetables are among the best dietary sources of folate. The active form of folate is abbreviated 5-MTHF.
  - » Cobalamin (vitamin B_{12}): Of the many forms of vitamin B_{12}, methylcobalamin helps a little more in the detoxification pathways.
  - » Vitamin D_3: Take enough vitamin D_3 so that a blood test shows a level between 50 and 75 nanograms/milliliter (ng/ml). In my opinion, maintaining the right level of vitamin D_3 is the most important marker of your health, and it should be checked every year during your physical examination.
  - » Fish oil: The good fats in fish oil do so many beneficial things for the body. They are needed to create brain cells, thus increasing

brain function; stabilize cholesterol levels; turn the genes on to heal intestinal permeability; and reduce and, in some cases, reverse autoimmune diseases.

- Adopting an intermittent fasting routine for weight loss and detoxification (biochemistry)
- Turning your wireless router off at night in your home while you sleep (electromagnetic)
- Putting your cell phone on airplane mode while you sleep, even if you need the alarm clock (electromagnetic)
- Improving sleep; if you need help, try taking melatonin supplements (2 to 5 milligrams at night) (mind-set)
- Actively reducing stress through meditation (mind-set)

ADOPTING A LIFESTYLE FOR CELLULAR REGENERATION

Here's a "truth-response" type of question: On a scale of 1 to 10, if 10 is the amount of energy, vitality, and health you *should* have, and 5 is half as much, now take your wishful thinking out of the equation—where do you fall on the scale? What's your number?

We all want to be a "10," and we often think that we're doing "pretty good" or "fine." But being asked to take our wishful thinking out of the equation brings up what I like to call a reality check, and we acknowledge that we're functioning as a 5 or a 6 or a 4, something less than acceptable (7.5 or above by my definition). So what does it really take to get to be a "10"?

A basic premise in biology is that when a cell reproduces, it reproduces an exact duplicate of itself. Inside our cells, our DNA carries the blueprints for optimally healthy genetic expression, a "library of blueprints" for our perfect self. This means we already have the potential to be a 10. This understanding is the premise of using stem cells to stimulate new, healthier tissue. I'm not getting into politics here about using stem cells; I'm just saying what our anatomy contains. So why don't we reproduce perfect skin cells or brain cells or blood vessel cells on our own? Why aren't we already a 10? Why are we functioning at a 6.2? After all, our genetics don't change. We have the "blueprint" to be a 10. Why aren't our new cells a 10? The answer? The environment of inflammation that's affecting the functionality of your cells.

Let's say you're 35 years old. You're doing pretty well in life regarding your health—not quite what you were at 22, but doing fine. You lived through your late teens and early twenties with maybe a little too much partying, but you're not really the worse for wear or having any problems to complain about. Your blood tests are "normal" in your annual physical—there are no alarms going off. Perhaps your brain is functioning at a 6.4 on a scale where 10 is optimal. Yet what that means is that you're barely getting by: On occasion you ask the question, "Where are my keys?" or you see someone and you have to dig deep to remember their name, or your mind wanders off when someone is talking to you.

Your cellular function is determined by what is happening around the cell, the "epi-cell," if you will. (I just made up a new word, but I hope the visual is clear for you.) Epigenetics means the environment around a gene determines whether that gene gets turned on or not. The epi-cell is the environment around the cell that determines how that cell functions and reproduces. So if the environment you created around this cell is full of inflammation, your cell is functioning as a 6.4, and life goes on.

But if you continue to live the same lifestyle, meaning eating foods that you have a sensitivity to or eating junk foods, drinking too much, and breathing bad air, you are taxing your brain further. Pretty soon your brain will begin functioning as a 6.3. When that cell reproduces, you reproduce a 6.3. If your current lifestyle continues with the same or even greater inflammatory triggers, you begin functioning as a 6.2, and that cell reproduces as a 6.2. With the same lifestyle, you begin functioning as a 6.1, and that cell reproduces as a 6.1. Due to the continual inflammation, the body continues to break down over the years and reproduces weaker cells as determined by the function of those cells. This process of getting old is technically referred to as *catabolism*.

However, once you make the changes to create a healthier internal environment by applying the principles in this book, your brain function will improve. Dr. Bredesen and others have proven this again and again. The inflammation that was affecting you on a cellular level reduces and your body stops making elevated antibodies. Your body wants to be healthy, so it's trying to regenerate a healthier body by creating healthier cells. Your cells are now able to reproduce newer, healthier cells as long as you continue to provide a healthier environment by eating more nutrient-dense, less inflammatory foods and mitigating environmental toxins. Instead of being a 6.1, you begin functioning as a 6.2. When that cell reproduces, it reproduces as a 6.2. You continue your healthier lifestyle, and you begin functioning as a 6.3. And those cells reproduce as 6.3s. You continue and begin functioning as a 6.4. When that cell reproduces, you reproduce a 6.4. And the body continues to rebuild over the months and reproduces stronger-functioning cells determined by the epi-cell (the environment that you have supplied around the cell). As your cells regenerate as healthier, stronger cells that can better communicate with one another, your brain will light up just like adjusting the dimmer switch from low to high. You'll start feeling less tired, less anxious, less confused. And one day you'll realize that your brain is working better than it has in years. This process of getting younger and stronger is technically referred to as *anabolism*.

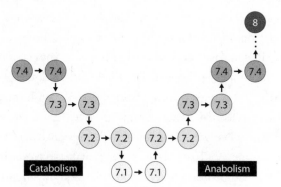

Reinvigorating brain function is a step-by-step process as you move from a catabolic state of degeneration to an anabolic state of producing stronger and healthier cells.

Dr. Bredesen has demonstrated that when there is so much tissue damage that a person has received the diagnosis of Alzheimer's, they begin feeling better within a few months of implementing the program, but it takes as long as 5 years to reverse the cognitive decline. The reason that it takes so long is that your internal environment is a mess. Brain cells take longer to regenerate than other cells in the body, and you will be rebuilding the brain one cell at a time. This is why you have to create and maintain an ideal anabolic environment in the brain (optimal nutrition, less inflammation) so that every day you are building new, healthier brain cells. Again, base hits win the ball game. As you shift from a catabolic state to an anabolic state, transitioning from the mechanism of getting older to one of youth, vibrancy, and better health, you regenerate healthier brain cells and the dimmer switch comes off.

BENEFITS YOU CAN EXPECT

As you implement the principles in this book, you can expect to experience two subtle but impactful changes to your body and brain: The first is that you are going to lower inflammation, and the second is that you will regenerate a healthier microbiome.

The first step in reducing systemic inflammation, always, is to stop throwing gasoline on the fire. When you're applying the principles that follow in the next few chapters, you will by default decrease inflammation immediately. It doesn't matter whether or not gluten or any other environmental toxin you have been exposed to is still in your system, because your symptoms are primarily related to the inflammation, not the toxin. The endotoxins we discussed throughout the book cause inflammation, but the stronger influence is your current lifestyle. That's why we address lifestyle first. And when you do, you start noticing a change rather quickly. The stored toxins in your body are an emergency brake to getting healthier, but as the inflammation comes down, your body will naturally flush them out more easily. Depending on the types and levels of toxins in your body, you may need some help flushing them out. There are a myriad of great detox programs out there. My favorite can be found in Dr. Joseph Pizzorno's book *The Toxin Solution*. It is the most comprehensive, and safest, program I've seen.

Within 24 hours, you'll begin to balance your microbiome. As your microbiome is rebalanced, your energy comes up (if it's been low) and your brain hormones (the neurotransmitters) become more balanced, resulting in a range of good feelings from reduced anxiety to less depression. Your blood pressure calms down, and your sleep improves. Your body and brain now have a chance to address whatever imbalances you have been dealing with.

All of these wonderful improvements will put you on the path to better health. They don't mean you're necessarily cured or your symptoms will completely disappear. However, you certainly should notice that they're reducing, or that you are seeing benefits like a decrease in brain fog.

While you can change your microbiome in as little as 1 day, it will take a bit longer for the inflammation to subside completely and for your immune system to get the message to stop attacking you. Even when you remove the antigens, the immune system continues to create antibodies for a couple of months. You may not be able to see the change yourself on a daily basis because the base hits—the daily wins of food selection creating a healthier environment around your cells—are small. But they're cumulative. And pretty soon you realize, "Wow, this is working."

I truly believe that almost everyone will benefit and see positive changes in their body function and how they feel by implementing this Transition Protocol. Regardless of whether or not you are sensitive to gluten, dairy, or sugar, these are toxic foods that take you closer to your threshold, or body burden.

You might find that some of your symptoms will go away earlier than others. This is because most of us have more than one weak link, and very few individuals are suffering from only one autoimmune disease. Technically, this is called *co-morbidities*—having more than one imbalance. For example, you may be feeling forgetful, and your spouse might be telling you that you seem more irritable than ever. When you remove gluten from your diet, your memory might improve, but your spouse may still think you're a pain in the ... Have patience; eventually all of the areas in your brain will respond with lower inflammation, your irritability will subside, and brain function is likely to improve overall.

WATCH OUT FOR WITHDRAWAL SYMPTOMS

People occasionally report that they experience withdrawal symptoms when they stop eating gluten and dairy. They might feel tired, depressed, or nauseated. Some don't want to exercise, and some have headaches (just like with coffee withdrawal). This is especially true of those who in their blood tests have elevated levels of the peptide in wheat called gluteo-morphins or elevated levels of the peptide in dairy called casomorphin. These are the poorly digested peptides we talked about in Chapter 3 that can stimulate the opiate receptors in the gut and brain. Opiate receptors trigger the production of hormones called endorphins and enkephalins that produce a "feel-good" response. Just as addicts may have withdrawal symptoms when they stop their drug of choice, such may be the case with gluten and dairy withdrawal.

My friend William Davis, MD, author of *Wheat Belly*, even came up with a name for it: wheat withdrawal. The same may be true for removing dairy. Dr. Davis believes that wheat withdrawal can be quite unpleasant for close to 40 percent of the population. That has not been my clinical experience. Our number has been closer to 10 percent, which is still a substantial number. You may have a friend or family member who has tried to go gluten-free and has told you, "My body must need wheat. It's been 3 days since I've had anything made of wheat, and I feel awful!" This response can be scary. But remember, it's not that the body needs wheat; it craves it. This is just the body craving a toxic substance that it has gotten used to having. Don't worry: The symptoms will disappear quickly. And best of all, the cravings will subside, and then you feel wonderful!

To lessen withdrawal symptoms:

- Stay well hydrated. There is a diuretic effect when you stop eating wheat, dairy, and sugar. If you lose weight the first week, about half that will be water from excess inflammation.
- Season your food with a little more salt than usual (sea salt is preferred). Some people experience leg cramps, and a bit of sea salt can prevent this. Nothing major: Just an extra pinch of salt per day will do the trick (unless your doctor has told you otherwise). Try putting the salt directly on your tongue. If you are sodium deficient and can get past the belief that "any salt is bad for you" (which is the furthest thing from true), you may notice that it tastes really good and you'd like a little more. The pleasant feeling of fulfillment with a little bit of salt is your body saying "thank you."
- Stay calm. Start this program when life is not at the peak of stressfulness. Don't begin this new routine the same day you start a new job or end a relationship. Giving yourself permission to launch this new program when you feel comfortable can lessen your body burden and reduce your withdrawal symptoms.
- Keep moving. Exercise will take your mind off your symptoms and create the endorphins you are looking for in a much healthier way.

ENCOURAGE YOUR KIDS TO FOLLOW ALONG

The earlier people can clean up their diets, the better. You'll have much better luck being compliant if everyone in your family is on board. Rodney Ford, MD, is a pediatrician, gastroenterologist, and allergist, and he puts children on this type of eating plan all the time. He told me during a Gluten Summit interview that for kids, "going gluten-free is not such a biggie. Children who come to my clinic are sick, tired, and grumpy. They've got sore tummies, acid reflux, migraine, other headaches, maybe vomiting, diarrhea, constipation, eczema, rashes, and more. They are predominantly irritable children, lethargic, lacking energy, and have poor sleep. Some are hyperactive and diagnosed already with attention-deficit disorder or ADHD. Most of them don't test positive for celiac disease. But when I put them on a gluten-free diet, most of them get better."

Even if the symptoms your child may be experiencing are vastly different from your own, the source of the problem may still be one of these three inflammatory foods: gluten, dairy, or sugar. The difference again is where the weak link in your chain is. Your child may have a weak link different from yours, but you can both reverse the damage of autoimmunity.

ACTION STEP WEEK 6: CONSIDER OTHER LIKELY SUSPECTS

If you're still not feeling well after following the guidelines of the Pyramid of Health, there may be a hidden trigger that will require a thorough "investigative doctoring" approach. At this point, I would suggest finding a certified functional medicine practitioner. You might find that your inflammation is related to a microbiome so far out of balance that more than just a change of foods is necessary. You may have a candida growth or a viral infection or Lyme disease. My Web site (theDr.com) has information about these common triggers.

THE BASE OF
THE PYRAMID:
ADDRESSING YOUR
STRUCTURE

THE REASON STRUCTURE sits at the base of the Pyramid of Health is that it is the foundation that all health is built on. A crooked or sagging foundation equals crooked or sagging health, particularly for the brain.

If mechanical problems are the primary insult creating the inflammatory cascade (pushing you over the waterfall), then you must address them, which is how you'll get yourself out of the pool of symptoms. Mechanical problems are usually associated with posture and are controlled by the function of your bones, muscles, and nerves. Addressing biochemistry with anti-inflammatories, whether pharmaceutical or nutritional, will help (a little), but the problem remains. Addressing your mind-set by seeing a therapist will help a little, but the problem remains. Putting a cover on your cell phone that diminishes EMFs will reduce inflammatory cytokines and decrease inflammation, helping you feel a little better, but the problem remains. These are all life jackets if you are not addressing the structural imbalance.

Abnormal structural function creates inflammation at the site as well as at other places throughout the body. For example, when you sprain your ankle and compensate by walking funny for a few days, your hip can start hurting because you're putting a new kind of pressure on it, which then causes inflammation. While the ankle pain can usually be treated with medication, if you don't address the root cause of the hip pain, the imbalance may not go away and will manifest somewhere else. You might even get a headache or neck pain, or create oxidative stress just from the same sprained ankle.[1, 2, 3] Worse, the over-the-counter anti-inflammatory medications—aspirin, ibuprofen (Advil), acetaminophen (Tylenol), naproxen (Aleve), and acetaminophen/aspirin/caffeine combinations (Excedrin)—are all great life jackets, but they have side effects that can begin after just one dose. In fact, according to a 2012 study, a single dose of two regular-strength aspirin can cause a leaky gut,[4] starting the entire autoimmune response and leading to a leaky brain and B4. Spinal care—chiropractic, physical therapy, massage, etc.—may be the safest approach and has turned out to be the perfect response for literally tens of millions of people over the years.

Imagine that you're driving down the road, and all of a sudden, your car's right front tire hits a pothole. Ka-boom! A bone-rattling thump. You're startled at first, and then fearful this is a blowout. "Oh no, I don't have time to change a flat tire," you think as you pull over to check the tire. You get out of the car and take a peek: Everything seems okay, so you get back in your car and continue driving, grateful that the tire did not blow. In a minute or two you forget about the incident, thinking everything is okay. But 6 months later, that right front tire has worn down because it was knocked out of balance and was driven for 6 months not sitting straight on the road.

That's what happens to our spine when we are out of balance, when the structure is off and we're not sitting straight with gravity. This scenario isn't always caused by a major trauma, although it could be. We can also become imbalanced from seemingly minor traumas, including poor posture, the way we sleep, the way we sit, or if the heels on our shoes are worn. All these habits contribute to your joints not being aligned with gravity and not being able to move as freely as they should. And because you're using your joints all day, every day, the imbalance causes inflammation, wearing down your cartilage first, then the bones, then causing the beginning of arthritis (bone spurs) that can develop anywhere, most commonly in your neck.

That's when the real trouble begins. Here come the symptoms of arthritis, a condition in which your joints become inflamed and eventually become malformed. This can result in stiffness, soreness, and, in many cases, swelling. This is the mechanism of osteoarthritis (OA), the most common form. The inflammation of OA results from wear and tear from imbalances such as poor posture (wobbly tires) contributing to poor joint function that activates an immune response. Neck dysfunction caused by this kind of imbalance plus inflammation is marked by neck pain. But inside, the problem is even bigger. Improper function of the joints in the neck creates pain, and bloodflow to the brain is compromised: The greater the pain, the more limited the bloodflow.[5] Remember when we talked about hypoperfusion in Chapter 2? This is one mechanism that creates B4. Now come the brain health symptoms: forgetfulness, anxiety, poor sleep, poor attention, etc.

MEET ANNA

This story is not about one of my patients, although it is near to my heart. I have kept a copy of the original study in every one of my examination rooms since it was released in 1990, because it explains the whole platform of why musculoskeletal care can help with so many different health issues.[6] I have shown this study to hundreds and hundreds of patients. You can read the original at theDr.com/study.

The write-up that follows features a 39-year-old woman who came to see her doctor complaining of chronic pelvic pain and problems with urination. Let's call her Anna. Her pelvic pain had started years before, back when she was just 18, shortly after falling down a flight of stairs. The pain started on her right side and gradually also appeared on the left. Her first doctor assumed that she was having an appendicitis attack, so Anna had an appendectomy. But the pathology report afterward showed her appendix was normal, and the pain in her pelvis remained.

A few months later, her menstrual cycles became severely painful, her pelvic pain continued, and she began having continuous diarrhea. As a result, she was hospitalized for evaluation and treatment, and her symptoms were diagnosed as "Irritable Bowel Syndrome secondary to stress." Now, excuse me, but what kind of a diagnosis is that? *Secondary to stress* implies that these symptoms were psychiatric in nature. But there was nothing wrong with her head; it was her bowels that were irritated. When she was released from the hospital, there was no change in her bowel function, and Anna was told that this might be something she would have to live with, or find a way to reduce her stress.

Two to three years later, Anna experienced vaginal discharges and recurrent bladder and vaginal infections. Treatments for these with multiple courses of antibiotics provided only temporary relief. She began to experience genital pain radiating on both sides of her labia and her clitoris. Sexual relations were extremely uncomfortable, and orgasm was not possible. Menstruation, which had been intensely painful, became even more severe and irregular, with excessive bleeding. Anna was prescribed estrogen therapy for regulation of her menstrual cycles, but she had no significant improvement.

When she was 26, Anna became pregnant. She began to experience low back pain and intermittent thigh pain in both thighs, as well as numbness and tingling. The pregnancy ended in a prolonged labor with the delivery of a normal healthy boy.

Two years later she became pregnant again, but at 5½ months the pregnancy was terminated by a spontaneous miscarriage. A few months later she became pregnant again, with all of the same symptoms. This time she was able to carry the pregnancy to 7 months and delivered a girl prematurely.

Because her pelvic and pubic pains had been continuous, following this delivery, the doctors performed the first of three exploratory abdominal surgeries to see what was causing the chronic diarrhea and a relatively new symptom, consistent total urinary retention, meaning she couldn't urinate at all. This exploratory surgery failed to reveal any abnormal findings that would explain her symptoms, and Anna agreed to have a partial hysterectomy in the hopes that some of the symptoms would diminish. After her hysterectomy she was discharged from the hospital with no change in her bladder function or her loss of sensory feeling around the vagina.

Over the next 10 years all of these symptoms continued, and worsened. With the exception of during her pregnancies, Anna had not experienced any pain attributed to the low back. But when she ran out of options provided by traditional medicine, a friend recommended that she see a chiropractor. Upon the very first exam, the chiropractor put her through ranges of motion, and she started to experience some low back pain. When the exam was over, the chiropractor concluded that Anna had an asymptomatic but well-defined L_5 disk bulge. If anyone had bothered to x-ray her back, they would have seen the disk problem.

Anna took to the treatments well and was committed to getting better. Almost 25 years of pain was gone in 4 weeks. Her recurrent bladder infections ended, and her urinary retention returned to normal. The chronic diarrhea was gone, and she was able to enjoy sexual relations with her husband without pain and with full function.

What did this doctor do? Some very gentle traction and spinal adjustments in the low back. What was the cause of her problems? They all could be traced back to the time when she was 18 and fell down a flight of stairs. The fall knocked her back out of balance (ka-boom), even though it didn't produce back pain. It affected the messages the brain was sending through the nerves down to her pelvic region.

Look at how this woman suffered for decades. She lost a pregnancy. She spent more than 20 years of her life in pain and dysfunction. All because she had knocked her back out of balance and none of the doctors she had seen had ever thought to look at her spine.

Every cell in your body is controlled by a nerve. The brain provides direction to every cell, telling it what to do. If the message gets interrupted for whatever reason, that cell is not going to receive the message clearly, potentially resulting in symptoms like all of those that Anna experienced. Once Anna's spinal imbalance was addressed, the messages from the brain that are carried by the nerves down the spine through the openings in the joints could get through clearly, so the brain's messages were relayed

Pelvic Pain and Organic Dysfunction Symptoms at Presentation

	D (In Years)	I (In Weeks)	N (In Weeks)
Pelvic Pain			
Inguinal (lower front abdomen pain left/right)	25	2	4
Suprapubic (above the pubic bone in very lower front center of abdomen)	25	2	4-6
Coccygeal (tailbone)	8	2	4-6
Rectal	22	2	4-6
Genital	8	2	4
Dyspareunia (difficult or painful sexual intercourse)	13	4	6-8
Pelvic Organic Dysfunction			
Recurrent bladder infections	22	None	
Urinary retention	10	2	4
Vesicle sensory loss (can't feel when urinating)	10	1	4
Enuresis (involuntary urination, especially by children at night)	2	2	4
Inability to contract urethral sphincter (bladder leakage)	10	2	4
Diarrhea	22	2	4
Excessive flatus (gas)	22	2-4	6-8
Decreased rectal sensory perception	22	1	4
Rectal bleeding	8	2	8-10
Rectal mucous discharge	22	2	8-10
Nocturnal encopresis (soiling of the underwear with stool)	8	2	4
Decreased genital sensory perception	Always	4	8-10
Anorgasmy (Failure of a male or female to achieve an orgasm)	13	4	30
Pain on orgasm	13	8	19
Loss of libido	10	5	8-10
Deficient precoital lubrication (not adequate lubrication to have relations with her husband)	10	8	12

D = duration in yr, I = initial improvement was noted in weeks, N = normalization in weeks.

correctly. The "dimmer switch" was turned up to full power, and the "juice" from her brain was being carried at its full potential. And she healed.

It would be silly to say that chiropractic care can fix everything. Yet it's very rational and scientific to say that chiropractic care may fix anything. Dr. Daniel Palmer founded the chiropractic profession in 1895, at a time when there was very little scientific evidence that could explain why chiropractic care produced the results it did. Dr. Palmer was the first to show that an imbalance of the spine could affect the function of another part of the body, away from the spine. Since then, tens of millions of people have received chiropractic care, resulting in improvements ranging from reversing back pain, headaches, brain dysfunction, and muscle pains to reversing organ dysfunction. Once again, if mechanics are the imbalance in your Pyramid of Health, regardless of where you're experiencing the symptoms, you must fix the mechanics.

THE ANATOMY OF OUR STRUCTURE

In all of our conversations about the brain, we've really stayed inside the boundaries of the head. Now we're going to connect the brain to the rest of the body. To do so, you need to understand how the central nervous system (CNS) and the peripheral nervous system (PNS) operate. The CNS consists of the brain and the spinal cord. The PNS is the network of nerves connecting the spinal cord to the rest of the body. The brain creates messages in the CNS, and these messages are delivered by the PNS. These messages tell the body what to do and when to do it (move your hand away from the stove; jump over that rock in front of you, etc.). The message from your brain to get your finger out of the flame on the stove is pretty close to instantaneous. But it's the temperature receptors in your fingertips that have to send the message up your hand, through your arm, up your neck, and to the brain. Your brain has to receive the message, process it, make a decision as to how to respond, and then send that message down your neck, through your arm, and to your hand muscles that says "get outta there." How quickly does that happen? Hopefully, fast enough that you don't get burned.

Imagine that you are a contractor building a new subdivision. You're creating 100 new homes. The first thing you do is lay down the underground cables that will service each house. There will be one big trunk that comes into the subdivision, and it has 100 wires in it. At the first intersection of the subdivision, the trunk splits in two, with 50 wires attached to each cable. These wires branch out to the streets, and then again to each home.

That's the way our spine works. If you think of the subdivision as your entire body, the single trunk leading into the subdivision is your brain connected to your spinal cord, and each wire is a nerve. This is how the brain sends messages to the rest of your body. When you have inflammation in

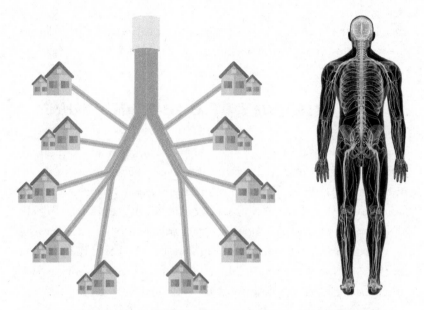

Just as damaging the trunk of the electrical wires leading into a subdivision may create a disruption of service in a single house blocks away, irritation causing inflammation at the spine can create a disruption of nerve transmission elsewhere in the body.

your neck, it could affect the messages going to your eyes, ears, tongue, tastebuds, or even your heart. Sometimes people have digestion problems and heartburn that get resolved when they address the message coming from the spine.

Inflammation can sometimes cause damage to one of the wires. When this happens, the houses in the far back right corner might not have phone service or cable, but the rest of the subdivision is fine. And if you damage the main cable coming into the subdivision (the brain), it may be the house over in the far right (your kidneys) that has a problem; or it could be a house over on the far left (your gallbladder). This is just one more reason why it is critical to maintain optimal brain health—including that of your CNS and PNS—especially as you age.

Do you want to know how sophisticated the human frame is? Here's how all the parts come together to provide you with a smooth ride. There are more than 7 trillion nerves in the human body. There are 31 pairs of *spinal nerves* that are split into five groups: 8 pairs of nerves in your neck,

12 pairs of nerves in your mid- and upper back, 5 pairs of nerves in your lower back, 5 pairs of sacral nerves, and 1 pair of coccygeal nerves. All of these nerves connect up to the brain and form the nervous system.

Next, there are 206 bones in every adult human body, and between every two bones is a joint, 7 ligaments, and 7 muscles (which condense into tendons that hook into the bones). The joint separates the bones with a cushion called a *disc*, which needs to stay plump in order to maintain proper alignment for the bones (like having enough air in your tires). Every joint in the spine has 7 different lines of movement; other joints are designed a little bit differently, and they can't move in quite as many directions, yet all of your joints are designed to maintain a balanced alignment that is supported by its stabilization package: the muscles, ligaments, and tendons.

This stabilization package acts like the lug nuts holding the tires on a car. Lug nuts hold the tires in place so that you experience a smooth ride. If you have only one lug nut on a wheel, instead of five, your tire is going to wobble, the ride won't be as smooth, and the tire will eventually wear down. When your muscles, ligaments, and tendons are too tight, caused by stress or poor posture, they prevent your joints from moving in a balanced range of motion, which causes your body to respond like a wobbly tire, creating excessive wear and tear. Here comes arthritis in your senior years.

Nerves exit the joints through a *foramen*, which acts like a sliding glass door. When your bones are in alignment, there is plenty of room for the nerves to transmit their messages—the sliding glass door coasts smoothly on its track. If you have an imbalance in the spine, the sliding glass door of your foramen is much smaller, more like a bathroom window. It's not as easy for the nerves to transmit their messages, and as the messages try to squeeze through, it puts pressure on the nerves. The ensuing inflammation produces what happens when you have a "pinched nerve." Think of Anna from the case study in the last chapter. That's exactly what happened to her, and because it wasn't addressed, she had 13 surgeries and years of misery.

A diminished nerve message from the brain can affect any tissue of the body. Poor posture or tight muscles limits the joints from working properly, causing inflammation and impacting the messages coming out of the nerves. Your gallbladder doesn't get a full message of what to do, or your gut muscles don't get the full message for peristalsis to move the waste along, and what you get is constipation. That's why a chiropractor can make an adjustment on the lower back and the patient's bowels start working like they haven't worked in years.

What's more, your spinal health directly influences your brain function. First, chronic low back pain, which is so very common, can activate increased brain inflammation,[7] leading to collateral damage in the brain and, as we've seen earlier, potentially creating B4. Some of this damage is highly localized. For instance, one 2017 study showed that 25 percent of

DR. TOM'S AT-HOME BIOMARKERS

Here's a way of telling if your disks are getting worn down. You are testing to see if they are able to stay plump and lubricated throughout the day.

Get into your car in the morning, and before you start the car, sit comfortably and adjust your rearview mirror so that when you look in it, the top of the rearview mirror is aligned with the top of the rear window. Now start the car and drive away.

At the end of the day, when you get back in your car, sit comfortably and take a look to see if you need to adjust your rearview mirror because it is no longer aligned with the top of the rear window. Almost everyone needs to make this adjustment. What that means is your spine has shrunk a minuscule amount during the day. You've lost water from your disks—they've been squished. Don't worry: When you lie down to go to sleep, you rehydrate your disks and they puff back up. This cycle goes on day in and day out for years. If the lifestyle habits and environmental exposures that have been slowly wearing you down continue, however, you'll keep losing a minuscule amount of height. Then, a decade later, when you're at the doctor's office for a routine physical, the nurse will check your height, and you'll realize you're 1¾ inches shorter than what it says on your driver's license.

But if you take care of your structure by following the tips later in this chapter and addressing the rest of the Pyramid of Health, you'll notice that you shrink less. You'll be able to tell a year from now when your disks are in really good shape, because your rearview mirror stays the same every time. You won't have to adjust it.

people with chronic low back pain also have multiple dysfunctions within their brain and central nervous system[8] affecting the fear-memory center called the *amygdala*. The amygdala, referred to as the reptilian brain, is the most ancient and primitive part of the brain. It serves an important role in evaluating fear and negative emotions, and it's where we create pain memories that can increase feelings of apprehension and anxiety. The brain dysfunction side effects of chronic low back pain will not go away with a couple of Tylenol. If the misalignment in your spine is still affecting your nervous system, it will continue to affect brain function.

Will better spinal alignment increase your memory and attention? You bet. Sleep deprivation caused by pain and discomfort impairs *cognitive flexibility*,[9] a fancy Scrabble word for decision making. Anxiety caused by amygdala damage also pushes on your ability to remember. By addressing your structure, you are automatically improving your brain function.

THE ROLE OF YOUR NECK WHEN IT COMES TO YOUR NERVES

We are supposed to have a curve in our neck where the head comes back over the shoulders. It's called a *lordosis*, and it is meant to distribute the weight of the head over the neck and shoulders. When your neck is positioned properly, the lines of communication through the nerves are completely open. But if you have a straight neck, or you have a reverse curve called a *kyphosis*[10] (when your head is in front of your shoulders), the weight distribution is off, the sliding door becomes a bathroom window, and the messages carried by the nerves are affected. Surprisingly, 23 percent of people with neck pain and 17 percent of everyone without neck pain have a kyphosis: Almost half the population have a reversal of how the bones are supposed to sit in the neck.

For instance, Larry is a CEO of a big company, and he was having a hard time coming up with words for things that he knows. Before coming to see me, he had been to 17 different doctors, and no one was able to figure out why this was going on. His hypoperfusion (lack of bloodflow, causing shrinking of the brain) was severe. Every blood and urine test had come back negative as to why this was happening. He traveled hundreds of miles to see me as a last resort.

The minute I saw him I suspected what at least part of the problem was. When Larry is standing, his head is 3 inches in front of his shoulders. That strain on his neck—the mechanical problem—is likely contributing to his symptoms. His posture was the clue for me to ask if he had been in an accident, and Larry told me that he was in fact in two motorcycle accidents, and the second one required spinal surgery to fuse two joints. I asked him to fill out a Living Matrix health history and was startled to learn that someone as bright as Larry was smoking cigars every day. Since I knew that smoking causes an inflammatory response,[11] I wondered aloud why none of his 17 other doctors put these clues together or instructed him to quit as a way of reducing this inflammatory trigger.

I then ordered simple x-rays (a full cervical series) that can record the movement capability of individual joint motion. We learned that a few of Larry's joints were locked up—not moving at all. This motion restriction created inflammation in the tunnel that holds the nerves within the spinal cord (foramen). It also was the likely cause of his neck pain and the trigger for his hypoperfusion into the brain.[12, 13, 14]

There is a specific treatment within chiropractic care that is designed to alleviate pain in fused necks (the Cox Flexion-Distraction technique). I found a chiropractor near Larry's home who was certified in this work. Within a few visits, Larry reported back to me that he was already noticing that his pain was reduced and his word retrieval was beginning to improve. I told him that this was great news and he was on the right path, but it would take some time—as much as 2 years—to complete this very focused treatment. His brain has to rebuild new neuronal circuits, and his neck muscles, tendons, and ligaments have to relax more to adapt to better function. Larry told me he would do whatever it takes to ensure that his brain works properly again. I told him that since he is willing to do anything besides seeing his new chiropractor, he would have to give up his daily cigar, which was also contributing to his inflammation. Larry wasn't happy, but he agreed.

DR. TOM'S TIP
TAKE A SELFIE TO FIND A KYPHOSIS

How can you tell if you have a kyphosis? Just take a selfie of your side profile. If your ears are in front of your shoulders, you likely have a kyphosis. You should be able to draw a straight line through your ankles, knees, hips, elbows, middle of your shoulders, and ears. Most of us are off from that. Some of us, way off.

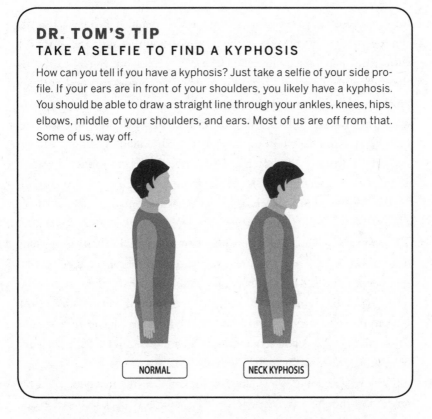

NORMAL   NECK KYPHOSIS

GRAB ONTO THE LADDER: WHAT YOU CAN DO TO IMPROVE YOUR STRUCTURE

While I strongly believe that everyone should see a chiropractor as part of their overall health-care program, there are a few simple yet critical changes you can make that will improve your spine's health and increase the effectiveness of your brain's messaging system. In this case, addressing how we sleep and how we sit are the base hits.

PILLOW YOGA

We sleep for 6 to 8 hours a night on average. We should make it nourishing and not detrimental. Sleeping with your head on a pillow tilts it forward and tucks your chin in, automatically creating a kyphosis. But you can train your spine to sleep in the right position that supports your neck correctly. It may take 6 months to a year to resolve, but you'll be opening the sliding glass door so that all of your nerve's messages come through more clearly. The result is better function out of your eyes, your heart, your gallbladder, your liver, and your thyroid. Your brain is working a little more clearly. You have a little more energy at the end of the day. You're not crashing in front of the television. All these things are subtle, but when addressed together, they're base hits helping to stabilize your structure.

The best position to sleep in for your back is on your back. Take the same pillow you've been resting your head on and tuck it under your knees. That immediately takes the pressure off your low back. Then take a small hand towel and roll it up. Secure it with a couple of rubber bands and put it under your neck. That's your pillow. You lie like that, pillow under your knees, hand towel under your neck, for 10 minutes. If you don't fall asleep in 10 minutes, throw the hand towel on the floor, go back to your old position, and go to sleep. Every night you give it 10 minutes with the same positioning. Eventually, you'll fall asleep that way.

What you're doing is encouraging the muscles, the ligaments, and the tendons of the spine and the neck to relax and move back in the direction they're built to be in. Gradually, you'll move from the small towel to a larger towel, creating a greater lordosis. Then you can transition to an orthopedic pillow that has a curve to it. That curve is reproducing the same position as the rolled-up hand towel, but now for a more pliable neck willing to keep moving toward normal. In 6 months you're sleeping with an orthopedic pillow under your neck and a regular pillow under your knees, and you're sleeping more soundly than you've slept in years, because your neck is now in the right alignment. It's like doing yoga for your neck.

MOVE YOUR CAR SEAT

Most people drive their cars with their seat's backrest leaning backward. This is another position that forces your neck in front of your spine. Try this. Sit in a chair, scoot your bottom forward like you sit in the car, extend both legs to the imaginary pedals, and put both arms out like you're holding the steering wheel. Now, where's your head compared to your shoulders? This should be an "aha" moment if you did it properly: Your neck is way ahead of your spine.

So let's change this, okay? It's a big base hit. May even be a double. The next time you get into the car, move the back of your seat one click forward. Do that every month, one click forward toward creating a 90-degree angle for your back and legs. Take your time. One click on the first of every month, until you replicate the 90-degree angle found in every seat in your house—at the kitchen table, at your desk, and so on.

Now add a lumbar pillow in the low back area. Your backrest might have one you can adjust, but if not, any small pillow can work. Another base hit. Together, these two adjustments will take a great deal of pressure off your nerve communication pathways.

BE CONSCIOUS OF YOUR POSTURE

It's not possible to think your way into having straight posture. As soon as you start thinking about something else, your brain's directive to those muscles will relax and you'll go back to the old posture. But it is possible to train your muscles, and I've had great results teaching this particular technique to many of my patients.

Imagine that two large helium balloons are floating above you, attached to your chest. These balloons are so powerful that they can lift your chest up toward the sky. When you walk this way, or sit this way, it automatically squeezes the muscles between your shoulder blades together as you lift your chest, and that automatically brings your head back a little bit over your shoulders.

You can check if you are making better progress by seeing if you can walk in a straight line. Close your eyes in an area where you have lots of room to walk without running into anything. Take 20 steps, then open your eyes. Did you walk straight or not? So many people cannot do this, but with training and better posture, you will be able to.

It's almost easier to check someone else's posture when you are upside

DR. TOM'S TIP
LOOK AT THE BACK OF YOUR SHOES

If your heels are worn down on the outside, which is so very common, you're going to wear your spine out faster, create inflammation, and get arthritis much earlier in life because your foot mechanics are way out of balance. Every time you step, you're throwing your joints suddenly and consistently out of balance, all the way up to where your head sits on the top bone in your neck.

The fix: See a chiropractor, but in the short term, get new heels on your shoes, or get new shoes.

down. There's a yoga position called Downward Facing Dog, where you balance yourself on your hands and feet with your hips raised in the air, and you are looking through your legs. Try this near a running path and watch someone running up toward you. Even the best runners can seem very awkward in their running from this position. The point of the exercise is to see that we're preconditioned, and that we make assumptions when we look at the world from the right side up. When you look at a runner right side up, he or she looks smooth and normal. When you look at the world from Down Dog, you see much more clearly the truth about somebody's biomechanics and how out of balance they are because they're running awkwardly.

When I saw a runner one day from that position, it made me realize we all have preconceived notions that influence the way we see the world. Look from Dog Down and what you thought was "normal" is so obviously out of balance. I believe that's the level of change we all have to experience to change the direction our world is going in. We all have to "Down Dog" our lives and stop accepting environmental toxicity, pharmaceutical advertising manipulation, and poisoned foods as normal. We have to change what we will and will not accept, and make those changes in base hits. For example, stop using plastic bags that are toxic to our environment. Just keep a few canvas bags in the car, and when you're going shopping, bring them into the supermarket with you. It's a base hit that costs almost nothing but can change the world.

DR. TOM'S TIP
STRUCTURE'S ROLE IN FUNCTIONAL MEDICINE

There are a number of disciplines that emphasize structural care, and every one of them has hundreds to thousands to tens of thousands of miracle result stories. Osteopathy, massage, cranial-sacral therapy, Feldenkrais therapy, Rolfing—they all have value. Make sure you have a functional medicine practitioner with a great overview of structure as part of your health-care team.

EXERCISE PROTECTS YOUR SPINE AND YOUR BRAIN

We all know that exercise is important for the body, but it is also critical for maintaining good structure and supporting brain health. Aerobic exercise in particular, to the point where you're sweating, is key for increasing circulation that will flush out the endotoxins in your cells. And like intermittent fasting, it will help you burn fat and eliminate stored toxins. You have to move this stuff out that doesn't belong in your cells.

It doesn't matter what type of aerobic exercise you choose—walking, swimming, exercise classes, dance classes, bicycling, etc. Whatever you choose, make it enjoyable, because you will need to work up to 30 minutes, 6 days a week. I get my aerobic exercise each day by doing hot yoga, which gets my pulse up to 125 beats per minute very easily.

There are two measurements you can take to see if your exercise program is working. Forget about your waistline for now. Instead, we're going to focus on how many steps you take each day and your pulse.

By carrying a smartphone when you exercise (with the right case that you'll learn about in Chapter 11), you can track how many steps you take a day. The goal is to reach three times what you are currently doing within a year. At first, that means parking your car out at the end of the parking lot instead of trying to find the closest spot at the supermarket or the mall. Walk in. Walk out with your cart of groceries. Walk the cart back to the building. Walk back to the car. Took you all of an extra 3 minutes to do that. You're "Down Dogging" your mind-set. Build from there, and make your exercise count.

I also recommend wearing a pulse monitor that has an alarm function built in. They're quite inexpensive nowadays. First, set the pulse monitor for your aerobic range, which is 180 beats per minute minus your age, plus or minus 5 points. If your resting pulse is below 72, subtract the difference from 180, and then if you have a diagnosed disease, take another 5 points off.

For example, I'm 65 and healthy, so that would mean 180—65, plus or minus 5 would be my aerobic range. Thus, my aerobic range is between 110 to 120 beats per minute, and the goal is to maintain that range during my 30 minutes of exercise. But wait, my resting pulse is 58 beats per minute.

DR. TOM'S TIP
MAINTAINING STRONG BONES

Despite what you may have heard, calcium supplements alone are not enough for keeping your bones strong. A family of supplements is needed, including calcium, magnesium, boron, strontium, vitamin K, and vitamin D.

In nature, calcium and magnesium usually occur together at a 1:1 ratio. The only time our ancestors would have higher percentages of calcium was during breastfeeding. When Far Eastern cultures adopted a Western diet, over a single generation, the incidence of osteoporosis skyrocketed. Throughout the world, one out of every two women over the age of 50 will have an osteoporotic-related fracture in her lifetime, with risk of fracture increasing with age. Of senior citizens who suffer a hip fracture, 20 percent die within 1 year.

In a study, all patients with osteoporosis (or its earlier stage, osteopenia) who had a sensitivity to wheat (celiac disease) had elevated antibodies to bone—an autoimmune mechanism.[22] And as it was reported in 2000 in the journal *Gastroenterology*, after 2 years on a gluten-free diet, these patients were no better. You have to do more than just eliminate the inflammatory foods.

The good news is that with appropriate nutrition and physical activity throughout life, individuals can significantly reduce the risk of bone disease and fractures. Never argue with your coach, and stop throwing gasoline on the fire.

THE BASE OF THE PYRAMID: ADDRESSING YOUR STRUCTURE | 185

I have to subtract 14 from 180 (assuming a baseline pulse for this formula is 72). Okay, 180 minus 14 = 166, minus my age 65, plus or minus 5 = 96 to 106 is my aerobic range. That's the range I'll want to hit for 30 minutes 6 days per week.

Use your pulse range as your coach. Set the alarm to your goal range. When you exercise and you're in your pulse range, the monitor is silent. If you're too low, it will remind you to pick up your pace. If you're too high, it will remind you to slow down. Here's the rule, though: *Never argue with your coach.* Even if you think you can exercise harder or faster—and most of us want to—that's not the goal here. We're creating a good habit that will burn fat and maintain well-being for a lifetime. This is the enhancing type of exercise that your body will thrive on, regenerate from, and build stronger tissue from. It's another base hit. You want to be spry in your eighties? You want to have the 20-somethings all joke with their friends that they want to be like you when they get "that old"? Never argue with Coach.

Exercise in your aerobic pulse range enhances and protects brain function by:

- Enhancing learning and *neuronal plasticity*,[15, 16, 17] the key mechanism that allows us to continue to adapt and learn as we age
- Delaying onset of and decline in several neurodegenerative diseases, including dementia[18]
- Slowing the functional decline after neurodegeneration has begun[19]
- Protecting individuals with the ApoE4 genotype (called the Alzheimer's gene)[20]
- Increasing the number of new neurons, and promoting survival of these new cells[21]

Lastly, don't forget to hydrate before, during, and after exercise. Drinking clean, filtered water is critically important for maintaining an anti-inflammatory lifestyle. Be sure you drink a minimum of ½ ounce per pound of body weight. Hydrate, hydrate, hydrate to flush, flush, flush. Get the toxins out!

ACTION STEP WEEK 7: WORK ON YOUR CORE

This week, work on strengthening your core—the muscles that support your spinal structure. Not only will your body thank you now, but when you're in your eighties and people are still commenting on your perfect posture and elegant stride, *you* will thank you! We are designed to stand and walk, but a lifestyle of sitting encourages a weak core. This happens over time when we drive with our car seats leaning back too far, or when we slouch in a recliner or on a sofa for hours watching TV. This creates weak core muscles, which is the basis of so many of the musculoskeletal problems that we have today.

Over time, working on strengthening your core muscles will eliminate a slumping, slouching posture. You can work on your core anytime, anywhere. The trick is to be conscious of the little points of muscle activation. Here's a great exercise to keep in mind: Before walking up the stairs, squeeze your glutes together and tuck your pubic bone up toward your navel. Now, very slightly lean forward as you walk up the stairs, holding the squeeze and tuck. Your muscles will let you know how they feel. Wherever you feel a bit of tightness, discomfort, or fatigue, that's where you've been overcompensating for a weak core. Keep working at this, and within a few days you'll notice that all of your walking muscles are becoming more balanced and stronger. You're well on your way to becoming a babe or a hunk in your eighties!

THE POWER OF
MIND-SET

Our beliefs are our destiny.
—MAHATMA GANDHI

IN 2016, THE National Academies of Sciences, Engineering, and Medicine convened a workshop of pharmaceutical industry leaders, doctors, and public health policy experts. They met to solve a single problem: Compared with other disease areas, central nervous system disorders have had the highest failure rate for new medications in advanced clinical trials. Most of the drugs that are meant to treat diseases associated with the brain, including Alzheimer's, Parkinson's, MS, and even depression, fail.[1]

This is the truth of 21st-century medicine. We cannot count on a single pill to solve most of our brain health problems. The medications we have available are, at best, the life jackets that will keep us afloat. However, this does not mean that we are destined to live with poor brain health. While big pharma continues to look for a better life jacket, I believe that one of the critical ways for changing our brain health is changing how we think about brain health, including our mind-set, i.e., the way we think about the possibilities of transformation, and the attitude and awareness we carry as we take care of ourselves. As we move away from the hope that one pill, one drug, will fix a lifetime of brain degeneration, we can approach regenerating our brain health as an everyday effort, where the base hits of lifestyle changes—diet, exercise, and holding onto a calm and present mind-set—can really make a difference.

From Day 1 in my training, addressing the mind-set has been an integral part of the Triangle of Health, and now, the Pyramid. How we think about our health—how we rationalize the foods we choose to eat ("I can have a little once in a while"), how we choose between going to bed to catch up on sleep or getting worked up late at night watching the evening news (which is all stress-enhancing, terrible information)—has a great deal to do with the types of brain hormones we produce, and which of our two nervous systems is dominant. The difference is whether we are in an anxious mind-set all the time, or a more relaxed, health-promoting state.

The sympathetic nervous system is exclusively designed to be used as a response to stressful, life-or-death situations. We know this because its nerves are quite thin compared to parasympathetic nerves. As an analogy, sympathetic nerves are the width of your pinkie, while the parasympathetic nerves are the width of your thumb. Both sets of nerves run parallel to each other, connecting the brain to every organ in your body.

Any electrician will tell you that the more current you send through a wire, the hotter the wire gets. So when we look at our two nervous systems, the thin sympathetic nerves and the thicker parasympathetic nerves, it makes common sense that the thicker parasympathetic nerves are supposed to run most of the time. Hans Selye, MD, PhD, who first associated the concept of "stress" with health concerns back in the 1950s, told us that the parasympathetic nerves are supposed to be running 90 to 95 percent of the time. That's why the parasympathetic nerves need more insulation so they don't overheat.

An electrician will also tell you that the thickness of the insulation affects the speed at which the electrical current travels. The parasympathetic nerves carry messages much slower than the sympathetic nerves. Why is that important? Because when our ancestors heard the growl of a saber-toothed tiger behind them, they had to immediately jump out of the way. If there was a delay from the time the brain recognized the threat and sent the alarm message to the muscles to move, those early humans were unlikely to be around for another day. That's why the sympathetic nervous system has very little insulation, so that the messages from the brain can travel quickly down the nerves to save your life, compared to the parasympathetic route.

We're supposed to rely on the lifesaving response of the sympathetic nervous system only in times of emergency. The problem is that we are living in a constant state of stress, so we are collectively stuck in a sympathetic-dominant state. How do I know? When the parasympathetic nervous system is dominant, we have deep breathing, relaxed muscles, good digestion, and a calm mind. When the sympathetic nervous system is dominant, we have quick, shallow breathing; an increased heart rate; tight, tense muscles; dilated pupils; limited digestive ability; and an alert, anxious, paranoid mind trying to determine the source of the stress. Which of these two descriptions sounds more like the way you live?

One reason that health problems occur is that our systems were not designed to be in a sympathetic-dominant state all of the time. Without the proper insulation, when overused, the thin sympathetic nerves literally start to burn out, creating inflammation. And the longer this goes on, the more inflammation occurs, along with its side effects. When this happens, you are much more likely to have elevated antibodies to your brain, nervous system, or wherever the weak link is in your chain. Our nervous system goes from parasympathetic dominance (our birthright) to sympathetic dominance. When this goes on long enough, and we start to wear down these thin wires because they're used way more than they're supposed to be, we go from sympathetic dominance to sympathetic fatigue— that feeling of being tired much of the time. If the stress continues, we go from sympathetic fatigue to sympathetic exhaustion, and finally as the "fight, fright, or flight" response continues, we go from sympathetic exhaustion to sympathetic depletion.

Degenerative diseases occur in a sympathetic-depleted state. Without the mechanism to return to a parasympathetic-dominant state, you become extremely vulnerable to developing any disease, depending on your weak link. At this point stress affects you much more and more frequently. If you're feeling burned out, it's because you are. And so is your brain's ability to be resilient, making it harder to adapt to what life throws at you.

As a medical student, Hans Selye observed that patients suffering from different diseases often exhibited identical signs and symptoms; in his words, they were "stressed." His definition of stress was anything that activates a sympathetic nervous system response, whether it's chemical, physical, or emotional. Dr. Selye was the first to point out that stress induces hormonal autonomic responses and that, over time, if these hormonal changes are excessive, they can lead to physical manifestations. He was the first to identify that excess stress wears your body out and causes disease. In a 1955 article in the medical journal *Science*, Dr. Selye showed how arthritis, stroke, and heart disease are all affected by a stress-induced, overworked, and worn-out sympathetic nervous system.

What organ controls the entire relationship of how our bodies respond to the stress of life? You might think from this discussion that it is the brain. Doctors used to believe that, until just a few years ago. Now we know that the microbiome is the central computer directing the microbiota-gut-brain (MGB) axis. The microbiota sends chemical messengers to the brain along the spinal cord and through the bloodstream. These messages instruct the hypothalamus how to respond to perceived stress. The hypothalamus tells the pituitary gland which stressors are the priorities, and the pituitary gland then sends the organs messages that tell them what hormones to produce. A healthy microbiota will ensure that you are more resilient during this stress response. The more emotionally resilient we are, the less we'll get worked up when faced with common stresses. So resilience is a good thing.

However, if your microbiota is out of balance, the anxiety you woke up with won't go away and may even increase because your ability to be resilient is dampened. You don't have the support in your gut needed to keep your brain calm.[2] Once you start balancing your microbiome, which you can do with the foods and supplements we'll review shortly, your brain hormones will begin to shift to a more balanced, parasympathetic-dominant state, allowing for less stressful thinking, less anxiety, more creative thinking, and a more open and resilient mind. You'll be in a more peaceful state, which is exactly where you need to be to begin working on your mind-set. And over time, those moments will lengthen and become more frequent. People will say, "You've changed. You're so calm now."

THE MOST POWERFUL BRAIN THERAPY: A POSITIVE OUTLOOK

The influence having a positive mind-set has over our health has been quantified in a variety of studies that investigated the placebo effect. The word *placebo* comes from the Latin phrase "I shall please" and was first used as a medical term in 1811, when it was defined as "any medicine adapted more to please than to benefit the patient." Although this definition has a derogatory implication, even then it did not imply that the remedy had no effect. Twenty years earlier, the first to recognize and demonstrate the power of the mind was English physician John Haygarth.[3] He set out to expose a popular medical treatment, "Perkins tractors," which were expensive metal pointers supposedly able to draw out disease. Haygarth compared the results of two different models and found that a wooden set was just as useful as the expensive metal ones. In his words, he showed "to a degree which has never been suspected, what powerful influence upon diseases is produced by mere imagination."[4] And as early as 1920, the placebo effect was connected to the use of medications. In a published paper in the *Lancet*, T. C. Graves wrote that "the placebo effects of drugs" demonstrated the power of belief in symptom resolution, where "a real psychotherapeutic effect appears to have been produced."[5]

Even as recently as 2015, in an effort to acknowledge the legitimacy of this phenomenon, the *New England Journal of Medicine* reported: "Placebo effects rely on complex neurobiologic mechanisms involving neurotransmitters . . . and activation of specific, quantifiable, and relevant areas of the brain (e.g., prefrontal cortex, anterior insula, rostral anterior cingulate cortex, and amygdala in placebo analgesia)."[6] This means that not only can we measure the effects of placebos on the brain, but they activate the same pathways that are affected by medication. Most of the "bad-mouthing" of placebo effects comes from the pharmaceutical industry trying to prove their drugs are more powerful than doing nothing at all. The reality of the situation is that what you think about, how you think about it, and your general outlook on life has a "most-powerful" effect on what hormones you produce, and you will have all the downstream benefits, or complications, of those hormones. Produce stress hormones and get the wear and tear of high stress. Produce relaxing parasympathetic hormones and your heart rate calms down, breathing is deeper, and brain waves of a peaceful nature are more prevalent. This is the basis of the benefits of meditation, which has been used for thousands of years (you'll learn more about it later in the chapter).

The question, then, is why. How is it that we can imagine an outcome that actually changes the way our body or brain works? This is another reason why we can say our genes are not our destiny. If we believe we can get better, we can affect our health. There have been scientific studies that have examined health outcomes based on this power of belief. In a 2007 study, 84 hotel attendants with cleaning responsibilities were divided into two groups. Half were told that their daily work satisfied the surgeon general's recommendations for exercise as part of a healthy lifestyle. The other half were told nothing. The first group showed a decrease in weight, blood pressure, body fat, waist-to-hip ratio, and body mass index, supporting the researchers' hypothesis that exercise affects health in part or in whole via the placebo effect.[7] Just thinking that their cleaning duties were exercise led to real, tangible health benefits as opposed to the group that saw their activity as only work.

When it comes to brain health, our attitude is just as critical. In 1998, a meta-analysis of 19 trials that had been used to test the efficacy of antidepressants was conducted. Only 25 percent of the measured therapeutic response was attributable to the actions of a drug, while there was a 75 percent placebo effect noted across studies. This study was followed up by a 2008 review, which required an appeal to the Freedom of Information Act to obtain access to unpublished studies on antidepressants; the pharmaceutical industry had tried to bury the studies. The review found that when these omitted studies were included in the data, antidepressants outperformed placebo in only 20 of 46 trials. The authors summarized: "... the benefit (of antidepressants versus placebo) falls below accepted criteria for clinical significance."[8] This review shows that antidepressants do not work often enough to validate recommending their use, and that's not even taking into consideration the harmful side effects many experience: weight gain, loss of sex drive, reduced blot clotting, and increased risk of stomach and uterine bleeding.[9] But we live in a world of greed and self-serving policies that benefit corporations and not the individual.

So many studies show us how our beliefs directly shape our life experience. Nicholas Gonzalez, MD, a world-famous pioneer in cancer therapy, believed that fear is an infectious disease that can destroy the most effective medical protocol, and that faith can heal with no protocol at all. A positive attitude toward your own treatment, and faith in your body's ability to heal, is a critical component in reversing disease. Kelly Brogan, MD, a clinical psychiatrist and functional medicine practitioner, writes in her bestselling book *A Mind of Your Own* that if we can look upon our health journey with curiosity, introspection, and an acceptance of the invitation to respond to what is out of balance, then we can shift our energetic focus away from the state of being ill, and toward a healthier new version of ourselves. She believes, as I do, that the power to transform our health lies within each one of us as long as we believe it is there.

That's why I shared earlier in the book that when patients come to me and they say, "I've been to Mayo Clinic, and they don't know what's wrong," my response is always the same. I tell them, "That's great! That means you do not have a disease. Because if you had a disease, Mayo

READ MORE ABOUT THE SCIENCE OF THE PLACEBO EFFECT

You Are the Placebo, the latest book by Joe Dispenza, DC, is a fascinating read into this topic. There are dozens of exercises you can try to see for yourself how powerful mind-set can be.

Clinic would find it. You have dysfunction. Something's not functioning right. Let's focus there." By responding this way, I've shifted the patient's thinking, hopefully removing a little of the panic and the fear and replacing it with an inquiry. Then, when their tests come back and we get together again, the patient is always worried what the results will be. I purposely do the added excitement thing again (they think I'm a little crazy anyway), and I say, "Good news. You're a mess!" They smile a little and have a quizzical look that says "does not compute." Then I explain which biomarkers are out of balance and how they are correctable. "Now, let's get to work," I tell them. One step at a time. Base hits win the ball game. We have to stop expecting a home run. Your body, and life, does not work that way.

UNCOVERING YOUR THINKING

The kinder we are to ourselves, the healthier we'll be. If you are eating gluten-free bread because I told you to, but you really want the bread you've always enjoyed, the gluten-free bread is not going to be a healthy food for you. But, if you eat the gluten-free bread with gratitude, because you are so happy to have found out that wheat was a problem for you, and you realize that you do feel so much better when you take it out of your diet, and you're so ready to have the bread that's almost as good as the one you used to love, you will have a very different result. This shift in thinking is referred to as *intentionality*, which means to be purposeful in word and action. Being intentional means you actively interact and engage with your life.

The key to all behavioral change is awareness. The calmer we can be, living in a state of gratitude, the easier it is to be aware of our current health and set goals for our future health. We need to create an awareness of reality in a nonjudgmental way. For example, an awareness about eating gluten-free means being aware that instead of putting something into your body that is a minor poison, and that the tests confirmed your immune system is trying to protect you from, your new selections are going to nourish you. Instead of seeing it as a punishment or obligation, it's a validation

EMOTIONAL ENERGY

The brain and heart send a variety of messages to each other, ranging from regulating our heartbeat to regulating our emotional state. We know that our emotions affect our heart rate: When you're scared, your heart races. They also affect the electromagnetic field we emit. Have you ever sat next to someone on a bus or a train, and you could sense their personality and actually feel it affect you? What you're feeling is their electromagnetic field. Coherent, relaxed states emit smooth, consistent wavelike patterns. Negative emotions are emitted as jagged, erratic patterns. They tax the heart a little bit more, whereas living in a state of appreciation is much easier on the heart.

that you're worth putting healthy fuel in your body. Awareness means understanding how your body behaves, from understanding your heartbeat to understanding the benefits of eating gluten-free. It's not just being more aware of the decisions you make. It's being aware of the physical state of your body, and holding that awareness with empathy and kindness.

OUR THOUGHTS
CREATE OUR ENERGY

A few years ago, I met a British woman at one of my lectures, and we hit it off right away. It wasn't but a few months later that she moved to San Diego to be with me, and we started planning and visualizing our future family. She was a brilliant nutritionist and lecturer who, like me, talked frequently about wheat sensitivities with or without celiac disease. Our plan was that she would go to naturopathic school in San Diego, and toward the end of her education, we would have the first of four or more kids. I would retire and she would open her practice, specializing in autoimmune conditions. She would go out on the lecture circuit carrying our message to the world. I would be the House Dad, the primary parent raising the kids. The plan seemed like paradise.

We had just come back from a lovely weekend with another couple,

which included a great deal of laughing and speaking of intimate friend-
ships and the joy of life. The next day I flew to Austin to teach, and I called
her cell phone before going on stage just to say hello.

"Hi, how's everything?"

"Good, but I have to tell you something."

"Okay, what's up?"

"I'm going home."

"Where are you?"

"I'm at the house. But I'm going home."

"I don't understand."

"I'm going back to England. I don't love you, and I'm going home."

"What? When?"

"Tomorrow."

"What? What?"

That was it. When I got back to San Diego, she was gone. The house
was empty, as if she had never been there. Suffice it to say my world was
rocked: A category 8 earthquake destroyed my psyche. My heart was broken, but even worse, my mind would not stop. "What's wrong with me?
Am I not lovable? What did I do wrong? How could this happen so
abruptly? I can't trust anybody," I thought.

Day after day my thoughts were always negative; there was no "joy of
life," no reason to be happy. I plodded along and did my work, but my
personal life was in shambles. My energy was bad, and I was tired most of
the time. I didn't want to do anything but watch action movies at night. I
had no social life whatsoever. This went on for months.

Finally, about 8 months later, I began to see that my thoughts were
creating my reality—I was stuck and spiraling down. I knew I needed
some help. Friends I trust had told me about a psychic who was incredible.
I had never done anything like that, but I decided to give it a try: Maybe
knowing my future would help me figure out how to move forward in the
present. I made an appointment with her assistant without saying who I
was, and I did not tell anyone I was going—even I thought this was going
to be too private and too weird.

When I walked in the door, the psychic was sitting on the other side of the room and was talking on the phone. She greeted me with a smile and waved me in to have a seat. Then she took a second look at me and started giggling, and then she pointed at me and started laughing. She told the person on the phone to "hold on," with deep belly laughter. She caught her breath and said to me, "You what? You were going to be a House Dad? Your angels are laughing their heads off. They're all around you, just laughing hysterically. They weren't going to let you be a House Dad; there are millions of people waiting to hear what you have to say."

Needless to say, I was dumbfounded. There was no way she could have known my work. In that moment, in that one moment, all of the negative thoughts that I had been living with, all of that negativity creating the aura around me of being morose, being unworthy, being unlovable—all of that went *poof*, gone in an instant, and I was back to my old self, ready to go out and tell the world what the scientists are saying about where disease comes from. My energy returned. My mind was clear. Within 18 months, I met my future wife, I wrote my first book, *The Autoimmune Fix*, and my wife and I launched a Web documentary, *Betrayal: The Autoimmune Disease Secret They're Not Telling You*.

I can't explain what happened with the psychic that day. I have no idea how what happened, happened. But I do know the result. My negative thinking created a funk that I couldn't move past, yet in an instant, it was gone without my making one other change to my lifestyle. That's the power our thoughts have, and the influence they have over our health.

GRAB ONTO THE LADDER: WHAT YOU CAN DO TO BUILD AWARENESS

The more focused we are on being aware, the better our immune system works. It also increases a positive outlook and decreases anxiety. For instance, Seattle Seahawks coach Pete Carroll practices meditation with his entire team. He has found that meditation profoundly changed the attitude of his players. And since beginning this practice, the team has been to the Super Bowl twice.

It is possible to address health concerns with a calm mind-set rooted in mindfulness, a mental practice that cultivates an open and accepting awareness of whatever is occurring in the present moment, without re-acting to or being absorbed by the experience. The aim of mindfulness training is not to explicitly change the content of an experience, but rather to change one's relationship to it. If we can't change the triggers causing the stress in our lives, we can change the way we react to those triggers, which changes the effect the triggers will have on our brain and body. Mindfulness is a useful intervention for a broad range of chronic disorders and mental health problems; for example, research has shown that it can lead to a decreased rate of relapse in chronic depression, and improvement in outcomes in first-time treatment of anxiety and depression.[10]

The US Marine Corps Resilience Training Program has demonstrated that mindfulness techniques reduce stress by allowing individuals time to regroup, thereby reducing the physical and mental responses to stressful events. One powerful 2012 study compared mindfulness to other health enhancement programs (diet, exercise, medications, etc.) and showed that mindfulness training results in a significantly smaller inflammatory response[11]—you will produce less inflammation, even though you are still producing the stress hormones in response to the trigger.

CONSCIOUS BREATHING

Rapid, shallow breathing accompanies stress. Conscious breathing en-courages a parasympathetic-dominant state of well-being. In one study, 29 patients noted significant improvements in anxiety and physical symp-toms, abdominal pain, and quality of life when they were conscious of their breathing.[12]

MEDITATION

Meditation is one way to begin to focus on yourself so that you can heal. During meditation, you learn to put the outside world aside and create a space in which you can experience your feelings without reacting to them or being consumed by them. You can acknowledge them with an attitude of self-acceptance and self-compassion.

An ongoing meditation practice can lead to increased development of several key areas of the brain, especially those related to higher-order cognitive functions. When we meditate, we increase the hormone BDNF (which stands for brain-derived neurotropic factor). This hormone is necessary for regenerating healthy brain cells. It has also been proven to increase brain activity and improve attention and concentration. According to Jon Kabat-Zinn, PhD, of the University of Massachusetts Medical School and author of *Full Catastrophe Living*, meditators can shift their brain activity to different areas of the cortex. For example, brain waves in the stress-prone right frontal cortex can move to the calmer left frontal cortex. This means that those who practice meditation can actually change their brains to make themselves calmer and happier.

Scientists also think that meditation can assist in neurogenesis. In a 2009 study from the UCLA School of Medicine, researchers used high-resolution MRIs to determine that long-term meditators had significantly larger gray matter volumes in areas of the brain that have been connected to emotional regulation and response control. This can mean that successful meditators are able to control their stress levels better, reducing anxiety and improving overall mood.

Meditation also helps us to be present and aware. Many of us have a habit of "living in our heads," where we have hundreds, if not thousands, of disparate thoughts going on all day. Unfortunately, we sometimes get entangled in all these thoughts: We occupy our minds very easily, and we determine that certain things are more real or more important than others. The benefit of meditation is that it will bring peace into that same mind that's spinning at a million miles an hour, allowing you to let go of as many distractions as possible and pay attention to a few thoughts at a time so that you can have peace. With practice, you'll be able to significantly quiet the mind. It gives us the opportunity to relax and feel whole. Base hits win the ball game.

Meditation allows you to take a moment to sit quietly or to ponder. It brings a state of profound, deep peace that occurs when the mind is calm and silent, yet completely alert. Yet meditation is not an act of doing; it is a state of awareness or simply being. You can meditate in your office as effectively as you can if you were sitting in the lotus posture on the top of a mountain. The point is not to be attached to what's happening on the outside, but to focus on the inside.

Meditation for me is like the sun in the sky. There are often clouds, but the sun is still there. There's often brain chatter racing in your head, but peace of mind is just on the other side. Sometimes I have trouble making my brain stop when I meditate, and I quite honestly sometimes feel frustrated and want to say to my brain, "Be quiet!" Then I catch that thought and laugh inside at how silly I'm being trying to tell myself to not think. When I can laugh at it and take a deep breath, my heart rate slows down. That's the ball game right there. Now I'm getting the benefits of taking this quiet time.

Don't put too much pressure on yourself to master meditation. If anything, meditation is an exercise in patience. That's why it's called a meditation *practice;* it takes time to learn how to quiet the mind. When you first learn how to meditate, you may actually feel more agitated instead of relaxed. This happens because you may be getting in touch with what you're really feeling for the very first time, and it might bring up negative or difficult emotions. This is actually very healthy. As you practice and become more in tune with your authentic self, you'll learn to laugh at yourself a bit more often, and you'll be able to release some of your pent-up energy and relax. Over time, you'll learn how to tap into your place of peace.

A MEDITATION PRACTICE

You can meditate wherever you are most comfortable. Sit comfortably in a chair or on a couch. You can sit cross-legged or with your feet flat on the floor. Make sure to hold your head and neck upright. It helps to imagine the helium-balloons-on-your-chest vision. If you find that you are too restless to sit in meditation, get up and take a walk, do a chore, or run an errand. Then come back and try again. Usually you'll feel calmer and more able to sit comfortably.

Wear comfortable, nonbinding clothing, and find a quiet space where you can turn off as many distractions as possible. Some people like to create a special place in their home to meditate. I don't suggest meditating on a bed—you might fall asleep—or in a room filled with other people (unless you are engaging in group meditation). Some people like to meditate in silence. Others enjoy listening to soft music or chanting. White noise that features the sounds of waves, rainfall, or other natural rhythms can also be effective. You might also like to record the instructions for the meditation so that you can play them back during your practice.

It helps if the lights are dimmed. Some people like to light candles during their meditation. If you are so inclined, I remind you to use them safely, and always place candles on a flat, fire-resistant surface, such as a ceramic dish. Once you're in your space, unplug. No TV, no cell phone, no computer. The point is to carve out some time for quality silence. Have a goal of meditating for 20 minutes a day, but you may need to build up to this level. My good friend Deanna Minich, PhD, features some lovely

OTHER MIND-SET ACTIVITIES FOR BUILDING AWARENESS

You don't have to sit cross-legged on the floor to activate your mind for healing. Here are other methods that help bring your mind into the present and help to create a healing state:

- Affirmation (positive self-talk)
- Biofeedback
- Breathing exercises
- Energy therapies
- Expressive therapies: journaling, art therapies, poetry, humor
- Hypnosis
- Movement systems: e.g., Alexander technique
- Prayer
- Psychotherapy
- Qigong
- Visual imagery
- Yoga

meditations on her Web site that I often use, and I encourage you to check them out at theDr.com/wholedetox.

ARE YOU READY FOR A TRANSFORMATION?

There's a difference between change and transformation. Change is what we need to do to move from one way of living to another, such as moving from poor health to excellent health. Transformation is a significant alteration in the way we think about our lives. Transformation is not necessary for short-term benefits. Just change your habit (i.e., stop eating wheat and your headaches go away). But transformation is required for long-term benefits ("I'm so grateful to finally have done the right test and found out why I continued to have headaches. I'm not going to throw gasoline on the fire anymore."). Both change and transformation are necessary for improving lifestyle and addressing the underlying mechanisms that are making you sick: We need to transform in order to change habits for the long term.

You can be the architect of your future, not its victim. Change is not just about entertaining new ideas; it's about transforming old ideas. As John Maynard Keynes said, "The difficulty lies not so much in developing new ideas as much as escaping from the old ones." And in our lifetime, Oprah Winfrey has said, "The greatest discovery of all time is that a person can change his future by merely changing his attitude."

We have to be able to adjust and adapt; this is the basis of neuronal plasticity, the ability of our brains to adapt. You certainly can force yourself to change and still think the same way, but there's not much mileage in that. You'll feel a little better but not really on the path to vibrant well-being.

I know that change is not easy, but it also is not impossible. The lifestyle changes outlined in this book take commitment and patience. Base hits are all you need. You probably bought this book (thank you!) because something in your life is not working. Just remember that change is an ongoing process.

More than 20 years ago, alcoholism researchers Carlo C. DiClemente, PhD, and James O. Prochaska, PhD, introduced a model to help professionals understand their clients with addiction problems and motivate them to change. Their model is based not on abstract theories but on personal observations of how people went about modifying lifestyle behaviors, specifically for smoking, overeating, and drinking. Functional medicine practitioners use this model, as it is quite relevant to making lifestyle changes that can enhance health.

In their book *Changing for Good*, Drs. DiClemente and Prochaska and John C. Norcross, PhD, described what they learned when they studied more than 1,000 people who were able to positively and permanently alter their lives without psychotherapy. They found that change does not depend on luck or willpower. Instead, it is a process that can be successfully managed by anyone who understands how it works. Once you determine which stage of change you're in, you can create a climate where positive change can occur right where you currently are and not where you think you should be.

The five stages of change are:

- Pre-contemplation: Individuals in this stage are not even thinking about changing their behaviors. They haven't seen that their lifestyle is a problem affecting their health and well-being.
- Contemplation: Individuals in this stage are willing to consider the possibility that they have a health problem, and the possibility offers hope for change. However, in this stage, people are often highly ambivalent. They are on the fence. What lets me know if someone in this stage will ultimately be successful is if he or she shows skepticism ("I don't believe this, but I'm willing to look at more information") rather than cynicism ("I don't believe this; it's untrue"). Contemplation is moving in the right direction toward change, but it is not a commitment.

- Determination: Individuals in this stage will make a serious attempt to improve their lifestyle behaviors in the near future. They are ready and committed to action because they have garnered enough information (say, from reading this book) and are now convinced that behavioral change may improve their health.
- Action: Individuals in this stage put their plan into action. In a few weeks, they start to see results, and nothing succeeds like success. A person who has implemented a plan begins to see it work and experiences a positive change in health.
- Maintenance: I tell my patients all the time that humans are the only species on the planet that finds something that works and then stops doing it. Permanent change requires building a new pattern of behavior over time and sticking to it. It's common that when you're feeling great after giving up gluten for several months, you will be tempted to have a piece of birthday cake or a blueberry muffin, even though it's not gluten-free.

However, after you eat it, I will bet that you won't feel so great anymore, and the value of maintenance will become obvious. It's human nature to blow it and go back to bad habits or old treats. Then we feel lousy, get back on track, and feel better. As you fall down and pick yourself back up again and again, the temptation of the birthday cake ("I'll just have a bite") will dissipate. After 6 months of maintaining your new lifestyle choices, you'll find that old lifestyle habits no longer pose a significant danger or threat.

Taking the Ready-to-Change Quiz (which you can access on my Web site at theDr.com/readyquiz) will help determine if you are truly committed to transformation. I've found that the most successful people come to this point in the book at the determination stage: They're ready and excited, but they need guidance. The quiz allows you to gauge your desire, receptivity, and commitment to improve your health.

Your score lets you know your starting point. Then you'll make a conscious (hopefully) choice to continue or not. If you say, "I'm not ready for this right now," it doesn't mean that you're not destined to get better. You'll choose when the time is right for you. However, if you say, "This is a bunch of garbage" and put the book down, then you're definitely not ready for a transformation. Hopefully, you'll come back when you are, because you can't argue with the science. This is your health journey, or as my mentor, Dr. George Goodheart, would say, "This is your football." Get a realistic overview of where you currently are, accept it, and choose to move forward when you are ready.

ACTION STEP WEEK 8: TRY A CONSCIOUS BREATHING EXERCISE

My friend Pedram Shojai, OMD, bestselling author of *The Urban Monk* and *The Art of Stopping Time,* created a terrific beginner's exercise in conscious breathing. To some this will sound ridiculous, to others outright idiotic. But I hope to enough it will sound like "I'm willing to give that a shot."

This week, set your alarm to go off once an hour while you are awake. When the alarm goes off, just pause for a moment with whatever you're doing, think of one thing you're grateful for today, and take five deep breaths. Sounds silly, but watch what happens after a few days. Life looks a little softer around the edges—not so rigid, not so abrasive to get by. Let me know what you discover; I truly would like to hear from you on this. There's a Facebook page for theDr.com, or you can send an email to info@ theDr.com, and they'll forward your message to me.

9

BIOCHEMISTRY: FOOD AS MEDICINE

JUST A FEW years ago, the new thing in health was to "detox." There were fasting cleanses, juice cleanses, cayenne pepper and maple syrup cleanses, even banana cleanses. But detoxes are really not all that new: People have been talking about cleanses and detoxing since the days of Hippocrates more than 2,000 years ago. These programs are supposed to push toxins out of your body and restore equilibrium and better health. It's a valuable tool in cleaning up one's internal environment. Nowadays, including "detoxing" as part of your regular routine is a vital component of a healthy lifestyle. By now I imagine your jaw has dropped more than once when you realized the amount of toxins you and your family are exposed to every day.

If a detoxification program creates an "aha" moment as we flush out the accumulated debris of food sensitivities, PCBs, dioxins, heavy metals, and BPA, and we feel better, it will hopefully reinforce that we need to do this again, and again, and again. For the rest of our lives. I hope you can see that this world we live in is unavoidably toxic to our bodies, triggering brain dysfunction and so much more.

Besides detoxing, you need to identify the foods to which you are sensitive and eliminate them from your diet. By doing so, not only do you stop throwing gasoline on the fire, reducing the inflammatory cascade, but your body also begins flushing out the stored toxins in your fat cells. Good news: Here comes weight loss! That's why it is critically important to drink ½ ounce of water per pound of body weight every day; you have to have good transport to get this crud out of your body when it's released from the fat cells. If you are not drinking enough water, circulating toxins have an affinity to redeposit back into your brain cells. And here comes brain inflammation from the immune response. But if you are drinking lots of water, you'll naturally lower your toxic load, which by definition means less endotoxin. With less endotoxin comes less internal "gasoline on the fire"—less inflammation. With less inflammation from internal endotoxin irritation comes burning of more fat cells, more trimming of the spare tire on your waist, and a happy, brighter you.

Couple these benefits from a lower toxic load with the intermittent fasting that we discussed in Chapter 4. Now you have a lifestyle that is hitting base hits every day: burning fat, turning the genes on for a more parasympathetic-dominant state of relaxation or "easy living," and modeling a way of life for your family, being as busy as you want to be. That is life-enhancing instead of life-depleting. Your brain cells function better. Every cell, every tissue in your body begins functioning better as you transition into an anabolic state. When you get the results you're looking for, as I expect you will, then you will know that you can't follow this eating plan for 3 weeks and then go back to your old ways. Look at this as a chance to upgrade your ride: Treat your body like the Lamborghini you deserve instead of dragging it around like your dad's 20-year-old pickup truck.

THE SIGNS OF EATING TOO MANY INFLAMMATORY FOODS

My mentors are the pioneers who had the courage to speak out about what they saw every day, and who thought "outside the box" and shared their insights with their seminars, their books, and their newsletters. Dr. Doris Rapp, Dr. George Goodheart, Dr. Jonathan Wright, Dr. Jeffrey Bland, and Dr. Aristo Vojdani were giants in the field of holistic health care who didn't set out to be different; they just had the courage to stand their ground. Dr. Doris Rapp passed away recently. She was at the forefront of connecting behaviors with foods, particularly with children. I had a chance to finally meet Dr. Rapp 2 years ago and thank her for her decades of service to all of us following in her footsteps. She looked at me and matter-of-factly said, "What else could I do?"

Below are some of the physical signs of inflammation, simple indicators to tell if your body burden is too great and you have "crossed the line" where the foods you are eating are presenting a health concern not just for your body, but for your brain. Just look for these signs of inflammation:

- Are your cheeks rosy red? Do you have broken capillaries on or around your nose? Do people assume you're a heavy drinker? Is your face generally red all over? Is it most noticeable on your forehead and cheeks? There's often a strong correlation between red faces and low stomach acid production, which produces inflammatory peptides of poorly digested food molecules. Maybe you even suffer from medium to large acne-type bumps. Your dermatologist has probably diagnosed it as acne rosacea and put you on medication. If your response is "I've always had red cheeks," you likely have always been inflamed. Adult acne is such a common inflammatory response to food sensitivities; we have seen literally hundreds of cases of skin clearing up when the person goes gluten-, dairy-, and sugar-free for a few months. After the skin has cleared up, if people try these foods again, they consistently "cross a threshold" and these foods will cause the acne to come back.
- Many people over age 50 have a slightly yellow tone to their facial skin. Most of us just chalk this up to getting older. But there is something you can do to get back the rosy glow of your youth. Vitamin B_{12} injections have been found to help restore the healthy pink-red tones to the face and even support the health of the ner-

vous system. A lack of B_{12} frequently is due to an older stomach that also isn't making the amounts of hydrochloric acid and pepsin that it once did, which causes more inflammation.

- A brownish yellow discoloration on the front of your legs. This is very often an early warning sign of the inflammatory cascade of insulin problems and eventual development of diabetes.
- Rough, bumpy skin on the backs of your arms often points to a deficiency in vitamin A or of the category of good fats called essential fatty acids; both substances are critical fire extinguishers of inflammation in the body. Without them, you are at much greater risk of developing the inflammatory cascade.
- Eczema—patchy red, cracking, itchy skin—is the end result of chronic inflammation.
- Skin "tags" under the arms, behind the neck, and in the groin area are associated with a distant warning sign for type 2 (maturity-onset) diabetes.
- Dry skin is a sign of long-term inflammation robbing the "good fats" from your cells.
- Wrinkles that run vertically across your forehead and are accompanied by abdominal pain are an early warning sign of a duodenal ulcer, most commonly caused by a bacterial infection accompanied by inflammation.
- Easy bruising (black-and-blue marks) is a likely sign of long-term mild inflammation that has weakened your blood vessels, causing them to rupture too easily.
- Cracked feet and heels are a "slam dunk" indicator of a deficiency of essential fatty acids (EFA). A dry, flaky scalp at any age reflects a diet too high in refined sugars and lacking in EFAs. Having a deficiency of EFAs is like having bone-dry twigs piled up and tossing a lit match on them—there's going to be a fire (inflammation) any minute.
- Having diagonal creases in the lobe of the ears has been associated with a fivefold increased risk of cardiovascular disease.[1]
- Have a sensitive scalp? Does your head feel a bit tender when

you brush your hair? Every time this has happened to me over the years, it's been a reminder that I've been forgetting to take my vitamin D (in my mind, *the* most important vitamin to take). Within a few days of taking 50,000 IU of vitamin D, I find that my scalp is fine and I can brush away. Low vitamin D makes the body much more susceptible to intestinal permeability and chronic inflammation.

- Hair loss or thinning in middle age is often caused by low hydrochloric acid (HCL) and may be reversed over 6 months or so by supplementing with HCL. As we age, we develop more of the results from eating a diet full of inflammatory foods. One result is that our stomachs stop producing adequate levels of stomach acid and pepsin. This leads to poor digestion of essential proteins, creates inflammation, and impedes the growth of new hair. By supplementing your diet with hydrochloric acid–pepsin capsules, you'll begin to digest and absorb protein properly, and your hair loss might stop.

- Hair loss on your lower legs and especially an abnormal loss of underarm or pubic hair frequently indicates that you have seriously low androgenic hormone (DHEA and testosterone) levels in your body. And when you have low hormone levels, your immune system can't function properly. Inflammation runs amok; the natural fire extinguishers have run out of fuel; and wherever the weak link is in your chain, that's where the low-hormone-related symptoms can show.

- Gum bleeding when brushing your teeth or rinsing (gingivitis or periodontal disease) is a clear indicator of substantial inflammation. Any "-itis" (gingivitis, periodontitis, arthritis, bursitis, etc.) is a name for excessive inflammation in specific tissue.

- A scalloped tongue is strongly suggestive of food allergies. Get this checked immediately by an allergist, because those foods are "gasoline on the fire" whether or not they are causing allergic symptoms.

- If you have cracks in the corners of your lips every once in a while, you likely are not getting enough B vitamins—a crucial "fire extinguisher" in your body designed to calm the inflammatory cascade.

- Dark circles under your eyes? There's a reason why they're called allergic shiners.

- Horizontal creases on the lower eyelids (called Dennie's lines) often indicate serious food allergies.

- Weak fingernails that bend, chip, and crack easily point to a problem in your stomach involving low acid and pepsin production.

- White spots on the fingernails almost always point to a zinc deficiency in the body. For some people, white spots can mean low levels of pancreatic enzymes or wheat sensitivity causing inflammation in the intestines and poor absorption.

- Joints ache often? Perhaps first thing in the morning, and you have to get in a hot shower to "loosen up" enough to move without pain? Many people have found that eliminating the nightshade family of vegetables (tomatoes, potatoes, peppers, eggplant, and tobacco) from their diets for several months results in a dramatic improvement. Pain is always an inflammatory biomarker. When you stop throwing gasoline on the fire (and for some, it's the nightshade family), the inflammation reduces and your arthritis symptoms drop dramatically.

- When you take your socks off, do you have sock marks on your legs? Or elastic band marks from where your underwear was on your waist? Now, it's certainly possible that your socks are too small or your underwear is too tight. Just put on a pair tomorrow morning that you know is not too small and see what happens by the end of the day. The marks are often indicative of edema (water retention), which can be from eating foods your body says are toxic, and so your body becomes edematous to dilute the toxicity of that food.

- Gently run your fingernails across your abdomen three times—not gouging or scraping the skin, just gliding your nails across your abdomen in the same line three times. Now wait 30 seconds and look at your abdomen. Can you see red streaks where your nails were gliding? That's suggestive of a histamine reaction. Elevated histamine levels tell us that something is not right. The question is, why does your body make elevated levels of histamines?

THE RIGHT DIET MAY PROTECT YOU FROM ENVIRONMENTAL TOXINS

In Chapter 4 we discussed many different types of pollution and some food-related remedies for them. But there are big-picture environmental toxins that affect us, and there is little we can do to avoid them. I'm referring specifically to air pollution. Our air quality has come a long way since the 1970s, when both the government and individuals took a "no more" stand. However, industrial accidents, wide-scale fires like those we see in California, and the small daily exposures that we might not notice—smelling fuel when you pump gas (benzene), the formaldehyde that is released from the pressboard of your kitchen cabinets, the toxic compounds in Scotchgard that protects your furniture from stains, or flame retardants found in your couch cushions, your child's car seat, or your mattress (organohalogens)—are still part of our lives and can affect brain health. For instance, one flame retardant, chlorinated tris (TDCPP), was removed from children's pajamas in the 1970s amid concerns that it may cause cancer, but now it's a ubiquitous addition to couch cushions. It can easily migrate from the foam into household dust, which children often pick up on their hands and transfer into their mouths. Tris is actually the most commonly used flame retardant in the United States; it's found in nap mats, car seats, strollers, nursing pillows, furniture, and more.[2]

When avoidance is impossible, a more healthful diet will protect us from the toxins floating in the air. Remember, toxins in the air go through our lungs, into the bloodstream, and right up to the brain, causing inflammation and B4 (leaky gut, leaky brain, or as you see here, leaky lungs: it's all the same mechanism). We know this because zonulin, the antibody associated with a leaky gut, is also produced when you have a leaky lung[3] or a leaky brain.[4] According to a 2017 *New York Times* article, a small but growing body of research suggests that taking the right supplements, in combination with a Mediterranean diet, which is very similar to the one I propose (focusing on fruits, vegetables, fish, and nuts), is the key. The foods on my plan cannot shield the body directly like a mask, but they can help us by reducing the damage. The emphasis in our plan is on fruits and vegetables that are high in phytochemicals and polyphenols that produce an anti-inflammatory effect. This occurs both for turning off the genes producing inflammation, and for turning on the fire extinguisher genes that put out the inflammation. The scientists in this 2017 study seem to agree:

> While a sedentary lifestyle and/or poor dietary habits can exacerbate the deleterious effects resulting from exposure to toxic chemicals, much emerging evidence suggests that positive lifestyle changes (e.g., healthful nutrition) can modulate and/or reduce the toxicity of environmental pollutants. Our work has shown that diets high in anti-inflammatory bioactive food components (e.g., phytochemicals or polyphenols) are possible strategies for modulating and reducing the disease risks associated with exposure to toxic pollutants in the environment. Thus, consuming healthy diets rich in plant-derived bioactive nutrients may reduce the vulnerability to diseases linked to environmental toxic insults.[5]

In addition to whole foods, supplements can play a laser-focused role when it comes to combating environmental pollution. For example, drinking broccoli sprout juice increases urinary secretion of benzene by 61 percent. When cooking fats burn, they produce a toxic compound called acrolein, and this juice increases secretion by 23 percent.[6] Broccoli sprouts contain sulforaphane and glucoraphanin, which act like magnets and pull toxic chemicals out. These sprouts contain much higher quantities of these vital compounds than the mature broccoli we typically eat, making a juice a better option.

Three grams of fish oils a day, which are high in omega-3 fatty acids, protect against the adverse cardiac and cholesterol effects associated with air pollution exposure. In one study from the Environmental Protection Agency (EPA), participants who were exposed to 2 hours of particulate pollution and given fish oil supplements had no significant reaction to the particles entering their bodies, making the pollution less dangerous.[7]

Vitamins can play such an important role in preventing damage from air pollution that one team of researchers from top medical research institutions around the world came out with the following statement: "B vitamin supplementation (2.5 milligrams per day of folic acid, 50 milligrams per day of vitamin B_6, and 1 milligram per day of vitamin B_{12}) [is] an attractive pharmaceutical intervention to counteract the PM effects (fine particulate matter)."[8] In another study that looked at children with asthma, the most vulnerable population to air pollution, in Mexico City,

DR. TOM'S TIP
GROW YOUR OWN SPROUTS

Broccoli sprouts have been known for at least 20 years to be a highly potent anti-inflammatory food, even against certain cancers. Here's a great family project that I've been recommending for years. All you need are the seeds and a large Mason jar. You won't be able to grow enough for a full glass of juice, but they are great to add to any meal. Follow these steps:

1. Add 2 tablespoons of broccoli sprouting seeds to a wide-mouthed jar.
2. Cover with a few inches of filtered water and cap with a paper towel.
3. Store in a warm, dark place overnight.
4. The next morning, drain the liquid off and rinse with fresh water, making sure to drain all the water off. Leave the jar inside a soup bowl with the open end angling down; this will help drain all the water away through the paper towel. Repeat this twice a day.
5. After a few days, the seeds will start to break open and grow. By the time sprouts are an inch long, they will have yellow leaves.
6. Move the sprouts out into the sunlight. Continue to rinse them daily until the leaves are dark green. This whole process will take about a week. They are great to add to salads, soups, and sandwiches, and as an ingredient in smoothies.
7. Once they are ready, replace the paper towel with a standard Mason jar lid and store in the refrigerator.

one of the most toxic cities in the world, vitamins C (250 milligrams per day) and E (50 milligrams per day) were found to be protective against ozone on lung function. Interestingly, the study stated that "the protective effect appeared to be greater among children with moderate asthma than among those with mild asthma."[9] The worse the children were, the stronger the effect of the vitamins.

THE MECHANISM OF FOOD TOXICITY

There are two major ways your food selections can be toxic to your body. If your immune system says, "We've got a problem," it does not matter what you "think" about the food; your body is saying no and will create an inflammatory response that can cause a myriad of symptoms. Second, the offending food directly impacts your microbiome and is now recognized as a primary modulator for resistant weight loss.

The relationship between weight gain and inflammatory food exposure is straightforward: The more environmental toxins you are exposed to in your food selections, the more weight-retaining microbiota you feed, the more inflammation your body responds with, and the more weight you gain. When you're exposed day after day to toxins (like gluten, dairy, and sugar), there are a number of consequences.

First, these foods overwhelm your response system, triggering and feeding the "survival bacteria" in the gut. Decades of less-than-ideal food choices have created a microbiome that has a will of its own, and it wants to survive. If you have a calorie-hoarding microbiome, it will send out chemical messengers to your brain that say, "I want more" of whatever the food is that feeds the obesity bacteria (such as high volumes of bad fats or sugar or allergenic foods or simple, processed carbohydrates).

Second, with excessive inflammation, in this case from poor food selections, you increase the storage capacity of white fat cells, which accumulate as the "spare tire" around the waist that is difficult to get rid of through dieting alone. There are 17 hormones that can be produced by white fat cells, and 15 of them produce inflammation.[10] You don't increase your white fat simply from eating too many calories. The body also produces excessive white fat cells as a protective mechanism to keep toxins that you've been exposed to away from the brain. If your detoxification capabilities are overburdened and you can't eliminate these toxins through your liver, bowel movements, urine, and skin, then in order to protect the brain, these chemicals get stored in the body and can create more white fat cells. Excessive amounts of white fat create more inflammation, which manifests as fluid retention (edema).

Once the body has created these toxic fat cells and swelling, it's not so willing to release them. A toxic body may intentionally hold on to excess body fat or fluid to prevent being reexposed to the same toxins during elimination. In other words, your body may be protecting you from toxic exposure by keeping these toxins out of circulation so they cannot get to the brain, in effect forcing you to hold on to excess weight.

When you end your exposure to the foods you are sensitive to, your body is better able to focus on getting rid of the excess fluid it has been retaining and to start burning the fat where the toxins are stored. Best of all, because you will be avoiding the most undesirable, calorie-dense, nutrient-poor foods and replacing them with more desirable nutrient-rich options, you're likely to drop more than a few pounds if you need to. This is one reason why thousands of people have reported losing as much as 15 to 30 pounds within 60 to 90 days on a gluten-free diet.

NEW RULES FOR CHOOSING FOOD

You can begin the process of optimal healing by eliminating the primary foods that your immune system may recognize as toxic. When you remove the three most common inflammatory foods at once—gluten, dairy, and sugar—both your digestive and immune systems have a chance to calm down, heal, and reset. But remember, when you stop pouring gasoline on the fire, you still have a fire to deal with. No matter where you are on the spectrum, along with reducing inflammation, we need to rebuild the damaged tissue so that we can create a better, healthier intestinal environment for good bacterial growth and to heal a leaky gut and leaky brain.

I consider the following suggestions to be an autoimmune eating style featuring food selections and vital nutrients meant to calm down inflammation and reverse the autoimmune cascade. A full autoimmune diet is a highly restricted food plan that eliminates all potential triggers. But clinically, I've seen that not everyone requires a full autoimmune diet. Instead, I've found that by eliminating the three primary triggers—gluten, sugar, and dairy—more than 80 percent of my patients feel dramatically better and begin reversing the autoimmune cascade. If your test results from Chapter 5 show that you have elevated antibodies to your own tissue, then you and your doctor can explore if you are experiencing molecular mimicry related to your diet. Are there other foods besides gluten, sugar, and dairy that are triggering antibodies to your own tissue? If so, you'll have to avoid those foods as well.

I want you to explore your health in baby steps so that you can continue eating the foods you love that don't affect your health. I've also found that the fewer foods that are restricted, the better the compliance.

You will be eliminating specific foods for a specific time and noticing the physical impact on your body and how you feel. This protocol is considered to be the best way to determine which foods are causing sensitivities. For the next 3 weeks, I will help you go completely dairy-free, gluten-free, and sugar-free. Instead of eating harmful foods that make you forgetful, anxious, and tired, you'll be enjoying all types of fruits and vegetables; clean meats, fish, and poultry; and healthy fats. The goal is simple. Take away the bad stuff, including highly processed foods, and add in the good stuff—whole, real foods that are easy to find and prepare.

The first thing people always ask me is what they can eat. The truth is, there's plenty to choose from, and as you'll see soon, I've listed all of the acceptable options. I don't want you to feel limited in any way. In reality, you can select from hundreds of options every day. And just wait until you try some of the recipes in Chapter 10!

You'll be eating the way people ate for most of human history. Plants (vegetables, fruits, nuts, seeds, and herbs and spices) and animals (meat, fish, poultry, and eggs) will represent the vast majority of your foods. Plants will be your main source of healthy carbohydrates and micronutrients (vitamins, minerals, antioxidants, and anti-inflammatory agents). Raw nuts, seeds, their derivative butters, and animal foods offer quality forms of healthy protein and fat. This is the big-picture view of making good food selections for the rest of your life. However, before we go there, you have to clean up some of the old damage and form better systems for how your bloodstream feeds your brain.

PREVENT AND REVERSE COGNITIVE LOSS BY ENHANCING KETOSIS

If you are already starting to get symptoms of cognitive loss or memory dysfunction (for example, if you often find yourself wondering where your car keys are), there's great benefit to adopting a ketogenic diet for a short period of time (1 to 3 months). Ketones, a by-product created when the body is breaking down fat for energy that occurs when food supply is low, can be an efficient backup system for supplying energy to the brain and the body. Burning off stored fat cells and creating ketones is how our ancestors survived if they had to go days to weeks without finding food. We can access ketones through a process called ketosis, which turns out to be a much easier, alternative way for getting fuel into brain cells, especially for those of us who already have poorly functioning blood sugar.

If you are having brain function symptoms, it is likely that your brain is reacting to an inflammatory trigger and has already lost some of its ability to use glucose as fuel—as much as 24 percent.[11] Your brain is literally starving, which creates even more inflammation and more loss of brain function. It's a vicious cycle. However, when you put your body in a ketonic state, studies have shown that not only are you better supporting your brain cells with fuel, but you are also enhancing your overall brain function and health.[12] We're turning up the dimmer switch, and the lights in your brain are burning brighter. Specifically, maintaining a ketonic state is known to improve both memory and cognition in Alzheimer's patients. It reduces hypoperfusion and increases bloodflow to the brain.[13]

A true ketogenic diet would have you avoid all carbohydrates. However, the human body is not designed to live without carbs forever. I suggest that you try it for 1 to 3 months, find out how incredibly good you feel, and then you can slowly transition back to a less restrictive diet. In order to maintain weight loss and the increased brain function you've been enjoying on a ketogenic diet, this would be a good time to introduce intermittent fasting (which we talked about in Chapter 4) as you add back healthier carbohydrate choices—making sure to avoid gluten, dairy, and sugar. Pay attention to how adding a small amount of carbohydrates back affects your brain function. If you are having symptoms again after reintroducing carbohydrates, or your enhanced brain function starts to dim, your body is not ready yet for the reintroduction of that amount of carbohydrates. Take them out of your diet again for another week or two, and then add in a smaller amount and see what happens.

The biomarker of insulin sensitivity, your HOMA score (which we discussed in Chapter 3), can be done every few weeks during this process. You should be seeing better results on every test. Depending on how beat up your glucose delivery system is, it may take a while before your HOMA score is in the normal range. Be patient, keep going for the base hits, and you will be able to get it back to normal.

While a ketogenic diet yields great results, it is only one element of this program. It's better than a typical life jacket of medications, but you will still need to get yourself out of the pool. Remember, you can't avoid carbs forever: Your body is meant to use them as a primary energy source. And unlike the roller-coaster ride of weight-loss programs (lose weight, gain weight, lose weight, gain weight . . .), what makes this brain health program permanent is that you will be going upstream and identifying the underlying causes, triggers, and mechanisms that put you in this state in the first place.

The way to make a ketogenic diet more likely to succeed and create permanent brain health benefits is to combine it with my pleiotropic nutritional approach outlined in the rest of the chapter. You'll also be addressing your food sensitivities, environmental toxin exposures, and the cumulative damage you've already accrued (B4 and leaky gut). Layering the right foods with intermittent fasting and supplementing with medium-chain triglyceride (MCT) oils and other crucial nutrients will yield the greatest results. For instance, a great deal of research has been done on MCTs, which are found in coconut and palm oil. However, palm oil isn't healthy for you: Never use it. MCTs supply easily accessible fuel to the powerhouse furnaces in every brain cell called mitochondria.[14] One MCT supplement that has been shown to enhance ketosis and provide benefits for addressing cognitive dysfunction is called NEOBEE.[15] A little more than 2 tablespoons of coconut oil provides the same dosage of MCTs found in NEOBEE.

MORE THAN A WORD ABOUT GMOs

One of my primary concerns when it comes to the health of our food supply is the prevalence of genetically modified foods and organisms, otherwise known as GMOs. These plants or animals are created in laboratories where their genetic makeup has been altered to create versions that cannot occur in nature or through traditional crossbreeding. Large-scale commercialization of genetically modified foods began in 1994. According to the FDA and the United States Department of Agriculture (USDA), today there are more than 40 GMO plant varieties, the three most prevalent being grains like rice, soy, and corn.[16] The graph below shows the rapid hijacking of agricultural diversity to genetically modified crops. By 2012, close to 90 percent of all corn, soy, and cotton produced in the United States were GMO varieties.

There are nine genetically modified (GM) food crops currently on the market: soy, corn, cotton (oil), canola (oil), sugar from sugar beets, zucchini, yellow squash, Hawaiian papaya, and alfalfa. GM grains are fed to the animals we eat and therefore affect dairy products, eggs, beef, chicken, pork, and other animal products. Some of these raw ingredients are also added to even the more "natural" processed foods, like tomato sauce, ice

Percent of GM Crops Grown in U.S.

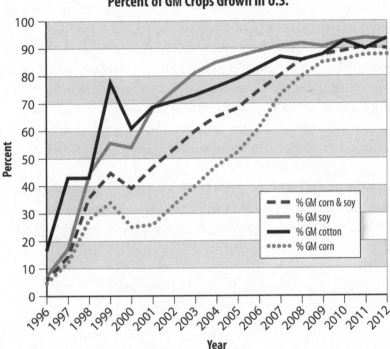

cream, and peanut butter. GM corn or soy is added to some spices and seasoning mixes, as well as soft drinks (in the form of corn syrup or the artificial sweetener aspartame, or the glucose, citric acid, and colorings such as beta-carotene and riboflavin). The ubiquity of soybean and corn derivatives as food additives virtually ensures that all of us have been exposed to GM food products. In fact, more than 80 percent of all processed foods, such as vegetable oils or breakfast cereals, contain some genetically modified ingredients.

GMO wheat will soon find its way into our kitchens. In the meantime, wheat has been hybridized through natural breeding techniques over the years to contain more gluten and other deleterious components such as fermentable carbohydrates, called FODMAPS. Like most GMO crops, wheat is sprayed with the weed killer called Roundup, whose active ingredient, glyphosate, is now authoritatively classified as a probable human carcinogen.[17]

The majority of US wheat crops are sprayed with Roundup a few weeks before harvest to kill the plant. There are two reasons for this. First, a dead field of wheat is easier to harvest because it won't plug up the combines. Second, the stress to the plant caused by the toxic chemical that's killing it causes the plant to suck up more nutrients from the soil in an effort to stay alive. Those nutrients go into the wheat seeds, creating plants that contain more gluten. Therefore, the majority of wheat products in the United States contain cancer-initiating glyphosate traces as well as more gluten.

Animal studies have suggested that GMOs might cause damage to the immune system, liver, and kidneys. Roundup has also been shown to alter the microbiota and create an environment of increased intestinal permea-

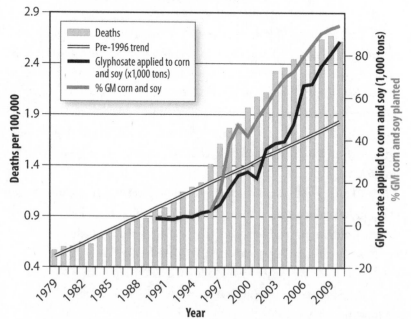

**Age-Adjusted Deaths Due to Stroke
(ICD 162.9 & 432.9 hemorrhage, non-embolic)**

Plotted against % GM corn and soy (R = 0.9827, p <= 1.354e-06)
& glyphosate applied to corn and soy (R = 0.9246, p<= 1.471e-07)
Sources: USDA:NASS; CDC

bility. Scientists are studying the interaction of this chemical with the detoxification capabilities of the liver, going as far as to say this is a "textbook example" of environmental triggers disrupting homeostasis and leading to an autoimmune response, including excessive inflammation in the brain's memory center, the hippocampus. It is also linked to gastrointestinal disorders, obesity, depression, autism, infertility, cancer, and Alzheimer's disease.[18] Take a look at the graph on page 222, which shows the increase in deaths due to strokes after glyphosate was introduced into our food supply.

I know this information is both shocking and upsetting, but it helps to explain the dramatic increase in so many diseases in the last 30 years. For more information, you can read the 13-page authoritative report I helped write: "Can Genetically-Engineered Foods Explain the Exploding Gluten Sensitivity?" (available on my Web site, theDr.com/gmofoods).

The scariest part about GMOs is that consumers don't know what they're eating, because GMO labeling is prohibited in the United States. Although most developed nations do not consider them safe, and labeling of GM food products is required in 64 countries, no labeling or restrictions are required in the United States. The only way you can avoid GMOs is by following these three simple rules:

1. Buy local produce. The simplest way to steer clear of GM crops is to join a local food co-op or CSA (community supported agriculture) or shop at local farmers' markets. Buy foods in their raw, whole, unprocessed state. You are more likely to find truthful answers from a local farmer or co-op compared to a major corporation.

2. Buy organic. Certified organic products cannot include GM ingredients. This includes both produce and meats, because if cattle have eaten GM feed, it alters the bacteria in their guts, which then affects both their meat and their milk.

3. Look for "Non-GMO Project Verified" or "USDA Organic" seals on single-ingredient packaged goods like flours, seeds, and nuts. And while you are doing that, make sure they all are marked as "gluten-free" somewhere on the label to reduce your risk of cross-contamination.

ENJOY YOUR FAVORITE FRESH FOODS

You can eat all forms of fruits, vegetables, spices, and nuts, especially when they are fresh and in season. I always recommend fresh fruits and vegetables when available, but for many, this isn't always possible. Frozen fruits and vegetables are acceptable because they are harvested when ripe and have had the opportunity to build a full repertoire of antioxidants and polyphenols. Choose organic produce whenever possible, and, if you can, find locally sourced varieties. Avoid canned fruits and vegetables that may have been preserved with sugar or salt. Roasted peanuts contain more resveratrol than do raw peanuts; resveratrol is the beneficial ingredient also found in red wine known to protect the brain and cardiovascular system. All other nuts should be eaten raw.

A number of fresh foods are known to heal the gut. These foods are healthy choices because they are anti-inflammatory by nature. Make sure to eat something from this list every day:

- Cinnamon
- Cruciferous vegetables (broccoli, Brussels sprouts, cauliflower, cabbage, bok choy), which contain a family of vital nutrients called glucosinolates that are potent polyphenols particularly useful for lowering inflammation in the intestines
- Dark-colored fruits with a high concentration of polyphenols, such as berries, cherries, and red grapes
- Green tea, which is also a prebiotic
- Omega-3 fatty acids. These must be acquired through diet because the body cannot produce them. Among so many other benefits they bring us, they turn on the genes that lower inflammation in the gut. Foods high in omega-3s include grass-fed beef, cold-water fish, seafood, black walnuts, pecans, pine nuts, chia seeds, flaxseeds, basil, oregano, cloves, marjoram, and tarragon.
- Parsley
- Tomato juice

These fresh fruits and spices are known to inhibit the production of amyloid plaques in the brain, and therefore are thought to be neuroprotective:[19]

- Cinnamon
- Dates[20]
- Ginger
- Ginseng
- Rosemary
- Sage
- Turmeric

INULIN IS YOUR FRIEND

There is a class of carbohydrates called *fructan* that act like fertilizer to support the good bacteria in our intestines. The best-known fructans are in the family called *inulin*. Inulin is a natural storage carbohydrate present in more than 36,000 species of plants. Inulin is also considered to be a prebiotic used as an energy reserve and for regulating cold resistance. Chicory root is a prebiotic that contains the highest concentration of inulin (our New Orleans readers will be happy to hear this, as it's a cultural addition to their regional cuisine). Other plants that contain this healthy bacterial fertilizer include wheat, sugar beets, leeks, asparagus, artichokes, onions, garlic, dandelion root, bananas, and plantains.

One of the potential pitfalls of a gluten-free diet is that most of us get more than 70 percent of our inulin from wheat. When we lose the wheat, whatever level of good bacteria we have in our gut, which has grown dependent on wheat as the major source of its fertilizer, begins to starve. Gluten-free products often are much lower in inulin. So in our efforts to fix intestinal permeability, we create a worse environment in our microbiome than we had before. This is why we must be sure to include inulin-rich foods as part of our daily diet (you'll see a list of these foods later in the chapter). Fermented foods will both inoculate and encourage the growth of gut-protecting families of bacteria.

Other high-fiber vegetables are equally important. We need butyrate to strengthen both the gut and the brain's blood barrier. Vegetables, especially root vegetables like parsnips, turnips, rutabagas, cabbages, sweet potatoes, purple potatoes, and multicolored carrots, contain insoluble fiber, which produces butyrate. I recommend that you eat one root vegetable every day.

FRUITS

Fruits are higher in sugar than vegetables, and some, like bananas, are very high on the glycemic index, which is a commonly used measurement to quantify how fast a particular food will raise your blood sugar. A banana has a glycemic index of 51 (that's a good number), and eating them once in a while is fine. But if we eat two bananas every day, along with other medium- to high-glycemic-index foods, the impact of too much sugar eventually sends our bodies down the path of roller-coaster blood sugar levels that lead to high-anxiety states ("going bananas") and diabetes.

Pure glucose is used as the base number for the glycemic index and is given a value of 100; all other carbohydrates are given values relative to glucose depending on how fast they get into the blood—the lower the index, the longer it takes, and the more stable your blood sugar remains. The higher the index, the more likely you'll feel the roller coaster of blood sugar peaks and drops.

Foods that have a high index (greater than 60) include ice cream, breads, all other flour products, white potatoes, raisins, potato chips, alcoholic beverages, and white rice. In fact, according to William Davis, MD, the bestselling author of *Wheat Belly*, the glycemic index of wheat products is among the highest of all foods. Low-glycemic-index foods (under 45) are considered more nutritious: It's no surprise that they include most other fruits, vegetables, and legumes.

The glycemic index can definitely help you make better food choices, and it points out several discrepancies of so-called healthy options. For example, just one slice of whole wheat bread is considered high on the glycemic index, coming in at 69; it's actually higher than a Snickers, which has a glycemic index of only 42, thanks to the peanuts in this candy bar. You can find the glycemic index of many foods on my Web site, theDr.com/glycemicindex.

Fruits that are considered low glycemic (apricots, plums, apples, peaches, pears, cherries, and berries) are excellent choices. Although some fruits, like berries, are great for you, because we're all guilty of eating way too much sugar, our blood-sugar-regulating systems are more sensitive than they should be. As you begin this program, listen to your body. A small amount of low-glycemic fruit is good for you, unless:

1. You have a known allergy or sensitivity to a particular fruit.
2. Your HOMA score (which we discussed in Chapter 3) shows that you have insulin sensitivity. Low-blood-sugar symptoms that affect your brain include brain fog, brain and body fatigue, and dizziness when standing. It is also related to depression, hyperactivity, anxiety, difficulty concentrating, and crankiness, headaches, and irritability.

All of these fruits are good choices to include in your variety:

- Acai berry
- Apple
- Apricot
- Avocado
- Banana
- Blackberry
- Black raspberry
- Blueberry
- Boysenberry
- Cantaloupe
- Cherry
- Coconut
- Cranberry
- Fig
- Goji berry
- Gooseberry
- Grapefruit
- Guava
- Honeydew
- Huckleberry
- Juniper berry
- Kiwifruit
- Kumquat
- Lemon
- Lime
- Loquat

- Lychee
- Mango
- Nectarine
- Olive
- Orange
- Papaya
- Passionfruit
- Peach
- Pear

- Persimmon
- Pineapple
- Plum
- Pomegranate
- Pomelo
- Quince
- Star fruit
- Strawberry
- Watermelon

NUTS AND SEEDS

Nuts and seeds are excellent sources of protein. Many of them are now ground into flours and butters that you can use instead of traditional wheat flour. There are no raw, commonly available nuts or seeds that are off-limits, unless you have a known allergy or sensitivity. Peanuts and coconut are both acceptable (I treat coconut as a superfood), although neither are technically nuts or seeds: Peanuts are in the legume family, and coconut is a fruit.

However, this is not an open invitation to eat every nut bar on the shelves. You must diligently read ingredients and labels carefully and avoid the bars made with sugar or dairy and those not labeled gluten-free. Organic and gluten-free processed foods are often made with unhealthy ingredients.

Good seed and nut choices include:

- Almond
- Australian nut
- Beech
- Black walnut
- Brazil nut
- Butternut
- Cashew

- Chestnut
- Chia seeds
- Chinese almond
- Chinese chestnut
- Filbert
- Flaxseeds
- Hazelnut

- Hemp seeds
- Indian beech
- Kola nut
- Macadamia
- Pecan
- Pine nut
- Pistachio
- Poppy seeds
- Pumpkin seeds
- Safflower
- Sesame seeds
- Sunflower
- Tiger nut
- Walnut

VEGETABLES

Vegetables are extremely adaptable. There are so many different ways to prepare them. You can eat most of them raw, lightly steamed, baked, or sautéed and enjoy them as a snack, side dish, or main dish. You can also add them to soups, chilies, stews, roasts, salads, stir-fries, and casseroles. Aim for buying the highest quality you can find, meaning organic, local, and farm fresh whenever possible.

The more vegetables you eat every day, the better. I recommend you include five different colors of vegetables per day. Each color provides a different family of antioxidants and polyphenols, which activate different genes that will keep you strong and healthy.

I know it can be a challenge to work vegetables into every meal, especially when you are cooking for children. My advice is to prepare vegetables in a way that your kids will eat them, which is more important than if they did not eat any vegetables at all. Strive for the least-altered way possible. It's a stretch to see the health benefits in deep-fried vegetables.

And the type of vegetable matters, too. The glycemic index of a yam is 37, a sweet potato 44, new potatoes 57, white-skin mashed potatoes 70, French fries 75, baked potato 85, instant mashed potatoes 86, and red-skin boiled potatoes 88. We always want to choose the foods with the lowest glycemic index that our children will eat. The glycemic load of food plays a subtle but determining role in the effects on our bodies of the foods we choose, so choose carefully.

There are no vegetables that are off-limits, unless you have a known allergy or sensitivity. The only caveat is nonorganic soy and corn. Practically all the soy and corn grown in this country is genetically modified, and that in itself can cause intestinal permeability. You need to read labels carefully and look for organic, which is always GMO-free.

Good vegetable choices include:

- Artichoke, globe
- Artichoke, hearts
- Artichoke, Jerusalem
- Arugula
- Asparagus
- Avocado
- Beans (all varieties)
- Beets and beet greens
- Bok choy
- Broccoli
- Broccoli rabe
- Brussels sprouts
- Cabbage
- Carrots
- Cauliflower
- Celery
- Collard greens
- Corn—organic only!
- Cucumbers
- Eggplant
- Fennel
- Fiddlehead ferns
- Garlic
- Jicama
- Kale
- Leeks
- Lettuce
- Mushrooms
- Mustard greens
- Onions
- Parsnips
- Peas
- Peppers (all varieties)
- Potatoes
- Pumpkin
- Radishes
- Rhubarb
- Romaine lettuce
- Rutabaga
- Sea vegetables
- Shallots
- Soy (edamame, tofu, etc.)—organic only!
- Spinach
- Squash
- Sugar snap peas
- Sweet potatoes (yams)
- Swiss chard
- Tomatoes
- Turnips and turnip greens
- Watercress
- Zucchini

THE DIRTY DOZEN AND THE CLEAN 15

You always want the cleanest food you can eat. As a general rule of thumb, buy organic and buy local. Local farmers use the most effective chemicals that they've been told are safe. Organic farmers don't use chemical pesticides on their crops at all. But when you buy produce from large commercial farming industries, their bottom line is tonnage per acre: how much they can produce. They will, without a doubt, use chemicals to get the results they are looking for: unblemished produce and lots of it. This is possible because the lobbying power of the agribusiness industry has gotten these chemicals approved as GRAS (Generally Regarded as Safe). I'd much prefer an asymmetrical apple that's safe for me to eat over a perfect apple that looks great but lacks in taste and is covered with harmful chemicals.

The vast majority of produce that you buy in the supermarket that is not labeled as either local or organic comes from these giant farms. And this means that those fruits and vegetables in the highest demand are often the most toxic. So what are they? The Environmental Working Group has published its list of both "The Dirty Dozen" and "The Clean Fifteen" every year.[21] Apples have topped the list 5 years in a row. The rest of the list includes strawberries, spinach, nectarines, peaches, pears, cherries, grapes, celery, tomatoes, sweet bell or hot peppers, and white potatoes. Of course, these fruits and vegetables are healthy choices, but when they are laced full of toxic chemicals, you are at risk of accumulating them in your body. Eventually, you will achieve a toxic threshold that triggers an inflammatory state.

This accumulation begins in utero, and you may cross the threshold at any age. Even children at birth may have already crossed the threshold of tolerance due to their parents' accumulative toxins and exposures before and during pregnancy. For example, a 2017 study published in the *International Journal of Cancer* showed that a mother's exposure to insecticides during pregnancy increases the possible development of childhood brain tumors by 40 percent.[22]

Accumulative toxins from pesticides can result in the same kinds of problems we know so well that occur with smoking cigarettes. We have known for quite a while that if a mom smoked during pregnancy, there is a 79 percent increased risk of the child developing asthma.[23] When fathers smoke cigarettes before conception, their children have a 68 percent increased risk of developing asthma.[24] As Joseph Pizzorno, ND, tells us from his research, "Advances in modern technology and science have left us with another problem—the accumulating effects of toxicity. The slow accrual of harmful chemicals in your body can gradually erode your organs and systems and lead to chronic disease."[25]

The Clean Fifteen include sweet corn, avocados, pineapples, cabbage, onions, sweet peas, papayas (non-Hawaiian, as many of them are GMO), asparagus, mango, eggplant, honeydew melon, kiwifruit, cantaloupe, cauliflower, and grapefruit.

If you can't find organic, shy away from the Dirty Dozen and go for the Clean Fifteen. And if you have only the Dirty Dozen, do what your mother told you to do and eat your vegetables anyway. It's all about the process of integrative health care, caring for your health in an intelligent fashion, and doing the best under whatever circumstances you face right now.

ANIMAL PROTEINS

Our first priority when choosing protein sources is to avoid eating animals that have been grain-fed. The best option comes from animals that have been grass-fed and pastured that you can buy directly from a local farm; the second-best choice is organic. For example, grass-fed beef has four times more omega-3s than corn-fed beef. For a source of good meat near you, contact a Weston A. Price Foundation chapter leader, or visit your local farmers' market. Another great resource for information is theDr.com/meat.

Grass-fed beef is healthier for you than corn-fed beef. There's no question about it. Cows have two stomachs for digestion because they are supposed to eat grass, not grains. They digest the chlorophyll in the grass and convert it to a kind of fat called conjugated linoleic acid, or CLA.

Grass-fed beef is high in CLA, while corn-fed beef is very low in CLA. CLA helps your body use cholesterol in a healthier way[26] and contributes to building the good bacteria in your gut to keep your weight down. CLA is also a supplement that you can take if you want to lose weight, as it contributes to the beneficial bacteria (lactobacilli and bifidobacteria) that help you burn up calories rather than storing them.[27] When you look at studies about obesity and the microbiome, you will find that people who take CLA build a healthier microbiome and lose weight. One study shows that you can lose up to one pound a month by taking this supplement.[28] Finally, grass-fed beef is unlikely to have the antibiotics and growth hormones of corn-fed beef.

When choosing proteins, a critical concept is the biological value (BV), the proportion of absorbed protein from a food that becomes incorporated into the proteins of our body. There is a reason why eggs are called the perfect food—their BV is 100 percent. That means that our bodies can use all of the protein in an egg (as long as we do not have an allergy or sensitivity to eggs). Cow's milk has a biological value of 91 percent; that's why it has always been considered a healthy option for children, as protein is the essential building block for growth. The problem, of course, is that the immune system can recognize milk as a toxin; it may be easy to use the protein, but it's not a food we are supposed to be eating.

Fish has a BV of 83 percent. Beef is 80 percent. Chicken is 79 percent. Soy is 74 percent. Wheat is 54 percent. The BV of beans is below 50 percent. These numbers point out how hard it is to get enough usable protein by following a vegetarian diet. This is one reason why vegetarians are often the sickest patients I see. They are typically protein deficient. However, the European Food Information Council has found that when two vegetable proteins are combined in one meal, the amino acids of one protein can compensate for the limitations of another, resulting in a combination of a higher biological value. That is why many different cultures serve nonmeat sources of protein together. Mexican beans and corn, Japanese soybeans and rice, Cajun red beans and rice, or Indian dal and rice combine legumes with grains to provide a meal that is high in all essential amino acids.

Whenever possible, avoid factory-farmed meats or fish that contains antibiotics and hormones. Unless you can make them yourself, avoid processed meats like hot dogs, bacon, sausage, jerky, and luncheon meats. Often these foods are flavored with sugar, contain gluten as a binding agent, and are laced with preservatives.

Eggs can be used for a wide variety of quick and healthy meals. Look for ones that are marked "free range and organic." Not only are these eggs healthier, they taste better and look a little different: The yolk has an orange tinge instead of a pure yellow color.

Good animal protein choices include:

- Beef
- Bison/buffalo
- Boar
- Chicken
- Duck
- Eggs (any variety)
- Elk (my personal favorite)
- Goose
- Lamb
- Pork
- Turkey
- Veal
- Venison

THE TRUTH ABOUT FISH

We've all heard how valuable fish is to eat. It has a high biological value, is loaded with the good fats that feed our brain exactly what it needs for optimum growth and function, and reduces our risk of cardiovascular disease. As a matter of fact, of all of the vitamins and minerals that you can take, nutritionists worldwide agree that it is the omega-3s found in high concentrations in cold-water fish that are the most ideal. They are cardioprotective, reduce high cholesterol, and are a primary raw material for healthy brain cells.

Yet fish is another casualty of environmental pollution. Persistent organic pollutants (POPs) is a collective designation for a group of environmental toxins that include dioxins, polychlorinated biphenyls (PCBs), brominated flame retardants, and pesticides. They degrade very slowly, are scarcely excreted, and therefore tend to accumulate in the body. Most of them are fat-soluble, and the highest concentrations in our diet are found in fatty foods, especially oily fish,[29] while breast milk is the main source for infants.[30]

The majority of scientists, the EPA, and the FDA are in agreement that pregnant women, women who might become pregnant, breastfeeding women, infants, and young children need to be extremely cautious in their fish selection and volume consumed. For babies in utero, there is convincing evidence of serious problems for the developing brain from mercury exposure (methyl mercury, to be exact), which continue after birth. The same type of brain and nerve development problems occur in infants and young children exposed to fish high in mercury. Dioxins and polychlorinated biphenyls present in contaminated and farm-raised fish may also increase the risk in both infants and young children for developing "poor expressive language skills"[31] and language delay.[32]

Salmon are relatively fatty fish that are high on the food chain (large fish like salmon eat medium-size fish that eat smaller fish that eat the plankton that accumulates the toxic chemicals in the ocean, which comes mainly from agricultural runoff and polluted rain). Thus the highest concentration of toxins accumulates in the fish that are at the top of the food chain. The healthiest choice is wild-caught fish; avoid the farm-raised varieties. In the largest-scale study done to date on salmon, scientists analyzed 2 metric tons of farmed and wild salmon taken from 39 locations around the world, looking for toxic PCBs, dieldrin (an insecticide), toxaphene (an insecticide), dioxins, and chlorinated pesticides. While there were no significant differences in mercury levels between farmed and wild salmon, contaminants including PCBs, dioxins, toxaphene, and dieldrin were found in threefold higher concentrations (on average) in farmed salmon compared to wild salmon. What's more, these were only 4 of the 14 contaminants found in farmed salmon that are known as "probable" or "possible" human carcinogens, according to the EPA.[33]

Farm-raised salmon has six times the omega-6 fats of wild salmon. We need a little, but not too much of the omega-6s. In excess, they may be linked to coronary artery disease. The studies suggest we lose about two-thirds of the cardioprotective benefits of healthy fats with farm-raised salmon.[34]

Just take a look at the summary statement from another study published in the *Journal of Nutrition:* "Young children, women of child-bearing age, pregnant women, and nursing mothers concerned with health impairments such as reduction in IQ and other cognitive and behavioral effects can minimize contaminant exposure by choosing the least contaminated wild salmon or by selecting other sources of (n-3) fatty acids."[35] Again, eat wild-caught fish or look for other sources of omega-3s—avoid the farm-raised fish.

The National Resources Defense Council (NRDC) has put together "The Smart Seafood Buying Guide: Five Ways to Ensure the Fish You Eat Is Healthy for You and for the Environment." Their guidelines include: Think small (smaller varieties of fish, such as sardines, have less mercury than larger varieties, such as swordfish), buy American, diversify your choices, eat local, and be vigilant. It's an excellent guideline to read.[36] You can find it at nrdc.org/stories/smart-seafood-buying-guide.

The safest fish I know of comes from Alaska, and Vital Choice Seafoods is my source. They have the safest canned tuna I've ever found; it's called Ventresca. My friend Randy Hartnell was a salmon fisherman for more than 20 years, and he realized that the smaller, younger tuna that are caught in the salmon nets are almost free of mercury contamination. The most remarkable fact about their tuna fish is the high concentration of brain food found in each can. The total omega-3s in one can of Ventresca is 7,000 milligrams, of which 1,680 milligrams are the anti-inflammatory good fat (EPA), and 4,860 milligrams are the raw material to build healthy brain cells (DHA). It's great for kids' tuna fish sandwiches on gluten-free bread. You can learn more about this great product at theDr.com/vitalchoice.

Here is a list of fish provided by the NRDC that is organized by mercury content. Personally, I would stay away from all fish outside of the first, "low-mercury," category. The only exception would be wild Alaskan salmon.

Low Mercury: Enjoy These Fish Often

- Anchovies
- Butterfish
- Catfish
- Clams
- Crab (domestic)
- Crawfish/crayfish
- Croaker (Atlantic)
- Flounder*
- Haddock (Atlantic)*
- Hake
- Herring
- Mackerel (North Atlantic, chub)
- Mullet
- Oysters
- Perch (ocean)
- Plaice
- Pollock
- Salmon (canned)**
- Salmon (fresh)**

* Fish in trouble! These fish are perilously low in numbers or are caught using environmentally destructive methods. To learn more, visit the Web sites of Monterey Bay Aquarium (seafoodwatch.org) and the Safina Center (formerly Blue Ocean Institute, safinacenter.org), both of which provide guides listing fish to enjoy or avoid on the basis of environmental factors.
** Farmed salmon may contain PCBs, chemicals with serious long-term health effects.

- Sardines
- Scallops*
- Shad (American)
- Shrimp*
- Sole (Pacific)
- Squid (calamari)
- Tilapia
- Trout (freshwater)
- Whitefish
- Whiting

Moderate Mercury

- Bass (striped, black)
- Carp
- Cod (Alaskan)*
- Croaker (white Pacific)
- Halibut (Atlantic)*
- Halibut (Pacific)
- Jacksmelt (silverside)
- Lobster
- Mahimahi
- Monkfish*
- Perch (freshwater)
- Sablefish
- Skate*
- Snapper*
- Tuna (canned chunk light)
- Tuna (skipjack)*
- Weakfish (sea trout)

High Mercury

- Bluefish
- Grouper*
- Mackerel (Spanish, gulf)

- Sea bass (Chilean)*
- Tuna (canned albacore)
- Tuna (yellowfin)*

Highest Mercury: Avoid Eating
- Mackerel (king)
- Marlin*
- Orange roughy*
- Shark*
- Swordfish*
- Tilefish*
- Tuna (bigeye, ahi)*

HEALTHY FATS

Coconut and coconut products are loaded with healthy fats and are shelf stable. Coconut's creamy texture is great for dairy-free cooking. Because of its high fat content, you can substitute coconut milk in any recipe that calls for a dairy equivalent. But besides its culinary flexibility, coconut-based products are great for brain health. Coconut oils contain medium-chain triglycerides (MCT), which are known to have neuroprotective properties. These are easily absorbed by the body and used for energy, easily metabolized by the liver, and converted to ketones, an alternative fuel for the brain (that's a good thing) so that we are less reliant on blood glucose for energy. The phenol compounds found in coconut prevent the accumulation of beta-amyloid plaque, a key step in the progression of Alzheimer's disease.[37]

The least processed options for cooking oils are clearly labeled as extra-virgin or cold-pressed. Look for oils sold in UV-protected bottles so they won't go rancid quickly. One of the primary cautions for cooking with oils is to make sure you do not heat them to smoking levels. When oils begin to smoke, they are becoming oxidized and produce high amounts of free radicals. So you want healthy oils that have a higher heating point before they smoke.

Good choices for healthy fats include:

- Avocado oil
- Coconut oil
- Ghee
- Macadamia oil
- Olive oil

FLOURS FOR BAKING

The following baking products are allowed on a gluten-free diet (unless you have a sensitivity to them) as long as the packaging is clearly marked as "gluten-free" and there are no added sugar or dairy ingredients (as in a pancake mix):

- Amaranth
- Arrowroot
- Buckwheat
- Gluten-free flours (rice, potato, bean)
- Hominy grits
- Millet
- Polenta
- Tapioca

FERMENTED FOODS

You benefit from eating a forkful of fermented foods every day. This is an excellent strategy for rebuilding and maintaining healthy gut bacteria: The foods themselves supply and produce probiotic bacteria that are then introduced into your digestive tract.

The typical sauerkraut that we get at the supermarket has sodium benzoate in it, which stops the fermentation. A few brands available at your grocer are genuinely fermented and free of sugars and additives. Look for some of my favorites, like Gold Mine Natural Food, Farmhouse Culture, Eden Foods, Wildbrine, and Bubbies. Fermented foods should be sold in airtight containers or purchased fresh at an olive bar in the grocery store. This type of storage allows the vegetables to ferment without producing mold that can trigger histamines that some people react to (including rashes, digestive upset, and inflammation).

Good choices include:

- Coconut kefir
- Fermented cucumbers (which are different from pickles, which are made with malt vinegar that may contain gluten)
- Kimchi
- Kombucha
- Olives
- Pickled ginger
- Sauerkraut

FOCUS ON PREBIOTIC FOODS

The microbiome is the primary modulator (hands on the steering wheel) of health throughout your body. What you eat will encourage (feed) more of the "good guys" or the "bad guys" in your gut. And this happens very quickly, in just 1 to 2 days. Prebiotics help the good guys grow.

Prebiotics can be classified in a few different categories. The most general category includes foods that increase the "families" of bacteria versus the individual species of bacteria, and the most well-known member of this family is green tea. Green tea is one of the most popular beverages in the world. Its beneficial health effects and components have been extensively reviewed, including its ability to increase *Bifidobacterium*, a family of good bacteria. The polyphenols in green tea act as antibacterials and go after the bad guys in the microbiome, including *Clostridium difficile*, *C. perfringens*, and *Streptococcus pyogenes*.[38]

Other well-known prebiotics that have this "general benefit" of increasing multiple families of bacteria include root vegetables, beans and legumes, bananas, cooked rice, cooked potatoes, chicory, asparagus, artichokes, onions, garlic, leeks, and soybeans as well as human breast milk.[39] When you make sure to include a few servings of prebiotics per day, you have a very good chance of rebuilding a healthier microbiome that favors weight stability (increasing it if you're too thin, decreasing it if you're carrying a spare tire around your midsection).

Here's a base hit with tremendous rewards: Eat a root vegetable every day. When I go food shopping, I always buy one or two of every organic root vegetable they have: parsnips, turnips, red beets, golden beets, rutabagas, carrots, or potatoes. Each root vegetable contains different building blocks for your microbiome, supplying excellent materials and helping to build stronger cells. I cook them all the same; I dice them up and sauté with olive, avocado, or coconut oil, add some spices and a little sea salt, and voilà, I'm good to go with satisfying veggies.

GETTING GLUTEN OUT OF YOUR DIET

A gluten-free lifestyle avoids the grains that contain gluten: primarily wheat, along with rye, barley, spelt, and kamut. Conventionally grown rice is known to be high in arsenic, so avoid that as well. There's no reason why you can't have organic rice or other organic gluten-free grains, unless you know you have a sensitivity to them.

Oats do not contain toxic gluten. However, when you buy oats off the shelf, it's very likely there is gluten in them because of cross-contamination. Either the fields where they were grown were contaminated (the farmer grew wheat in that same field in previous years), the trucks that transported the oats to the manufacturing facility transported wheat the previous week and the trucks weren't cleaned between deliveries, or the manufacturing facility processed both wheat and oats on their assembly lines. In a study published in the *New England Journal of Medicine* that looked at four different samples of oats from three different companies (one organic, one where the oats were manufactured in an oats-only facility so there was no chance of cross-contamination at the manufacturing site, and one very famous large manufacturer), only 2 of 12 samples were free from toxic levels of gluten.[40] There are companies that take pride in the fact that their oats are gluten-free; they take the extra step. Bob's Red Mill, GF Harvest (theDr.com/thrive), and Trader Joe's whole grain gluten-free rolled oats are some of my favorites.

I'm not going to lie: Going gluten-free is a challenge at first. Wheat is everywhere in our Western diet, including pasta, snack foods, breakfast cereals, most breads, condiments, and sauces, as well as thickeners and stabilizers used in soups, frozen foods, and processed meats. The following lists, and the recipes in Chapter 10, will make the transition easier. It just takes a bit of planning.

My friend Melinda Dennis, RD, is the nutrition coordinator of the Celiac Center at Beth Israel Deaconess Medical Center, a division of Harvard Medical School. She reminded me that it's important to replace the wheat you are leaving out of your diet with lots of healthy proteins and fiber-rich vegetables, as we listed earlier. She believes, as I do, that if you pull all wheat out of your diet, you lose a tremendous amount of prebiotic fiber, B vitamins, and iron. If you move from wheat to a gluten-free diet and you don't pay particular attention to what you are substituting, you're setting yourself up for failure with potential nutrient deficiencies and development of an unhealthy microbiome. You might even gain weight, depending on the gluten-free foods you choose.

AVOID THESE FOODS ENTIRELY UNLESS LABELED GLUTEN-FREE, DAIRY-FREE, AND SUGAR-FREE

Food manufacturers have jumped on the bandwagon with tons of gluten-free products. The problem is that they are usually just as bad as their gluten-containing counterparts, but for different reasons. These foods are often made with highly refined carbohydrates, sugar, and various chemicals. As is the case with fat-free foods, once the manufacturers take out one ingredient, they have to replace it with something else that offers similar flavor, consistency, or mouthfeel. Gluten-free products often contain large amounts of filler in an effort to add flavor. So as tempting as gluten-free pastries sound, we have to avoid them due to their high sugar content.

Here are gluten-containing store-bought foods you should avoid:

- Beer
- Bouillon cubes
- Bread
- Cake
- Candy
- Cereal
- Cookies
- Couscous
- Crackers
- Croutons
- Gravy
- Imitation meats and seafood
- Oats not labeled as gluten-free
- Pasta
- Pie
- Salad dressing
- Soy sauce

ALWAYS LOOK FOR A GLUTEN-FREE LABEL

The majority of packaged foods that are labeled gluten-free are in fact safe for you to eat. In a 2014 study appearing in the journal *Food Chemistry*, three FDA scientists demonstrated that 97.3 percent of gluten-free foods were correctly labeled.[41] This means that the guidelines are working at the industry level and the requirements by the FDA are being met. That sounds great. But if you're a person with celiac disease and you eat one of the nearly 3 percent of products that are contaminated with toxic levels of gluten, you may experience an immune reaction that you think comes out of the blue, and you will never know why you're having a relapse because you've been working extra hard at eating gluten-free.

According to this FDA directive, all packaged foods labeled as gluten-free must contain fewer than 20 parts per million (ppm) of gluten. However, in the same 2014 study referenced above, researchers found that among the foods that should naturally be gluten-free (not those labeled gluten-free), such as rice pasta, for which the ingredients are only rice, salt, and water, 24.7 percent still had toxic levels of gluten. That's one out of four foods that you may think are safe choices, yet aren't. This inadvertent exposure is a primary reason why some people don't heal even when they follow a strict gluten-free diet. In fact, only 8 percent of celiacs heal completely on a gluten-free diet; another 65 percent will heal the shags but will still have inflammation-causing intestinal permeability. The likely culprits are these types of inadvertent exposures to gluten. That's what makes this topic of hidden gluten so critical for those with a sensitivity; with every exposure, you run the risk of months of elevated antibodies destroying tissue wherever your weak link is.

Last, when a product has been labeled as gluten-free, the equipment used tests only for alpha-gliadin, the most common peptide fragment of poorly digested wheat. Yet alpha-gliadin is present in only 50 percent of wheat; the rest contain other peptides that may stimulate an immune response. The term *gluten-free* is therefore a misnomer in the industry. The accurate term would be *alpha-gliadin–free,* which makes foods labeled as gluten-free more than slightly suspect.

For all of these reasons, I highly recommend that you avoid as much processed food as possible. You are always better off preparing your own foods by using ingredients as they occur in nature, like fresh vegetables, fruits, and animal proteins.

The following list contains some of the tricky ingredients people don't always know to look for. All of these ingredients are wheat in disguise.

WHEAT IN DISGUISE		
Ale	Enriched bleached wheat flour	Pasta
Atta flour	Enriched flour	Persian wheat (*Triticum carthlicum*)
Barley	Farina	Polish wheat (*Triticum polonicum*)
Barley enzymes	Farina graham	Poulard wheat (*Triticum turgidum*)
Barley flakes	Farro	Roux
Barley grass	Filler	Rusk
Barley groats	Flour (normally this is wheat)	Rye
Barley (*Hordeum vulgare*)	Fu (dried wheat gluten)	Rye flour
Barley malt	Germ	Secale
Barley malt extract	Gluten	Seitan
Barley malt flavoring	Glutenin	Self-rising flour
Barley pearls	Graham flour	Semolina
Beer	Granary flour	Shot wheat (*Triticum aestivum sphaerococcum*)
Bleached flour	Hordeum vulgare extract	Sooji
Bran	Kamut (Khorasan)	Spelt
Bread crumbs	Kluski pasta	Sprouted barley
Bread flour	Lager	Steel-ground flour
Breading	Maida (Indian wheat flour)	Stone-ground flour
Brewer's yeast	Malt	Stout
Brown flour	Malted barley flour	Strong flour
Bulgur	Malted milk	Tabbouleh/tabouli
Bulgur wheat	Malt extract	Teriyaki sauce
Cereal binding	Malt flavoring	Timopheevi wheat (*Triticum timopheevii*)
Cereal extract	Malt syrup	*Triticale x triticosecale*
Chilton	Matzah meal	*Triticum aestivam*
Couscous	Matzo	*Triticum vulgare*
Croutons	Meripro 711	*Triticum vulgare* germ oil
Edible starch	Mir	*Triticum vulgare* (wheat) flour lipids
Einkorn (*Triticum monococcum*)	Nishasta	Udon noodles
Emmer (*Triticum dicoccon*)	Oriental wheat (*Triticum turanicum*)	Unbleached flour
Enriched bleached flour	Orzo pasta	

COOKING INGREDIENTS THAT MAY CONTAIN GLUTEN

Manufacturers introduce gluten to lots of foods you ordinarily wouldn't think twice about cooking with on a gluten-free diet. These are the type of questions we get all the time. (For example, "Is vanilla extract okay?" The answer: Some brands contain gluten—you have to check.) Some of these ingredients are used in the recipes in Chapter 10, so be sure to purchase versions clearly marked as gluten-free on the label. If you have to eat or use gluten-free packaged foods, avoid those with long lists of unfamiliar ingredients, especially if they contain any of the following terms:

Avena sativa	Additionally, may have been contaminated by other grains
Baking powder	May contain wheat starch
Bicarbonate of soda	May contain wheat starch
Bouillon	May contain gluten
Broth	May contain gluten
Brown rice syrup	May contain barley
Caramel color	May be derived from highly processed wheat or barley, usually gluten-free in North America
Caramel flavoring	May contain gluten, depending on manufacturing; usually gluten-free in North America
Carob	May contain barley
Cellulose	May be derived from gluten-containing grain
Cereal	May consist of gluten-containing grain
Cider	May utilize barley in production
Citric acid	May be derived from wheat (or corn/beet sugar/ molasses)
Clarifying agents	May contain gluten-containing grain or by-product
Codex wheat starch	A highly processed wheat starch with gluten removed
Crisped rice cereals	May contain barley
Curry powder	May contain wheat starch

Dextrimaltose	A highly processed starch that can be derived from barley
Dextrin	A highly processed starch that can be derived from wheat (or other starch)
Dextrose	A highly processed starch that can be derived from wheat or barley (or other starch). Gluten source does not need to be labeled in Europe.
Edible food coatings and films	May contain wheat starch
Edible paper	May contain wheat starch
Emulsifier	May be derived from gluten-containing grain
Fat replacer	May be derived from wheat
Flavored liquors	May contain gluten
Flavoring	May be derived from gluten-containing grain
Gin	Derived from a combination of distilled grains
Glucose syrup	A highly processed sweetener that can be derived from wheat (or other starch). Is usually derived from corn in North America. Gluten source does not need to be labeled in Europe.
Grain alcohol	May be derived from distilled gluten grain
Grain-based vodka	May be derived from distilled rye or wheat
Heeng/hing	Usually mixed with wheat flour
Herbal tea	May contain gluten in flavoring, such as barley
Hydrogenated starch hydrolysate	May be derived from wheat
Hydrolyzed plant protein (HPP)	May be derived from wheat
Hydrolyzed protein	May be derived from wheat
Hydrolyzed vegetable protein (HVP)	May be derived from wheat
Hydroxypropylated starch	May be derived from wheat
Kecap/ketjap manis (similar to soy sauce)	May contain wheat
Maltodextrin	May be derived from highly processed wheat
Maltose	May be derived from barley or wheat
Malt vinegar	Derived from barley, contains only traces of gluten due to fermentation process

Miso	May be made from barley
Mixed tocopherols	Commonly derived from wheat germ (or soy)
Modified (food) starch	May be derived from highly processed wheat
Mono- and diglycerides	Wheat may be used as a carrier during processing
Monosodium glutamate (MSG)	May be derived from wheat
Mustard powder	May contain wheat starch
Natural flavoring	May be derived from gluten-containing grain
Perungayam	Usually sold mixed with wheat flour
Pregelatinized starch	May be derived from gluten-containing grain
Protein hydrolysates	May be derived from gluten-containing grain
Rice malt	May contain barley
Rice syrup	May contain barley enzymes
Sake	May be derived from distilled wheat, rye, barley
Scotch	May be made from gluten-containing grain
Seasoning	May contain wheat starch
Smoke flavoring	May contain barley
Soy sauce/shoyu	May contain wheat
Soy sauce solids	May contain wheat
Spice and herb blends	May contain wheat starch
Stabilizers/stabilizing agents	May be derived from gluten-containing grain
Starch	May contain barley
Suet	Suet from a packet contains wheat flour
Tamari	May contain wheat
Textured vegetable protein	May be derived from gluten-containing grain
Tocopherols	Commonly derived from wheat germ (or soy)
Vanilla extract	May contain grain alcohol
Vanilla flavoring	May contain grain alcohol
Vegetable gum	May be derived from gluten-containing grain
Vegetable protein	May be derived from gluten-containing grain
Vegetable starch	May be manufactured using gluten-containing grain
Whiskey	May be derived from distilled wheat, rye, barley (or corn)
Xanthan gum	May be derived from wheat
Yeast extract	May be manufactured using gluten-containing grain

HOW TO GO DAIRY-FREE

The protein structure of cow's milk is eight times the size of the proteins found in human breast milk, which is why so many people have a hard time digesting cow's milk. The protein structure of goat's milk is six times that of human breast milk.[42] It's not as bad, but it's still not easy to digest. However, some types of animal dairy may be acceptable, if you can find them. According to a 2007 study published in the *Journal of Allergy and Clinical Immunology*, if the milk of an animal has a protein structure that's more than 62 percent similar to human milk protein, that milk is more likely to be nonallergenic.[43]

These options really do exist. Some ethnic specialty stores carry good alternatives to cow's milk: camel milk,[44] reindeer milk,[45] and donkey milk.[46] I tried camel milk just recently, and I found it to be wonderful without the typical mucus-producing side effects that I get with cow's milk. It's been a long time since I've been able to have a bowl of cereal (gluten-free or not) with animal milk; camel's milk fully satisfied that craving. You can learn more at theDr.com/camelmilk.

There are also plenty of animal milk substitutes. I'm not a fan of soy milk, even in its organic form. Although there are studies that show the pros and cons of soy, there is no question of its phytoestrogen impact. These plant-based, estrogen-like molecules from soy bind on receptor sites in the body and act like a weak form of the hormone estrogen. If you have an estrogen deficiency, consuming additional soy may be a good thing. Yet if you have adequate levels of estrogen, or excess levels of estrogen, this may be a bad thing, for both men and women. What's more, the studies that show the benefits of soy come from Asian institutes, where participants ate foods made from whole soybeans.

Key nutrients are lost in the process of creating soy and other substitute milks, and sweeteners, including barley malt (which may contain gluten), are added to enhance the taste. Additionally, gums are added as stabilizers. There is strong evidence that some people with food sensitivities also create antibodies to these gums that are added to processed foods.[47] Some triggers that have been identified as making people more vulnerable to an immune reaction to the gums in foods include drinking alcohol and exercise with the simultaneous intake of medicine, including aspirin, beta-blockers, and medications for high blood pressure.[48] According to Dr. Aristo Vodjani, one of my mentors and the pioneering world expert in the immune response to foods, the most common gums, listed here in order from most to least reactive, include:

- Carrageenan
- Mastic gum
- Locust bean gum
- Xanthan gum
- Beta-glucan
- Gum tragacanth
- Guar gum

My favorite milk substitute is coconut milk, which is rich in lauric acid, a heart-healthy saturated fat that improves HDL (good) cholesterol. You can also try nut or rice milks, but as a rule of thumb, always choose the unsweetened variety. "Plain" milk substitutes actually have 6 grams (1.5 teaspoons) of added sugar per cup. Flavored varieties can have anywhere from 12 grams (3 teaspoons) to 20 grams (5 teaspoons) per cup. You can get vanilla flavor without the added sugar if you look for the "unsweetened" marker on the label.

The Food Allergen Labeling and Consumer Protection Act requires that all packaged food products that contain milk as an ingredient must list the word "milk" on the label. However, you will still need to read all product labels carefully. Milk is sometimes found in products even if they are labeled as nondairy. Many nondairy products contain casein (a milk protein that would be listed on a label), including some brands of canned tuna. And some processed meats may contain casein as a binder. Exposure to casein has been linked to migraine headaches.[49] I've seen remarkable improvements when patients with migraines go gluten- and dairy-free. Many times, these patients, who may have suffered for years, will become migraine-free inside of a month or two.

Shellfish is sometimes dipped in milk to reduce the fishy odor. Many restaurants put butter on grilled steaks to add flavor. Some medications contain milk protein, so always ask your pharmacist when filling prescriptions and discuss with your doctor before you stop taking any medications.

Most people are not sensitive to the fat molecules in dairy but rather the proteins. If you've ever had lobster or crab legs served in a restaurant, it comes with clarified butter (also called ghee). Ghee is the fats of butter with the casein protein removed, which is why it is usually okay to eat, even for someone with a dairy sensitivity (ghee is on the list of healthy fats on page 240). You can use ghee in recipes in place of butter. The exceptions are those people who already know that they have antibodies to milk butyrophilin.

Avoid foods that contain milk or any of these ingredients:

- Artificial butter flavor
- Au gratin dishes and white sauces
- Baked goods
- Butter, butter fat, butter oil, butter acid, butter ester(s)
- Buttermilk
- Cake mixes
- Caramel candies
- Casein
- Caseinates
- Casein hydrolysate
- Cereals
- Cheese
- Chewing gum
- Chocolate
- Cottage cheese
- Cream
- Curds
- Custard
- Diacetyl
- Gelato
- Half-and-half
- Ice cream
- Lactalbumin, lactalbumin phosphate
- Lactic acid starter culture and other bacterial cultures
- Lactoferrin
- Lactose
- Lactulose
- Margarine
- Milk (in all forms: condensed, derivative, dry, evaporated, goat's milk, low-fat, malted, milk fat, nonfat, powdered, protein, skimmed, solids, whole)

- Milk protein hydrolysate
- Nisin
- Nougat
- Pudding
- Recaldent
- Rennet
- Salad dressing
- Sherbet
- Sour cream, sour cream solids
- Sour milk solids
- Tagatose
- Whey
- Whey protein hydrolysate
- Yogurt

THESE INGREDIENTS SOUND LIKE MILK BUT AREN'T

These ingredients do not contain milk protein and are therefore safe to eat:

- Calcium lactate
- Calcium stearoyl lactylate
- Cocoa butter
- Cream of tartar
- Lactic acid (however, lactic acid starter culture may contain milk)
- Oleoresin
- Sodium lactate
- Sodium stearoyl lactylate

HOW TO GO SUGAR-FREE

We are a sugar-crazed society: Seventy-four percent of food products contain caloric or low-calorie sweeteners, or both. Of all packaged foods and beverages purchased in the United States in 2013, 68 percent (by proportion of calories) contained caloric sweeteners and 2 percent contained low-calorie sweeteners.[50] In my Gluten Summit online interview with Liz Lipski, PhD, academic director of nutrition and integrative health programs at Maryland University of Integrative Health, she told me that the average American is eating somewhere between 130 and 145 pounds of sugar in the form of table sugar and high-fructose corn syrup every single year. That's more than many adults weigh. When I looked into this a little deeper, I discovered that the USDA says that each American consumes an average of 152 pounds of caloric sweeteners per year, which amounts to more than two-fifths of a pound—or 52 teaspoons—per day![51]

With all of the detrimental side effects of refined sugar, and its inclusion in most of the processed foods we eat, it begins to make sense where the unbelievable increased rates of obesity and diabetes come from in our country today.

Raw sugarcane actually has health benefits ranging from protecting the liver from toxic substances to lowering cholesterol to stabilizing blood sugar.[52] Yet when we take this plant with its many antioxidants and flavonoids, and we extract just the crystalline white powder we call sugar, we lose all the protection the plant could give us.

With only a few medical exceptions, we need little sugar in our diet. The sugars we do have are supposed to come in the form that they're found in nature, called complex carbohydrates. Refined carbohydrates are the sugars that feed cancer cells. As a matter of fact, there's an entire branch of chemotherapy devoted to reducing sugar's ability to get into cancer cells. Sugar is also a scrub-brush irritant to the intestinal lining, causing a great deal of inflammation (more gasoline on the fire). Excess sugar feeds the wrong kinds of yeast in our bodies and encourages the excessive growth of bad bacteria (dysbiosis), all of which increases gut inflammation, creating the leaky gut.

You will be avoiding all sugars, including zero-calorie sweeteners, which can be just as damaging as sugar. In a 2014 study published in *Cell Metabolism,* researchers found that the artificial sweetener Splenda dramatically increases the growth of the calorie-hoarding bacteria that triggers weight gain, kills beneficial intestinal bacteria, and blocks the absorption of prescription drugs.[53]

Sugar is as difficult to remove from your diet as gluten because it's as pervasive. To avoid sugar, you have to be diligent about reading ingredient labels on packaged goods: Even spice mixes and rubs sometimes contain sugar. Every fast-food item that I've ever checked includes refined sugar as a primary ingredient—even the salt. This is just another reason why I strongly suggest you use the recipes and meal plans in Chapter 10 and focus on eating only whole foods.

Beverages are one of the biggest hidden sources of sugar. It is loaded into sodas, fruit juices, and milk substitutes, as I mentioned above, so they must be avoided. A school education program for 7- to 11-year-old children that emphasized drinking more water over fruit juice and sweetened beverages produced a 7.7 percent reduction in the number of kids overweight or obese in 1 year.[54] Diet sodas are no better because of the artificial sweeteners that alter the gut bacteria and encourage more obesity.

Alcoholic beverages are basically liquid sugar—carbohydrates that may be either derivatives of wheat (see the lists above) or sugar (like wine or rum). In a symposium on the Medical Consequences to Alcohol Ingestion organized by the National Institute on Alcohol Abuse and Alcoholism, the Office of Dietary Supplements, and the National Institute of Diabetes and Digestive and Kidney Diseases of the National Institutes of Health, the main takeaway message was that alcohol exposure can promote the growth of Gram negative bacteria in the intestine, which may increase intestinal permeability (the leaky gut). For the geeks reading this:

> Alcohol exposure can promote the growth of Gram negative bacteria in the intestine which may result in accumulation of endotoxin. In addition, alcohol metabolism by Gram negative bacteria and intestinal epithelial cells can result in accumulation of acetaldehyde, which in turn can increase intestinal permeability to endotoxin by increasing tyrosine phosphorylation of tight junction and adherens junction proteins. Alcohol-induced generation of nitric oxide may also contribute to increased permeability to endotoxin by reacting with tubulin, which may cause damage to microtubule cytoskeleton and subsequent disruption of intestinal barrier function.[55]

Why did I include this quote? Because alcohol consumption damages tubulin (the scaffolding inside every nerve cell), which generates elevated antibodies to tubulin, which is one of the biomarkers of brain inflammation. Here is an example of a gut problem contributing to brain inflammation and B4.

Alcohol, even fine wines, damages the intestines, leads to intestinal permeability (the leaky gut), and unfavorably alters gut bacteria. If you are on a leaky gut repair protocol, it is important to completely avoid alcohol while your intestinal lining is healing. I recommend that you stay off the hard stuff for the first 3 weeks so you can give your body a break. Afterward, you can experiment with some of the gluten-free wines, beers, and distilled liquors. Or you might realize that you haven't missed them all that much. Now, I'm half Italian. And my grandfather would turn over in his grave if I said no to vino. But we all have to realistically evaluate what the triggers are that take us over the edge. If you add a glass of wine per day back into your routine and you notice your "feeling good" result is reversing because of the sugar in these drinks, you have to reevaluate the importance of that glass of wine.

Registered dietician Erica Kasuli, RD, CDN, director of nutrition for the world-famous Amen Clinics, taught me to think differently about this journey of tweaking what you eat. She gave me a great line that I use with my patients: "Don't erase. Replace." Little changes can lead to big results. So if you want to do some gluten-free baking, replace sugar with raw honey, which is very different from refined honey. Raw honey contains an entire family of nutrients and compounds: It's a whole food. Local raw honey is always preferred, as it has preventive characteristics to the local pollens you may be sensitive to.

To avoid hidden sources of sugar, look for any of the following terms in ingredient lists:

- Agave syrup
- Aguamiel
- All-natural sweetener
- Aspartame
- Barbados molasses
- Barbados sugar
- Beet sugar
- Brown sugar
- Cane sugar
- Cane syrup
- Caramel
- Caramel color
- Clarified grape juice
- Concentrated fruit juice

- Confectioners' sugar
- Cornstarch
- Corn sweetener
- Corn syrup
- Dark brown sugar
- Date sugar
- Date syrup
- Dextrine
- Dextrose
- Disaccharides
- Evaporated cane juice
- Fig syrup
- Filtered honey
- Fructose
- Fruit juice concentrate
- Fruit sugar
- Fruit sweetener
- Galactose
- Glucose
- Glycerine
- Granulated sugar
- Grape sugar
- Guar gum
- Heavy syrup
- High-fructose corn syrup
- Hydrogenated glucose syrup
- Invert sugar
- Invert sugar syrup
- Jaggery
- Lactose
- Levulose
- Light brown sugar
- Light sugar
- Light syrup
- Lite sugar
- Lite syrup
- Mannitol
- Modified food starch
- Monosaccharides
- Natural syrup
- Nectars
- Polysaccharides
- Powdered sugar
- Raisin syrup
- Raw sugar
- Ribbon cane syrup
- Ribose
- Rice malt
- Rice syrup
- Saccharine
- Sorbitol
- Sorghum molasses
- Sorghum syrup
- Soy sauce
- Splenda
- Sucanat
- Sucrose
- Turbinado sugar
- White sugar
- Xylitol

Glucose, a form of sugar, is the primary source of energy for every cell in the body. Because the brain is so rich in nerve cells, or neurons, it is the most energy-demanding organ, using one-half of all the sugar energy in the body. Brain functions such as thinking, memory, and learning are closely linked to glucose levels and how efficiently the brain uses this fuel source. If there isn't enough glucose in the brain, neurotransmitters, the brain's chemical messengers, are not produced and communication between neurons breaks down. In addition, hypoglycemia, a common complication of diabetes caused by low glucose levels in the blood, can lead to loss of energy for brain function and is linked to poor attention and cognitive dysfunction.[56]

This means that a little sugar is good, but a lot gives you the exact opposite effect. Most of us have seen what happens when you give a child a candy bar: First their blood sugar goes up from the bloodstream being flooded with the sugar from the candy bar; then wait 45 minutes or so and watch as their blood sugar takes a nosedive. This is also what happens to alcoholics when they've had too many drinks. My mentor, Dr. George Goodheart, used the analogy that there are two types of drunks:

- The one who sits in the corner and is morose, nonparticipatory, and doesn't talk
- The one who is aggressive, loud-mouthed, hyperactive, even violent

Today, we call that Attention-Deficit/Hyperactivity Disorder (ADHD). This is exactly what happens to kids (and adults). Adults just have a little more self-control in public than kids (sometimes).

PROTECT YOURSELF FROM INADVERTENT FOOD EXPOSURES

Inadvertent exposures—mistakenly eating gluten, dairy, sugar, or anything else you have a sensitivity toward—can stand in the way of your success. Sadly, inadvertent exposure is the primary reason why so many people don't feel better even when they are "strictly" following a gluten-free diet. It's not that people are cheating and eating gluten-containing foods every so often. Most of my patients with food sensitivities are really trying hard to live a clean life, yet they are still suffering from symptoms because they are ingesting gluten, often without knowing it.

In order for you to heal more completely, we need to give your body extra ammunition, and the most effective way to do this that I know of is by supplementing your diet with additional digestive enzymes. Digestive enzymes are naturally produced in the pancreas and small intestine. They break down our food into nutrients so that our body can absorb them. You can also supplement with additional, specific enzymes that will more fully digest inadvertent gluten. These enzymes protect you from the effects of an inadvertent exposure to any of the top eight allergens (wheat, dairy, soy, egg, nuts, fish, hemp, pea).

Take gluten-assisting digestive enzymes before every meal to make sure no traces of poorly digested gluten leave the stomach. That includes any time you're eating a meal that contains anything other than simply prepared meats and vegetables (because gluten, dairy, or sugar is often added to soups, sauces, seasonings, dressings, etc.).

While there are many gluten digestive enzymes on the market, I wasn't happy with their results. Over the years, a number of my patients were not responding as well as they should have from taking this extra step of using enzymes. The research showed that these enzymes were working in the laboratory, but not always in clinical practice. I started looking into why this approach wasn't working completely. I found researchers who had spent 11 years working on developing an enzyme to help digest gluten more completely and quickly. We spent 2 more years collaborating, figuring out what the unknown factor was. Then it hit us.

We realized that the immune system's sentries, designed to protect you, are standing guard in the first part of the small intestine (called the duodenum) right where it connects to the stomach. This area contains dendritic cells and antigen-presenting cells (the sentries). If any poorly digested protein molecules come out of the stomach, the sentries send out an alarm message activating our defense mechanisms. The immune system response produces a great deal of inflammation in the places we absorb most of our vitamins and minerals—the first part of the small intestine. This is where celiac disease begins. This is one main reason why people with adverse reactions to food have symptoms in so many different parts of the body. The reduced absorption of vitamins and minerals will demonstrate symptoms wherever the nutrient deficiency is showing itself.

Remember, once the immune system turns itself on, it can be active for 3 to 6 months from one exposure. Realizing that the alarm gets pulled just as food comes out of the stomach, we realized that we need to make sure these foods are completely digested before they get into the small intestine. We needed to create a digestive enzyme that would produce full digestion of all eight major food sensitivity offenders within 60 to 90 minutes, before the food you eat moves out of the stomach and into the small intestine. These digestive enzymes are called E3 Advanced Plus, and they are available on my Web site at theDr.com/e3advancedplus. Every other gluten-assisting digestive enzyme on the market may work, but they take 3 to 4 hours to digest gluten, which still allows partially digested peptides to come out of the stomach, activating the sentries standing guard, and starting the entire autoimmune cascade. So all of these gluten-digesting enzymes will help farther down the intestinal tract (3 to 6 hours after taking them), but you've already activated the inflammatory cascade in the first part of the small intestine.

E3 Advanced Plus enzymes support a healthy microbiome because they contain prebiotics that support our beneficial bacteria. This creates a balanced environment specifically in your small intestine, which is very difficult to do with any supplements. They also contain specially selected probiotics that have the dual result of reinoculation and will also assist in digesting gluten.

You can achieve a similar result by including varied fermented vegetables and prebiotics in your diet daily.

STOPPING LEAKY GUT AND LEAKY BRAIN IN YOUR MOUTH

The main bacterium that causes gum disease, *Porphyromonas gingivalis*, releases an extremely potent toxin that disrupts gut flora and has been shown to cause leaky gut. These bacteria can cause a little permeability in the mouth, allowing the bacteria to move from the mouth into the bloodstream.

One simple thing you can do to ensure that you have healthy flora in your mouth, in addition to brushing and flossing your teeth, is to swish around a little bit of coconut oil in your mouth every day. Some studies say swish for 10 minutes; some doctors recommend 30 minutes. I'm personally happy to get in 1 minute, believing that some is better than none. This is referred to as oil pulling. In one 30-day study using coconut oil swished in the mouth, a statistically significant reduction in plaque and an improvement in the health of the gingiva (the gums) was noticed after 7 days, and these two markers kept improving as the study went on.[57] Oil swishing or oil pulling will reduce bacteria and viruses in the mouth that shouldn't be there.[58]

I keep a small amount of coconut oil in a container in my shower, and I swish around about a teaspoon in my mouth and then spit it out. At first, the taste and the consistency are a little hard to get used to. Now I look forward to it because my mouth feels so fresh afterward.

NUTRIENTS THAT ATTACK INFLAMMATION AND HEAL AND SEAL THE GUT AND B4

To address an excessive inflammatory response, you need to modulate your inflammatory genetic expression by turning off as many genes as you can that are inflammatory activators, and turning on as many genes as you can that are anti-inflammatory activators. The safest strategy to modulate your genetic expression with the fewest side effects and long-term problems is twofold: First and most important, eat the highest-quality food, preferably organic. Second, supplement your diet with the right nutrients.

Natural vitamin and mineral anti-inflammatories are nowhere near as powerful or dangerous as pharmaceutical anti-inflammatories. It's not even on the same scale. It's David and Goliath, bicycles to Ferarris, rowboats to speed boats—you get the picture. Natural anti-inflammatory substances in the form of vitamins, antioxidants, polyphenols, and nutrient supplements—like epigallocatechin gallate (EGCG), the most powerful antioxidant polyphenol, which is found mostly in green tea, or lycopene in tomatoes, or the curcumin in turmeric, or vitamin C—activate some of the 1,100 genes associated with the inflammatory cascade by either dimming the inflammatory genes or activating the anti-inflammatory genes. They do not shut down the gene activity as completely as pharmaceuticals do. Pharmaceuticals work like an on/off switch, shutting down all inflammatory genes. That's not such a good idea, because inflammation is the way our "armed forces" protect us. It's *excess* inflammation that is the problem. When you shut down the entire inflammatory mechanism, that's when you may experience some of the side effects related to pharmaceutical anti-inflammatories, like autoimmune diseases, depression, anxiety, or even cancer. We need some inflammatory response capability to deal with all of the chemical assaults we're exposed to every day. Even though they're much weaker, natural anti-inflammatories are a critical part of a more effective strategy. It's another example of my *pleiotropic* approach that uses many safe, natural substances that activate multiple genes and provide multiple benefits to produce an anti-inflammatory effect.

Here's an example: Green tea has been shown to modulate genes to heal intestinal permeability and to protect from the damage of powerful pharmaceuticals that shut down TNF production (a powerful anti-inflammatory). And it's been shown to protect the elasticity of your blood vessels. Green tea can protect our thinking capabilities, as it is known to have a "neuroprotective action." One of the ways it does that is by reducing the formation of both beta-amyloid plaques in Alzheimer's disease and alpha-synuclein fibrils in Parkinson's disease.[59, 60, 61, 62] Green tea, and its active polyphenol, EGCG, is a beneficial food/nutrient because it modulates so many genes to produce an anti-inflammatory effect.

Is green tea *the* answer to all of our health concerns? Of course not. But is it a valuable contributor to a pleiotropic program? Of course it is. We do know that it activates many genes for an anti-inflammatory net effect. I have been trying to drink a little green tea every day. It's a base hit.

There are naysayers who focus on the facts that the supplement market is an unregulated field, and that some products do not contain what they say they do or the amounts they claim on the label. These complaints are valid. There are crooks in every discipline who will try to squeeze a profit any way they can. That's why you want to turn to trusted sources for your supplements. After reading hundreds of studies showing the benefits of nutrients influencing the genes of inflammation and healing, I have identified 22 different anti-inflammatory nutrients that work together synergistically to lower inflammation and restore the intestinal lining. I have taught this nutrient model to many doctors, who have used it with more than 10,000 patients. There are no side effects to this approach that I'm aware of.

The Gluten Sensitivity Support Packs™ are a powerful combination of six pills that contain these 22 different nutrients. My formula promotes the creation of healthy tissue in the intestines, the skin, the brain, the joints, the entire digestive system, and nearly every other organ system in the body, and it does not contain any wheat or gluten. You can find these supplements on my Web site at theDr.com/GSSP, or create your own support pack using the information provided below.

There are no contraindications for people who are currently taking prescription medications. I recommend taking the GS Packs (one pack per day) for a minimum of 6 months and then retesting through the bloodwork described in Chapter 5 to confirm if the abnormal biomarkers have returned to normal.

I also recommend colostrum—Mother Nature's cure for a leaky gut. At childbirth, the first 3 to 5 days' worth of breast milk is not milk at all—it's colostrum. Colostrum is produced by the mammary glands of all mammals during the birthing process. Colostrum contains antibodies newborns need to be protected against disease. Colostrum modulates genes like no other substance on the planet does, and we now know that it is the best remedy for all-around gut health. It contains growth factors and hormones designed to close the tight junctions for newborn babies (who are all permeable in utero). In adults, it turns the same genes on to help repair damage to the intestinal lining, restore gut integrity, close the tight junctions, and serve as a primary modulator of inflammatory genes in the gut. It also promotes recolonization of the bowel with good bacteria.

Roughly one-quarter of the total solids in colostrum are antibodies (IgG, IgE, IgA, IgD), which newborns need to colonize their microbiome. The IgGs in colostrum provide a baby with immediate protection from bugs, bacteria, viruses, mold, fungus, and parasites. For adults, colostrum will also provide protection from these same invaders. It also activates the genes that repair the microvilli so that you can regrow the shags that have been worn down if you have celiac disease. As Andrew Keech, PhD, a world-renowned authority on colostrum, said on my Gluten Summit, "There are many one-note players on the health food store shelves that can help heal damaged intestines; only colostrum plays the entire symphony."

We can supplement with colostrum from cows to help heal our guts. The peptides of colostrum are identical between cows and humans. In fact, the immunological part of the colostrum—these peptides—is exactly the same in every mammal. However, there is a difference in the quality of colostrums on the market. The product I endorse on my Web site is exactly the same product licensed by six governments in Africa as the first treatment of choice for HIV. That's how beneficial colostrum can be. Look for colostrum made by grass-fed cows that haven't been given antibiotics or bovine growth hormone. For most adults, one scoop per day of the powder is the recommended dosage. You can learn more at theDr.com/colostrum.

Even though colostrum can be considered a dairy product, it is typically very low in allergenic proteins and is extremely low in casein. However, if you have a dairy sensitivity, speak with your doctor before taking this supplement. Together, you can determine whether or not it's a good idea to try the colostrum and see if you notice any symptoms.

Whenever I discover a patient who has a true dairy sensitivity, I will suggest trying the colostrum for at least 2 months because it will turn on more genes to reduce inflammation and heal the intestines than anything else I could recommend. At the same time, I have the patient take all other dairy out of the diet. If you try this and find that you are having any symptoms of gas, bloating, abdominal pain, etc., then discontinue the colostrum. Clinically, I have found that 7 or 8 out of 10 patients with a dairy sensitivity will thrive on this protocol.

Other nutrients that play a major role in creating a healthy intestinal environment include:

Vitamin D: Vitamin D is exceptional for healing intestinal permeability because it supervises the function of the tight junctions, the spaces between the cells in your gut that could allow large, undigested molecules to pass into the bloodstream. The protein family called zonulin that holds our cells tightly together in the gut works like shoelaces that are supposed to be tied tightly most of the time. The usual mechanism is that the shoelaces loosen a little to let small molecules slide down between the cells to be screened and cleared by our immune system before being allowed into the bloodstream. This is how we're supposed to absorb the vitamins and minerals from our food. However, when the shoelaces are untied, larger food particles slide through the tight junctions into our bloodstream.

Vitamin D plays a critical role in the tying and untying of the intestinal shoelaces. Without enough vitamin D, the laces won't tie tightly. That's one reason why so many autoimmune diseases are much more prevalent in countries far from the equator—people in those areas have less exposure to the sun, and thus their bodies make less vitamin D.

Vitamin D is also the fuel for many different families of good bacteria in your gut. In fact, there are hundreds of benefits to vitamin D. Remember the receptor sites that act like a catcher's mitt? We've discussed how hormones traveling through the bloodstream are attracted to their own hormone receptor site. Testosterone will not enter a thyroid receptor site, insulin will not enter an estrogen receptor site, and so on. There are only two substances for which there are receptor sites on every cell of your body. That means that every cell of your body needs these two substances. One of them is thyroid hormone because that is the thermostat that controls the temperature and metabolic activity of every cell. The other receptor site is vitamin D. You want to take extra vitamin D every day because every cell in your body needs it.

The sun converts hormones in your skin made of LDL cholesterol. Many people think that LDL is the bad cholesterol, but this is not true. Excessive amounts of the wrong type of LDL can be bad, but the cholesterol in our skin gets converted into vitamin D by the sun.

The recommendation by experts is to spend about 15 minutes in the sun every day, around noon when the sun is the hottest. Get the sun on your arms and legs, and that is all you need. No reason to turn red—rather, consistent minor exposure will build up your vitamin D levels. There's one blood test that everyone should do every year, and that is the test for vitamin D. You want to do it in the spring because you will be coming out of winter, when you had the lowest amount of sunlight. This will help you determine how your body handled the lower amount of sunlight in the winter and help you find out if your levels are deficient. Remember, without vitamin D, our cells don't function. If you don't have enough vitamin D, it might affect your brain, or create intestinal permeability, or challenge your liver or your kidneys. Any cell of your body can manifest poor function because of inadequate vitamin D.

Glutamine: The gastrointestinal tract is by far the greatest user of the amino acid glutamine in the body; the epithelial cells that form the lining of the gut use glutamine as their principal metabolic fuel. Glutamine is known to help shield damaged intestines and turn on a number of genes that allow the gut to heal.

However, if you have a history of yeast infections, you will need to carefully monitor the amount of glutamine you are taking, because this amino acid may increase yeast growth. Glutamine is also a raw material for the immune cells that produce a healthy amount of inflammation in our intestines. But if you are already inflamed, glutamine may increase the inflammation (rarely, but it can happen). That is why, I always tell my patients, if you don't feel well taking the GS Packs, take the glutamine out for a couple of weeks, keep taking everything else to turn on genes and produce the anti-inflammatory effect, and after a few weeks, reintroduce the glutamine.

Fish oils: Fish oils are remarkably useful because they contain omega-3 fatty acids that turn on or off many genes to produce an anti-inflammatory effect. Fish oils are also known to reduce your risk of cardiovascular disease (mainly stroke and acute myocardial infarction), lower high blood pressure, and enhance brain function.

The primary ingredients in fish oils are eicosapentaenoic acid (EPA) and docosahexaenoic acid (DHA). EPA has anti-inflammatory properties: It can turn on the genes for anti-inflammation in the gut and turn off other inflammatory genes. DHA plays a major role in fetal brain development and the retina of the eye during the first 2 years of life. About 35 percent of the walls of your brain cells are made of omega-3 fats. If there is not enough of these good fats available to make good strong brain cells, the body will use whatever raw material it can find to use as a fat resource. If you eat French fries, or deep-fried foods, the body will use that as the raw material for your brain cells. However, those fats are much thicker and gooier, and they don't allow for easy transmembrane passage.

Your brain cells communicate with one another by sending chemical messengers produced in one brain cell right through the walls of the brain cell into the neighboring brain cell. But if your diet is full of the wrong kinds of fats, the message can't transfer seamlessly from one brain cell to another. That is why when you supplement with fish oils rich in omega-3s, you can raise a child's IQ by more than three points (that's substantial). Your brain will push out the bad fats in the cell walls and replace them with the good fats, and your brain starts working better.

Omega-3s can be acquired only through diet, as the body cannot produce them. Fish have high omega-3 values, but because so many are not safe to eat, high-quality fish oil supplements (tested for heavy metals and chemical contaminants) provide a perfect way to get these essential nutrients. Therapeutic dosages up to 3 grams for adults have been shown to be remarkably effective and safe.

Probiotics: Probiotic supplementation supports the microbiome in the same way that fermented foods do: They introduce beneficial bacteria. Thirty years ago, we knew it was important to give probiotics to our patients, but we were all working with limited scientific data. The best recommendation we could give was to "take some probiotics, the more the better." Today we know there are thousands of different strains of good bacteria in the microbiome that can positively react with probiotics, yet there are currently still many unanswered questions about what happens if you give a large amount of one or two types. Until we know more, it seems rational to take a moderate dosage of a number of different probiotics rather than a larger dose of one or two.

This is one of the reasons why I strongly suggest that you get your probiotics from whole fermented foods rather than supplements. Try to vary the fermented vegetables, because each vegetable can host different cultures and families of good bacteria.

I also recommend taking a mixed probiotic capsule along with your fermented vegetables. The families of bacteria I look for in a probiotic supplement include *Lactobacillus, Bifidobacterium* (they're the most common), *Bacillus subtilis* (which will increase the *Bifidobacterium* count by more than 500 percent), and *Saccharomyces boulardii*.

Adaptogens: One day in the spring of 2012, my sister called and said, "It's time." Our mother had been suffering from sepsis and now had been in a coma for 8 days, unresponsive to any stimuli. So I quickly threw some things in a bag, booked the next flight, and was on my way home to disconnect our mother from the IVs and monitoring devices.

I arrived at my sister's home at 2:00 a.m. Everyone was asleep, so I went into our mother's room, and there she was in the hospital bed, curled in a fetal position, eyes half-open, just looking miserable. I gave her a kiss and said, "Hi, Mom, I'm here." No response whatsoever.

I went to the guest room to go to sleep. When I opened my bag, there on the top was the bottle of the adaptogenic herb concentrate I had just begun taking a few weeks before. I had been impressed with my results after beginning these herbs—my energy was noticeably better. Something came over me and I said, "Why not?" I went back to my mother's room, tilted her head, and squirted a couple of drops of this herbal concentrate in her mouth. I went to sleep, but I woke up 2 hours later and gave her a few more squirts.

"What's that?" my sister asked when she saw me squirting the concentrate early the next morning.

"A new product I'm trying that is pretty impressive for energy. I thought I'd give some to Mom."

"Can't hurt," she responded.

Hospice came every morning at 8:00 a.m. to sit with Mother, bathe her, and play Frank Sinatra albums (we thought she'd like that). We left her in good care and came back about 4 hours later. We walked in the door, and there was our mother in a wheelchair.

"Hi-i-i-i, Te tommm."

There were no words for how we felt. My sister started crying, and I stared in disbelief and finally said what every good doctor in that situation would say: "Give her 3 ounces four times per day!"

I knew immediately what had happened, but I didn't think that it was possible. The herbs in this adaptogenic formula had turned on the genes in my mother's gut and brain to reduce inflammation and activate awareness—the dimmer switch was turned up, so the lights were brighter. Our mother was back from the brink. She lived another 6 weeks on the herbs from Sun Horse Energy. She had no pain and was wheeled into the kitchen to sit at the table for every meal. She engaged to some degree in the conversations, smiling at the jokes, and even got upset one time and barked!

As a direct result of this experience, when I got back to California, I found the formulator of this product and told him what happened. His jaw dropped. He had never heard of such a thing. I believe so much in this product that today I am the medical director of the company that produces it.

The term *adaptogen* was coined by the Russian scientist Dr. Nikolai Lazarev in the late 1940s following research done on eleuthero root. In 1968, Israel I. Brekhman, PhD, and Dr. I. V. Dardymov formally defined adaptogens as plants with three characteristics:

- Adaptogens are nontoxic: They can be safely taken for extended periods of time.
- Adaptogens produce a nonspecific biological response that improves the body's ability to resist multiple forms of stress, including

physical, chemical, and biological stressors. That means they are not "target-specific" like drugs, but beneficially impact the entire body.

- Adaptogens have a normalizing influence, meaning that no matter in which direction the stressors are throwing the body out of balance, adaptogens help to bring the system back into balance. If the system is functioning too high (i.e., anxiety), they calm us down. If the system is functioning too low (i.e., depression), they turn the lights on to brighten us up.

A 2017 study on adaptogens in the *Annals of the New York Academy of Sciences* uses this definition: "Adaptogens are stress-response modifiers that increase an organism's nonspecific resistance to stress by increasing its ability to adapt and survive."[63] Sounded pretty good to me. And in the last 4 years, I have seen so many unbelievable results with these adaptogens that I am now a firm believer of the indispensable role they can play in bringing us back to health. The product we launched at the Institute for Functional Medicine's Annual Conference is called Fog Cutter. And it is remarkable in helping the brain adapt to and survive the stresses you are facing. It comprises the following adaptogenic ingredients; see what the science has shown about each of them:

- Bacopa: Nine studies confirm 11.2 to 17.9 percent improved cognition and 9 to 12 percent faster reaction time in subjects taking a bacopa extract.[64] Another study showed advanced word recall and memory scores in the aged who took a bacopa extract.[65] It has also been shown to increase oxygen to the brain, reduce oxidative stress, and reduce stress hormone levels and nerve degeneration.[66]
- *Ganoderma lucidum:* This mushroom protects the hippocampus (memory center) when exposed to toxins, protects the neurons from dying due to inflammation, and improves cognition.[67]
- Ashwagandha: In a study of adults with mild cognitive impairment (MCI), 8 weeks of taking ashwagandha demonstrated "significant improvements in immediate and general memory, executive func-

tion, sustained attention, and information-processing speed."[68] A second study demonstrated ashwagandha's ability "to restore the levels of brain-derived neurotrophic factor" (that's BDNF, which you learned about in Chapter 8; it's a critically important hormone for brain vitality and cell growth), "as well as the expression of other synaptic regulators, which are highly implicated in synaptic plasticity" (meaning very important in our brain's ability to adapt and thrive).[69] In a third study of adult men taking ashwagandha for 2 weeks, scientists noted that "significant improvements were observed in reaction times with simple reaction, choice discrimination, digit symbol substitution, digit vigilance, and card sorting tests."

- Tulsi (Holy Basil): After reviewing all 24 studies on 1,111 humans for this herb, the researchers concluded: "All studies reported favorable clinical outcomes, with no studies reporting any significant adverse events. The reviewed studies reinforce traditional uses and suggest tulsi is an effective treatment for lifestyle-related chronic diseases, including diabetes, metabolic syndrome, and psychological stress." Brain improvements included cognitive flexibility and attention, improved working memory after day 15, reduction in stress-related symptoms, *significantly* lowered biological age score (getting younger-functioning cells), and decreased anxiety, stress, and depression.[70]

- *Cordyceps sinensis:* The herb protects the brain from the injuries of toxic assault (from chemicals, foods, etc.).

- *Centella asiatica:* It's known to revitalize the brain and nervous system, and increase attention span and concentration. A study demonstrated the protective effects of CA against beta-amyloid neurotoxicity (the plaque in Alzheimer's).[71]

- *Scutellaria baicalensis:* The authors of one study concluded: "These results confirm Scutellaria's anti-inflammatory effects and might be used to protect cells against beta-amyloid plaque."[72]

There are literally hundreds more studies on the 17 ingredients in Fog Cutter. To learn more about it, and as a way of saying "thank you" for purchasing this book, feel free to go to theDr.com/FogCutter and watch the video where I explain this product in much more detail. And you'll also receive a special thank-you gift.

READ SUPPLEMENT AND MEDICATION LABELS: AVOID PROBLEMATIC INGREDIENTS

Inside supplements, and even medicines, can be small, hidden exposures to gluten, dairy, or sugar. As with everything you put in your mouth, read labels carefully and look for clues that signal gluten contamination; current labeling regulations do not require gluten to be labeled in vitamins or medications. While supplements and medications are usually gluten-free, gluten can be added as a binding agent or other inactive ingredient. Often, glutens are the starches used to absorb water in the pills so they have a longer shelf life. When a product contains the word "starch," the source needs to be identified. The primary offender is maltodextrin, a starch that is typically derived from corn but can also be extracted from wheat, potato, or rice.

Tablets and capsules are the most likely potential sources of gluten contamination, as they often contain excipients, absorbents, protectants, binders, coloring agents, lubricators, and bulking agents that may contain gluten. Each of these additives can be made from synthetic materials or natural sources that are derived from plants or animals. While they are considered inactive and safe for human use by the FDA, they can still be a potential source of contamination.

Mannitol and xylitol are considered safe. These are sugar alcohols that are refined to the point where they're no problem for most people, even though some of them may be derived from wheat. Other safe additives that you might find in medication are titanium dioxide, lactose (unless you have a lactose sensitivity), gelatin, dextrin, and magnesium stearate.

A good rule of thumb is to always ask your pharmacist to make sure whatever prescription you are filling is gluten-free. A pharmacist will be able to review the patient package insert and let you know what's included in the medicine, or they can give you the paperwork so you can read the ingredients. They can also go online and check for you, or teach you how to contact the pharmaceutical manufacturer.

Unfortunately, it's not as easy to find the hidden sources of gluten with supplements. Although there are some health food store employees who are brilliant at what they do, the majority have no formal training in the composition of and additives to nutritional products. If you are lucky enough to have a health-care practitioner who recommends nutritional supplements to you, they will be able to answer your questions as a pharmacist would. And if they do not know the answer to the question about ingredients, they have the channels to find out. You can be assured that any products I recommend have been vetted more than once to make sure they're safe.

Treat every refill of a nutritional supplement or medication as if it's a brand-new product for you. First, companies often change their formulations, and generics do not have to be exact duplicates of brand-name medicines when it comes to the inactive ingredients. The same is true for over-the-counter medications. Read all labels carefully and avoid the following ingredients:

- Alcohol
- Alpha tocopherol
- Alpha tocotrienols
- Avena
- Avena sativa
- Barley
- Barley beta glucans
- Barley bran
- Barley grass
- Barley leaf
- Barley powder
- Beta glucans
- Beta glycans
- Beta tocopherol
- Beta tocotrienol
- Brewer's yeast
- Caramel color
- Cereal fiber
- Cernilton (rye grass)
- Citric acid
- Cross-linked starch
- D-alpha-tocopherol
- D-beta-tocopherol
- Delta tocotrienol
- Dextrate
- Dextrimaltose

- Dextrin (if source is not specified; the source is usually corn or potato, which is acceptable, but wheat is sometimes used)
- D-gamma-tocopherol
- Dietary fiber
- Gamma tocopherol
- Gamma tocotrienols
- *Hordeum distichon*
- *Hordeum vulgare*
- Maltodextrin
- Maltose
- Mixed tocopherols
- Mixed tocotrienols
- Modified starch
- Oat beta glucan
- Oat bran
- Oat extract
- Oat fiber
- Oat grass
- Pregelatinized modified starch
- Pregelatinized starch
- Rye grass
- Rye grass pollen extract
- *Secale cereale*
- Sodium starch glycolate
- Starch
- Tocopherol
- Tocopherol acetate
- Tocopheryl succinate
- *Triticum aestivum*
- Vitamin E
- Wheat bran
- Wheat germ extract
- Wheat germ oil
- Wheatgrass
- Wheat protein
- Wheat starch
- Wild oats
- Xanthan gum
- Yeast

ACTION STEP WEEK 9: PUT FOOD RECOMMENDATIONS ALL TOGETHER

This week, start working on your biochemistry. One of the most far-reaching, impactful changes we can make to our Pyramid of Health is to realize that what is on the end of our forks is the most common environmental trigger of inflammation we are exposed to. If you could address only one aspect of your health, the most effective would be to address your biochemistry, simply by avoiding foods that harm you and introducing foods that help you. As you begin to eliminate the foods that your body is sensitive to, you stop fueling the autoimmune inflammatory fire.

This side of the pyramid is about regenerating a healthier-functioning brain. In order to do that, we *must* do a few things:

- Stop throwing gasoline on the fire by avoiding gluten, dairy, and sugar.
- Get accumulated toxins out by choosing local and organic food whenever possible.
- Turn genes off to calm down the inflammatory cascade with supplements containing powerful antioxidants and polyphenols such as colostrum, fish oils, vitamin D, and green tea.
- Turn genes on to rebuild stronger, more vibrant, more resilient cells with adaptogenic herbs.

10

THE FIX YOUR BRAIN RECIPES

I'M A "PRETTY GOOD" COOK. Not great, but pretty good. It would be silly of me to think I know all of the great recipes to give you a wide variety to choose from and see which ones you and your family will like. So I sent out a request to many of my colleagues in the world of health, heath care, and education: "Send me one of each of your favorite breakfast, lunch, and dinner recipes, and I'll put them in my book and give you the credit." I explained that they need to fit these criteria:

- Easy to make
- Gluten-, dairy-, and sugar-free
- Family friendly (all members of a family will like it)
- Support the brain and brain function

Here they are. I've tried many of them, and they're fabulous. I hope you find a few that are "wins" for you and your family. Remember, these are not ordinary recipes, and they don't come from ordinary people. Two of the contributors, Dr. Stephen Masley and Lisa Stimmer, are also real chefs. The rest of the contributors are world experts in the field of health care who over the years have developed these recipes, targeting healthier brain function. I hope these recipes tickle your taste buds as they fuel your immune system and stimulate the rebuilding of healthier brain cells.

To find out more about the individual contributors, see the appendix for their bios. Enjoy!

BREAKFAST

BREAKFAST QUINOA

BY TREVOR CATES

SERVES 1–2

> 2 teaspoons coconut oil
> ½ apple, unpeeled, sliced or diced into small pieces
> ½ cup cooked quinoa
> 2 tablespoons pumpkin seeds
> 1 tablespoon coconut shavings
> Dash of ground cinnamon
> Dash of stevia powder

1. In a saucepan, heat the oil. Add the apple, coat with the oil, and heat until warm.

2. Add the quinoa, pumpkin seeds, coconut, cinnamon, and stevia. Stir and warm in the saucepan over low heat. Serve warm.

BRAIN BENEFITS
Pumpkin seeds may ease depression, because the seeds contain L-tryptophan, which raises levels of the mood-modulating brain chemical serotonin.[1]

PUMPKIN WALNUT CRUNCH PARFAIT

BY ALAN CHRISTIANSON

SERVES 2

¼ cup canned pumpkin
½ small organic pear, chopped
¾ cup unsweetened coconut yogurt
1 tablespoon chopped walnuts
1 teaspoon honey

In a bowl mix all the ingredients. Serve chilled.

BRAIN BENEFITS

There's a reason why **walnuts** are shaped like your brain. They are a good source of omega-3 fatty acids, which is essential to brain health. Walnuts also increase the diversity of the beneficial bacteria in the gut, which then increases the production of the necessary brain chemicals that originate in the gut, such as serotonin.

Pumpkin is one of the well-known gourds that has substantial medicinal properties. The dark orange color of its flesh contains health-promoting antioxidants. The flesh is thought to be anti-inflammatory.[2]

E3 ENERGY EVOLVED
CHOCOLATE CHIP PANCAKES

BY HEATHER AND DAMIAN DUBE

SERVES 2

1 cup flax meal
1 teaspoon raw cacao powder
2 scoops e3ee Approved Chocolate Non-Denatured Whey Protein
   Concentrate
2 eggs
½ cup organic lite coconut milk
⅛ teaspoon raw sea salt
2 tablespoons raw unsweetened cacao nibs
1 ounce walnuts, chopped
½ cup frozen organic blueberries
Organic unrefined coconut oil
Coconut Secret Coconut Nectar (optional)

1. Preheat an 8″ cast-iron or stainless-steel skillet on medium for 3 to 5 minutes.

2. In a bowl, combine the flax meal, cacao, and protein. Stir with a fork until combined.

3. Add the eggs and coconut milk and stir until fully mixed and no clumps are present. Stir in the sea salt, cacao nibs, walnuts, and blueberries.

4. Coat the heated skillet with the coconut oil. Using a soup ladle, add a ladle-full of batter to the skillet. Cook for 3 to 4 minutes, then flip with a spatula. (Cook times may vary.) Transfer the cooked pancake to a separate dish.

5. Repeat step 4 until all the batter is used. Top with the coconut nectar, if desired.

BRAIN BENEFITS
Whey protein decreases oxidative stress and increases mitochondrial activity in the brain.[3]

SALMON AND CAPER OMELET

BY SHANNON GARRETT

SERVES 2

    4 pasture-raised eggs
    2 tablespoons full-fat coconut milk
    Black pepper
    ½ cup flaked wild-caught salmon
    1 tablespoon capers, drained and rinsed
    2 teaspoons minced fresh dill
    ¼ cup plain Greek-style coconut yogurt
    2 tablespoons ghee
    1 avocado, sliced

1. Whisk the eggs, coconut milk, and pepper in a bowl and set aside.

2. In a separate bowl, combine the salmon, capers, dill, and yogurt and set aside.

3. In a skillet, melt the ghee over medium-high heat. When bubbly, add the egg mixture and reduce the heat to medium-low. When the eggs are set, add the salmon filling to the center and gently fold in half into an omelet. Cook a few minutes longer until the center is done. Serve immediately and enjoy. Garnish with the avocado.

BRAIN BENEFITS

Salmon is a rich source of anti-inflammatory omega-3 fats, which are essential for good brain health.

NOVA LOX BREAKFAST SALAD

BY RANDY HARTNELL

SERVES 2

- 1½ tablespoons organic extra-virgin olive oil
- ½ tablespoon fresh lemon juice
- ½ teaspoon Dijon mustard
- Salt and pepper
- 2–3 large handfuls of kale salad mix (or similar blend of healthy salad greens)
- ½ English cucumber, peeled if desired and thinly sliced in half-moons
- ½ avocado, thinly sliced
- 4 ounces Vital Choice Sockeye Nova Lox, thawed and cut into ribbons
- 2 organic eggs

1. In a large salad bowl, whisk together the oil, lemon juice, mustard, and salt and pepper to taste. Add the kale mix (or other hardy greens) and toss to combine. (With a hardy green such as kale, it's fine to dress it in advance and let it rest while the eggs cook.)

2. Divide the dressed kale mix between 2 large plates and top with the cucumber and avocado slices. Top each salad with half of the lox slices and set aside.

3. Add the eggs to a small saucepan and cover with water. Bring the water to a boil, then reduce the heat to just below a simmer. Cook for 6 to 10 minutes, depending on your preference. (I cook mine to somewhere between medium and hard-boiled.) Place the eggs in an ice bath for 2 to 4 minutes, then carefully peel.

4. Halve each egg and add it to a salad. Enjoy right away while the eggs are still warm.

BRAIN BENEFITS

Kale is a leafy green high in the antioxidants lutein and zeaxanthin, which are thought to improve visual and cognitive function throughout the lifespan. These plant-based nutrients have anti-inflammatory properties, can improve brain structure and development (particularly in children), and may be protective against eye disease. In adults, a higher amount of lutein in the diet is related to better cognitive performance.[4]

BLUEBERRY CHIA PORRIDGE

BY OCEAN ROBBINS

SERVES 2–4

½ cup chia seeds
2 cups cold organic or non-GMO-certified soy, almond, or rice milk
2 tablespoons maple syrup
1 teaspoon vanilla extract
2 cups fresh or frozen blueberries

1. Place the chia seeds in a pitcher and pour in the milk. Stir until all the seeds are fully immersed in the liquid. Place in the refrigerator and let soak for 8 hours or overnight.

2. Remove the pitcher from the refrigerator and stir in the maple syrup, vanilla, and blueberries. Pour into bowls or mugs.

BRAIN BENEFITS

Chia seeds are known to be high in omega-3 fatty acids. This important nutrient must be acquired through diet because the body cannot produce it on its own. Omega-3s turn on the genes that lower inflammation in the gut and in the brain.

Blueberries contain dietary flavonoids that are thought to protect the brain in many ways, including the potential to protect neurons against injury induced by neurotoxins, an ability to suppress brain inflammation, and the potential to promote memory, learning, and cognitive function. Therefore, the consumption of flavonoid-rich foods throughout life holds a potential to limit the neurodegeneration associated with a variety of neurological disorders and to prevent or reverse normal or abnormal deteriorations in cognitive performance.[5]

CAULIFLOWER HUMMUS AND CHICKEN BREAKFAST BURRITOS

BY ELAINE DE SANTOS

SERVES 4

1 large head cauliflower, cut into florets and steamed
1 teaspoon grated lemon zest (use a microplane to make zesting super easy)
½ teaspoon garlic powder
½ teaspoon ground cumin
2 tablespoons coconut oil, divided
Sea salt and freshly ground black pepper
2 boneless, skinless chicken breasts, cut into cubes
4 large green leaf lettuce leaves
¼ cup chopped fresh cilantro

1. In a food processor, place the cauliflower, zest, garlic powder, cumin, 1 tablespoon of the oil, and salt and pepper to taste. Pulse until smooth.

2. In a medium skillet over medium heat, heat the remaining 1 tablespoon of oil. Add the chicken and season with salt and pepper to taste. Cook for 10 minutes, or until cooked through.

3. In the lettuce leaves, layer the cauliflower hummus, chicken, and cilantro. Roll up the lettuce leaves and serve.

BRAIN BENEFITS
Cauliflower is known to maintain brain health and promote communication between nerve cells.

CHICKEN AND ZUCCHINI GRATIN

BY ELAINE DE SANTOS

SERVES 4

1 pound bacon, chopped
2 large boneless, skinless chicken breasts, cubed
1 medium shallot, sliced thin
2 cloves garlic, minced
2 cups frozen spinach, thawed and the liquid squeezed out, or 6 cups fresh spinach
1 cup canned full-fat coconut milk

1 tablespoon coconut oil
2 medium zucchinis, grated
Pinch of fresh grated nutmeg
Sea salt and freshly ground black pepper

1. Preheat the oven to 425 degrees.

2. In a large skillet over medium heat, add the bacon, chicken, and shallot. Cook for 5 to 10 minutes, or until the bacon is crispy, the chicken is browned, and the shallot is tender. Stir in the spinach, cover, and set aside.

3. In a large bowl, mix together the milk, oil, zucchini, nutmeg, and salt and pepper to taste. In a large baking dish, layer half of the zucchini mixture and then all of the bacon mixture. Top with the remaining zucchini mixture and place in the oven. Bake for 35 minutes, or until the zucchini is tender, the chicken is cooked through, and the mixture is bubbling.

4. Let rest for at least 15 minutes, then slice and serve warm. Enjoy!

BRAIN BENEFITS
Coconut oil is a healthy medium-chain triglyceride (MCT) oil, which supplies easily accessible fuel to the powerhouse furnaces in every brain cell called mitochondria.

5-MINUTE GLUTEN-FREE, DAIRY-FREE PALEO ENGLISH MUFFINS

BY LISA STIMMER

SERVES 2

1 egg or 2 egg whites (for a less eggy flavor)
1 tablespoon oil (melted coconut, almond, avocado, or grapeseed) or ghee, melted
1 tablespoon real maple syrup or agave nectar
2 tablespoons water
½ teaspoon vanilla extract
¼ teaspoon sea salt
3 tablespoons almond flour*
1 tablespoon coconut flour or almond flour
1 tablespoon psyllium husk powder or flakes
¼ teaspoon baking powder
Pinch of ground cinnamon (optional)

1. Whisk together the egg, oil or ghee, syrup or nectar, water, vanilla, and sea salt in a mixing bowl.

2. Add the flours, psyllium, and baking powder. Whisk until fully incorporated.

3. Transfer the mixture into 2 greased microwavable 3"-round ramekins. Microwave for 3 minutes on high. Remove from the ramekins, slice the muffins in half, and toast for 2 minutes.

*For a nut-free option, replace the almond flour with 3 tablespoons more coconut flour.

Note: Another option is cinnamon raisin English muffins. Just add ¼ teaspoon ground cinnamon and 2 tablespoons raisins or Craisins to the recipe.

BRAIN BENEFITS

Eggs contain choline, which is required to make the essential components for all membranes and plays an important role in brain and memory development.[6]

ARTICHOKE AND SPINACH GREEK OMELET

BY ISABELLA WENTZ

SERVES 4

10 eggs
1 cup chopped artichoke hearts, packed in water
1 large tomato
4 ounces fresh baby spinach, chopped
2 cloves garlic, minced
⅔ cup chopped green olives
½ teaspoon dried thyme
½ teaspoon dried oregano
Sea salt and freshly ground black pepper
2 tablespoons coconut oil

1. In a large bowl, whisk together all the ingredients except the oil.

2. Heat the oil in a large skillet over medium-high heat. Pour the mixture into the skillet. After 1 to 2 minutes, when the omelet has begun to brown, fold it in half and continue to cook for another 1 to 2 minutes on each side, until the center is cooked through. Serve immediately.

BRAIN BENEFITS

Spinach is a green leafy vegetable that is rich in phylloquinone, lutein, nitrate, folate, α-tocopherol, and kaempferol, all of which may help to slow cognitive decline.[7]

LUNCH

GARDEN GAZPACHO

BY NANETTE ACHZIGER

SERVES 4

> 4 or 5 Roma tomatoes, roughly chopped
> ⅓ cucumber, roughly chopped
> ½ red bell pepper, roughly chopped
> ¼ small onion
> ¾ cup garbanzo beans, cooked
> 1 clove garlic
> 1 tablespoon red wine vinegar
> A handful or two of ice
> Sea salt and freshly ground black pepper
> 1 or 2 dashes of ground cumin
> 2–3 tablespoons extra-virgin olive oil, plus extra to drizzle

1. Put the tomatoes, cucumber, bell pepper, onion, beans, garlic, vinegar, and ice into a high-speed blender (use a handful or two of ice to keep the gazpacho cold while blending). Blend until smooth, adding water to get a drinkable consistency.

2. Season with salt and pepper and cumin.

3. With the blender on low, drizzle in the oil to desired taste. Serve in small glasses with a drizzle of oil on top.

BRAIN BENEFITS

Garlic may help reduce the risk of dementia, including vascular dementia and AD, and is thought to protect the brain against neurodegenerative conditions.[8]

WILD SALMON WITH KALE

BY DAVE ASPREY

SERVES 2

   2 wild salmon fillets (sockeye salmon is great)
   1 teaspoon coconut oil
   Sea salt
   3 tablespoons ghee
   1 bunch (12 ounces) kale, stems removed and leaves torn into pieces
   1 tablespoon minced fresh chives, parsley, and/or dill
   1 lemon

1. Preheat the oven to 320 degrees.

2. Place the salmon on parchment paper on a baking sheet. Rub with the oil, season with salt, and top with 1 tablespoon of the ghee. Wrap the parchment around the salmon, folding the seams and tucking them to make sure the steam doesn't escape.

3. Bake for 18 minutes, or until the fish is medium-rare.

4. Meanwhile, steam the kale for 3 minutes, or until just wilted. Drain, then add the remaining 2 tablespoons ghee and season to taste with salt.

5. Place the kale on a plate. Put the salmon on top and sprinkle with the herbs and fresh-squeezed lemon.

BRAIN BENEFITS
Ghee has historically been used as a brain tonic to improve memory. It is said to promote all three aspects of mental functioning: learning, memory, and recall.[9]

CHICKEN–COCONUT MILK CURRY

BY HYLA CASS

SERVES 4

   1 cup organic unflavored, unsweetened coconut milk (pure, no
      additives)
   2 pounds chicken, cut into cubes (thighs or breasts, but I prefer thighs
      as they're more moist)
   1 cup chopped mushrooms

1 cup chopped broccoli

1 onion, chopped

4–5 cloves garlic, chopped

1 tablespoon curry powder

1 teaspoon minced fresh ginger

1. In a large skillet over medium heat, add the coconut milk, chicken, mushrooms, broccoli, onion, and garlic. Cook for 15 minutes.

2. Add the curry powder and ginger, reduce the heat, and cook for 15 to 20 minutes, or until done to taste. Serve over brown rice.

BRAIN BENEFITS

Mushrooms and their extracts appear to hold many health benefits, including immune-modulating effects. A number of edible mushrooms have been shown to contain rare and exotic compounds that exhibit positive effects on brain cells and may have an anti-dementia/AD effect because of these active compounds.[10]

Curry powder contains curcumin, which has antioxidant, anti-inflammatory, and anti-amyloid activity. In addition, studies in animal models of AD indicate a direct effect of curcumin in decreasing the amyloid pathology of AD.[11]

COOL CUCUMBER SALAD

BY TREVOR CATES

SERVES 2

2 cups cubed organic English cucumber

1 cup sliced radishes

2 cups minced parsley

½ cup grated carrots

3 tablespoons minced mint

3 cloves garlic, minced

3 tablespoons lemon juice

2 tablespoons extra-virgin olive oil

½ teaspoon Himalayan sea salt or Celtic sea salt

½ cup pumpkin seeds

Add all the ingredients to a large salad bowl and mix together. Serve chilled.

LENTIL AND BEET SOUP

BY ALAN CHRISTIANSON

SERVES 3

1 cup French green lentils
2 teaspoons cumin seeds
2 tablespoons extra-virgin olive oil
2 ribs celery, chopped
3 medium beets, cleaned and sliced
1 quart chicken or vegetable stock
Salt and pepper

1. Place the lentils in a medium bowl and cover with water. Soak for at least 2 hours, then drain.

2. In a large saucepan over medium heat, stir the cumin seeds in the oil until fragrant. Add the celery and beets and cook for 2 to 3 minutes.

3. Add the stock and lentils to the saucepan. Season to taste with salt and pepper. Simmer for 30 to 40 minutes.

BRAIN BENEFITS

Lentils have a unique ability to bind with brain-damaging toxins, such as arsenic, and remove them from the body.

Beets improve methylation reactions, helping the brain produce its brain chemicals more effectively. Beets are also high in folate (vitamin B), which may boost mood and alleviate depression. Cognitive decline and some forms of dementia, including Alzheimer's disease, are associated with lower folate levels.[12]

E3 ENERGY EVOLVED TACO SALAD

BY HEATHER AND DAMIAN DUBE

SERVES 3–4

2 tablespoons olive oil
1 pound boneless, skinless chicken breast, sliced into small pieces
½ teaspoon garlic granules
1½ cups coarsely chopped yellow onions

1½ cups chopped vine-ripe tomatoes
2–3 tablespoons ground cumin
1½ tablespoons chili powder
1 teaspoon dried oregano
2 teaspoons raw sea salt
1½ tablespoons minced fresh cilantro
½ lime
½ cup filtered water
6 cups shredded green cabbage
1 avocado, cut into small pieces

1. Preheat a large skillet over medium heat for 3 to 5 minutes. Once it's hot, add the olive oil and chicken and cook until nearly done.

2. Add the garlic and ½ cup each of the yellow onions and tomatoes and cook for 3 to 4 minutes, or until the onions are tender.

3. Reduce the heat to medium-low and add the cumin, chili powder, oregano, salt, cilantro, and lime juice, continuing to cook for 3 minutes, stirring frequently.

4. Add the water and simmer for an additional 3 to 5 minutes, stirring frequently.

5. Place the cabbage on dinner plates. Remove the taco mixture from the heat and spoon over the cabbage. Top with the remaining onions, tomatoes, and avocado and serve.

SUBSTITUTIONS

Replace the cabbage with 6 to 8 lightly steamed collard green leaves. Spoon the mixture in the center of the leaves. Add the remaining onions, tomatoes, and avocado. Fold the leaves to form a wrap/burrito and serve.

SPRING SHRIMP AND BLUEBERRY SALAD

BY ELAINE DE SANTOS

SERVES 4

1 pound shrimp, peeled, deveined, and grilled
½ cup radishes
2 heads romaine lettuce, chopped
1 small avocado, peeled, pitted, and sliced
2 tablespoons extra-virgin olive oil
¼ cup apple cider vinegar
1 tablespoon leeks, chopped
1 tablespoon fresh dill, chopped
3 cups blueberries
Sea salt and freshly ground black pepper

1. In a large bowl, combine the shrimp, radishes, lettuce, and avocado.

2. In a small bowl, whisk together the oil, vinegar, leeks, dill, blueberries, and salt and pepper to taste. Pour over the salad. Toss and serve.

BRAIN BENEFITS
Black pepper may improve memory impairment and neurodegeneration in the hippocampus.[13]

CURRY CHICKEN SALAD

BY SHANNON GARRETT

SERVES 4

4 organic boneless chicken breasts
1–2 bay leaves
½ cup chopped celery
½ cup chopped walnuts
⅔ cup avocado mayonnaise
2 teaspoons gluten-free Dijon mustard
1 teaspoon curry powder
Sea salt and black pepper
Mixed salad greens
2 teaspoons minced fresh parsley

1 avocado, chopped or sliced
Pomegranate arils

1. Wash and pat dry the chicken. Add water to a steamer (per manufacturer's instructions) and add the bay leaves. Place the chicken in the steamer basket and steam for 45 to 50 minutes. Do not overcook. Allow to cool, then shred or chop.

2. In a large bowl, combine the chicken, celery, walnuts, mayonnaise, mustard, and curry. Blend well with a fork and season to taste with salt and pepper.

3. Add the salad greens to plates and mound with the chicken salad. Garnish with parsley, avocado, and pomegranate arils. (If desired, drizzle salad greens with the juice of a lemon and extra-virgin olive oil.)

BRAIN BENEFITS

Pomegranate contains polyphenols that have been shown to improve mild memory complaints, including verbal and visual memory.[14]

ZUCCHINI BOATS WITH SAVORY TURKEY STUFFING

BY DONNA GATES

4 zucchinis, cut in half lengthwise, trimmed, cleaned, and blanched
2–3 tablespoons coconut oil
3 cloves garlic, minced
1 small onion, minced
2 ribs celery, minced
3 tablespoons chopped fresh parsley
1 teaspoon dried oregano
1 teaspoon paprika
½ teaspoon pepper
¼ teaspoon cayenne
¼ teaspoon Celtic sea salt
1 pound ground turkey
2 eggs, scrambled

1. Preheat the oven to 375 degrees.

2. Scoop out the centers of the zucchinis, taking care not to pierce the skins.

3. In a large skillet over medium-high heat, add the oil and cook the garlic, onion, and celery together until the onion is translucent. Add the spices and salt and cook a few minutes longer. Add the ground turkey and eggs and remove from the heat.

4. Stuff each zucchini boat with the mixture and place in a deep-sided roasting dish.

5. Bake for 30 minutes, or until the turkey is slightly golden on top and cooked throughout.

BRAIN BENEFITS

Parsley contains quercetin, which is thought to have a myriad of health benefits, including reducing the risk of neurodegenerative disorders related to its highly pronounced antioxidant and anti-inflammatory properties.[15]

SALMON CHOWDER

BY ANDREA NAKAYAMA

ANDREA LIVINGSTON FROM BETTERHOOD PDX,
CREATED FOR FUNCTIONAL NUTRITION ALLIANCE

SERVES 4–6

1 tablespoon ghee
1 medium onion, chopped
2 ribs celery, chopped
2 teaspoons dried dill or 2 tablespoons fresh
1 teaspoon dried thyme
1 medium turnip or parsnip, peeled and cut into small cubes
2 medium carrots, chopped
4 cups chicken, fish, or vegetable broth
1 can (14 ounces) coconut milk
1 pound wild-caught salmon fillet, skin removed, cut into cubes
Sea salt and pepper

1. In a large soup pot, heat the ghee over medium heat. Add the onion and cook until soft. Add the celery, dill, and thyme. Toss to coat and heat for 1 minute. Add the turnip or parsnip and carrots and cook for 3 to 5 minutes.

2. Add the broth and coconut milk. Bring to a boil, then simmer for 10 to 15 minutes, or until the vegetables are soft. Add the salmon and simmer for another 5 minutes. Season to taste with salt and pepper.

BRAIN BENEFITS

Turnips, parsnips, and **carrots** are all root vegetables that contain different prebiotic building blocks for your microbiome, supplying excellent materials and helping to build stronger cells.

SPINACH-APPLE-WALNUT SALAD

BY CYNTHIA PASQUELLA

SERVES 2

½ cup walnuts
2 tablespoons raw honey
4 cups baby spinach
½ Fuji apple, cored and chopped
2 tablespoons lemon juice
2 tablespoons olive oil

1. Heat the oven to 350 degrees.

2. Place the walnuts in a single layer on a baking sheet and drizzle with the honey. Bake for 10 minutes, stirring occasionally.

3. Place the nuts in a large bowl with the spinach, apple, lemon juice, and oil. Toss, serve, and enjoy!

SUBSTITUTIONS

Try substituting almonds for walnuts and a Granny Smith apple for the Fuji. This will result in a slightly tangy, fresh flavor. No honey in the house? Use 2 tablespoons agave nectar or blackstrap molasses instead.

BRAIN BENEFITS

Apples contain quercetin, which is thought to have a myriad of health benefits, including reducing the risk of neurodegenerative disorders related to its highly pronounced antioxidant and anti-inflammatory properties.[16]

Honey improves memory-related brain areas, reduces brain oxidative stress, and increases brain-derived neurotrophic factor (BDNF) and concentrations of the brain chemical acetylcholine.[17]

YOU CAN FIX YOUR BRAIN | 294

CREAMY CARROT CURRY SOUP

BY OCEAN ROBBINS

SERVES 4

2 cups chopped carrots
1½ cups chopped onions
3 cups water
½ cup raw or roasted cashews (if dry-roasted,
    use unsalted or low salt)
1 tablespoon organic or non-GMO-certified tamari
    or coconut aminos
2 teaspoons curry powder (or more, if you like it hot)
½ teaspoon turmeric
¼ cup chopped parsley

1. In a saucepan over high heat, combine the carrots, onions, and water. Cover
and bring to a boil, then reduce the heat and simmer for 10 minutes.

2. Place the vegetables and cooking liquid, cashews, tamari, curry powder, and
turmeric into a blender and blend until creamy.

3. Serve hot, garnished with the parsley.

MESCLUN SALAD WITH GRILLED
CHICKEN BREASTS AND PEAR VINAIGRETTE

BY LISA STIMMER

SERVES 4

CHICKEN
2 boneless, skinless chicken breasts (5–6 ounces each),
    pounded to ½" thickness
2 teaspoons grapeseed oil
Sea salt and pepper

SALAD AND DRESSING
5 tablespoons hazelnut oil or pecan oil (or avocado or grapeseed oil)
3 tablespoons pear vinegar or cider vinegar plus ¼ peeled pear,
    chopped and blended into dressing
1½ tablespoons pure maple syrup or agave

Sea salt
Pinch of cayenne
¼ cup hazelnuts or whole pecans, toasted
2 ripe pears, peeled, cored, and thinly sliced
½ pint fresh raspberries
12 ounces mesclun salad mix

1. To make the chicken: Heat the grill to medium-high. Rub the chicken with the grapeseed oil. Sprinkle with salt and pepper. Grill for 4 minutes per side, or until grill marks have formed and the chicken is cooked through. Remove from the heat and let rest for 3 minutes. Cut into ¼"-thick slices for presentation (20 slices total).

2. To make the salad and dressing: In a blender, blend the oil, vinegar, ½ tablespoon of the syrup or agave, salt, and cayenne. Adjust the flavor to taste.

3. Preheat the oven to 300 degrees. Toast the nuts for 10 minutes, or until slightly brown. Let cool, then chop. Remove to a bowl and immediately drizzle with the remaining 1 tablespoon syrup or agave, sea salt, and cayenne to taste. Stir well.

4. To assemble the salad, arrange the pears and raspberries around the outside edges of 4 plates. Toss the salad mix with half of the dressing and evenly mound it in the middle of the plates. Arrange the chicken slices like a star on the salad. Sprinkle the nuts over the top. Top with the rest of the dressing and serve immediately.

BRAIN BENEFITS
Pecans/pecan oil are known to be high in omega-3 fatty acids. This important nutrient must be acquired through diet because the body cannot produce it on its own. Omega-3s turn on the genes that lower inflammation in the gut and in the brain.

THE "SAM" SALAD

BY IZABELLA WENTZ

SERVES 4

> 4 (3–4 ounces) salmon fillets, cooked
> 1 avocado
> 1 ripe mango
> ¼ cup mayonnaise

Chop the salmon, avocado, and mango. Toss with the mayonnaise and serve immediately.

BRAIN BENEFITS

Mango polyphenols are antioxidants, a property that enables them to protect brain cells against damage due to oxidative stress.[18]

QUICK SAUERKRAUT SALAD

BY MAGDALENA WSZELAKI

SERVES 1–2

> 1 cup lacto-fermented sauerkraut
> 1 teaspoon cumin seeds, roasted
> ½ cup broccoli sprouts
> ½ avocado, sliced
> 1 medium carrot, grated
> 1 teaspoon black sesame seeds (optional)
> 2 tablespoons extra-virgin olive oil

In a serving bowl, combine the sauerkraut and cumin. Add the broccoli, avocado, and carrot. Sprinkle the sesame seeds, if using. Drizzle with the oil.

BRAIN BENEFITS

Sauerkraut is a fermented food, which is a type of food that grows bacteria in it or on it. That bacteria are some of the best detoxifying agents available. The beneficial bacteria in these foods are capable of drawing out a wide range of toxins and heavy metals in both the brain and body. They can contain 100 times more probiotics than a supplement. Every day, you need to eat just a little bit, such as one forkful of fermented foods like sauerkraut and kimchi, both made from cabbage.

DINNER

SANCOCHO

BY NANETTE ACHZIGER

SERVES 4

2 tablespoons extra-virgin olive oil
1 onion, diced
6 cloves garlic, minced
1 habanero, minced
4 cups chicken stock
2 ribs celery, sliced thin
1 carrot, sliced in half-moons
1 small cassava, diced
1 ripe plantain, sliced in half-moons
1 green plantain, sliced in half-moons
1 tomato, diced
1 teaspoon sea salt
Freshly ground black pepper
¼ cup chopped cilantro
2 cups diced, cooked chicken

1. In a large pot over medium heat, add the oil and onion and cook for 4 minutes. Add the garlic and habanero and cook for 1 minute more.

2. Add the remaining ingredients except the chicken and simmer for 25 minutes, or until the vegetables are tender.

3. Add the chicken and simmer another 5 minutes, then serve.

BRAIN BENEFITS

Cassava is a root vegetable that contains different prebiotic building blocks for your microbiome, supplying excellent materials and helping to build stronger cells.

LAMB CHILI

BY DAVE ASPREY

SERVES 2

1 leek, sliced
2 carrots, chopped
4 ribs celery, chopped
2 cups water
½ cup asparagus, thinly sliced
1 cup cauliflower, chopped
1 cup zucchini or summer squash, chopped
1 pound grass-fed ground lamb or grass-fed ground beef
1 teaspoon apple cider vinegar
1 teaspoon ground coriander
1 teaspoon ground cumin
1 teaspoon allspice
1 tablespoon dried oregano
1 bay leaf
1 teaspoon sea salt
¼ cup coconut oil
1 tablespoon Brain Octane Oil
Olive oil

1. In a medium pot, combine the leek, carrots, and celery and cook over medium-low heat for 3 minutes, or until fragrant and the leek is soft.

2. Add the water, asparagus, cauliflower, squash, meat, vinegar, spices, and salt. Cover and cook for 10 minutes.

3. Stir in the coconut oil and Brain Octane Oil until incorporated.

4. Serve in a bowl drizzled with the olive oil.

BONE BROTH PROTEIN MEATBALL SOUP

BY JOSH AXE

SERVES 8–10

- 1½ pounds ground bison or beef
- 2 eggs, whisked
- 1½ teaspoons sea salt
- 1 teaspoon smoked paprika or cayenne
- 2 tablespoons coconut oil
- 4 cups bone broth, or 3 scoops Ancient Nutrition "Pure" Bone Broth Protein Powder mixed in 36 ounces water
- 2 bay leaves
- 4 carrots, chopped
- 1 large sweet potato, chopped
- 1 cup green beans, chopped
- 1 cup green peas
- 2 tomatoes, chopped

1. Mix the meat, eggs, ½ teaspoon of the salt, and the paprika or cayenne in a medium bowl. Roll into small meatballs.

2. In a large pot, heat the oil over medium heat. Add the meatballs and cook for 5 to 8 minutes, just until brown.

3. Add the broth, bay leaves, carrots, sweet potato, and the remaining 1 teaspoon salt and bring to a simmer over medium-high heat.

4. Add the beans, peas, and tomatoes and simmer for 20 minutes, or until the sweet potatoes are done.

BRAIN BENEFITS
Bone broth contains a collagen that acts as a natural probiotic, meaning that it feeds the good bacteria and helps to seal a leaky gut.

SALMON WITH GREENS AND BLACK BEANS

BY TREVOR CATES

SERVES 4–6

SALAD
1 cup black beans, cooked
2 cups chopped organic baby kale
1 cup sliced carrots
¼ cup sliced green onions

DRESSING
¼ cup extra-virgin olive oil
¼ cup fresh lime juice
2 cloves fresh garlic, chopped or pressed
3 teaspoons chopped fresh cilantro
Himalayan salt or Celtic sea salt
Pepper

SALMON
1 tablespoon avocado oil
4 fillets (4 ounces each) wild Alaskan salmon

1. To make the salad: Combine the beans, kale, carrots, and green onions in a medium bowl.

2. To make the dressing: In a small bowl, combine the oil, lime juice, garlic, and cilantro. Season to taste with salt and pepper. Pour three-quarters of the dressing into salad. Set aside.

3. To make the salmon: Preheat the oven to 400 degrees. Coat a baking sheet with the oil and place the salmon skin side down. Bake for 5 to 10 minutes. Spoon about 1 teaspoon of the dressing onto each fillet. Place the warm salmon over the salad. Drizzle with the remaining dressing.

SARDINES WITH TOMATOES

BY ALAN CHRISTIANSON

SERVES 2

1 pint cherry tomatoes
1 tablespoon extra-virgin olive oil

1 can sardines packed in olive oil
½ teaspoon dried oregano
½ teaspoon dried thyme
Pinch of cayenne
1 clove garlic

1. Cut the tomatoes in half and add to a 2-quart saucepan. Add the oil and sauté the tomatoes on low heat for 1 hour, stirring regularly.

2. Drain the sardines and add to the saucepan, breaking them up. Add the oregano, thyme, cayenne, and garlic and cook for 10 minutes.

3. Serve on quinoa or spaghetti squash.

BRAIN BENEFITS
Sardines are high in omega-3 fatty acids, which are known for their anti-inflammatory effects. Various studies indicate promising anti-depression effects.[19]

E3 ENERGY EVOLVED COCONUT CURRY LAMB

BY DAMIAN DUBE

SERVES 2

12 ounces ground lamb
2 cups sliced zucchini
2 cups sliced bok choy
1 tablespoon curry powder
1 teaspoon turmeric
½ teaspoon cardamom
½ teaspoon raw sea salt
¼ cup organic original coconut milk
¼ cup organic lite coconut milk

1. Preheat a large skillet over medium heat. Add the lamb and cook thoroughly, mixing frequently with a spatula.

2. Add the zucchini and bok choy. Cook until slightly tender, stirring frequently.

3. Reduce the heat to low and add the curry, turmeric, cardamom, salt, and both coconut milks. Cook for 2 to 3 minutes, being careful not to burn.

4. Remove from the heat and serve.

CITRUS GLAZED MEATBALLS
WITH CRISPY SWEET POTATO NOODLES

BY ELAINE DE SANTOS

SERVES 4

> 8 tablespoons coconut oil, divided
> ½ large onion, minced
> 2 cloves garlic, minced
> 1 teaspoon ground ginger
> 1 pound ground beef
> 1 tablespoon chopped fresh thyme
> Sea salt and freshly ground black pepper
> ½ cup fresh orange juice
> ¼ cup coconut aminos
> 2 large sweet potatoes, peeled

1. In a large skillet over medium heat, heat 2 tablespoons of the oil. When it has melted and the pan is hot, add the onion and cook, stirring, for 8 minutes, or until translucent. Add the garlic and ginger and cook, stirring, for 1 minute, just until fragrant. Remove from the heat and place the mixture in a bowl. Set aside to cool for a few minutes.

2. When the mixture has cooled, add it to a large mixing bowl with the ground beef and thyme. Season with salt and pepper. Gently mix with your hands until everything is well incorporated. Form into 1½″ meatballs.

3. Add 2 tablespoons of the oil to the skillet used for the onion mixture and heat over medium heat. When the oil is melted and the skillet is hot, add the meatballs. Brown for 3 minutes on one side, flip, and add the orange juice and coconut aminos. Cook, covered, for 10 minutes, or until cooked through. Remove the meatballs from the pan and set aside.

4. Leave the remaining juices in the pan and increase the heat to medium-high. Cook for 5 to 10 minutes, reducing the sauce by about half. Set the sauce aside.

5. Using a vegetable peeler, peel the sweet potato into long, flat ribbons, or spiralize it with a vegetable spiralizer.

6. In another skillet, heat 2 tablespoons of the oil over medium-high heat. When the oil has melted and the pan is hot, add half of the sweet potatoes. Cook, stirring, for 10 minutes, being sure not to stir them too often to ensure that they

brown on the bottoms. Remove the first batch, then add the remaining 2 tablespoons oil and repeat with the remaining sweet potatoes. Serve the meatballs on top of the sweet potato noodles.

BRAIN BENEFITS

Ginger is considered to have anti-amyloidogenic activity and may suppress the development of plaques in the brain.[20]

CHICKEN BROCCOLI WITH COCONUT ALFREDO

BY ELAINE DE SANTOS

SERVES 4

¼ cup lemon juice
1½ teaspoons Italian seasoning
Sea salt and freshly ground black pepper
3 boneless, skinless chicken breast halves, cut into bite-size pieces
¼ cup almond flour
2 cups fresh broccoli florets
1½ tablespoons coconut oil
3 cloves garlic, minced (divided)
2 tablespoons ghee
¼ cup arrowroot flour
2 cups full-fat coconut milk
12 ounces cooked spaghetti squash

1. In a large bowl, combine the lemon juice and Italian seasoning and season with salt and pepper. Add the chicken and toss to coat well. In a small bowl, sprinkle the almond flour over the chicken.

2. Steam the broccoli florets until tender-crisp. Drain, chill with cold water, drain again, and set aside.

3. Heat the oil in a large skillet over medium-high heat. Add 2 cloves of the minced garlic. Add the chicken and cook, turning occasionally, for 10 to 15 minutes, or until browned. Remove from the pan.

4. Add the ghee and the remaining garlic to the skillet. Stir in the arrowroot flour and cook, stirring constantly. When bubbly, gradually stir in the coconut milk. Cook until creamy. Add the chicken and broccoli and stir to coat with the sauce.

5. Serve over hot spaghetti squash. Top with pepper.

BRAIN BENEFITS

Broccoli, with high levels of vitamin K and choline, will help keep your memory sharp.

SWISS CHARD SAUTÉ WITH COCONUT MILK

BY SHANNON GARRETT

SERVES 4

- 1 teaspoon coconut oil
- 1 onion, sliced
- 1 large leek, sliced
- ½ cup full-fat coconut milk
- 1 bunch Swiss chard, thinly sliced
- 1 teaspoon curry powder
- ½ teaspoon sea salt
- 1 teaspoon black pepper

1. Heat the oil in a large saucepan over medium-low heat and add the onion and leek. Cook for 5 to 7 minutes until soft.

2. Add the coconut milk, chard, curry, salt, and pepper. Cook for 3 minutes, or until the chard wilts.

3. Serve immediately and enjoy. Suggestion: Serve with poached or broiled wild-caught salmon drizzled with lemon juice.

TEX-MEX (OR ITALIAN) MILLET AND AMARANTH CORN CASSEROLE

BY DONNA GATES

- 1 tablespoon coconut oil or ghee
- 1 large onion, minced
- 1 mild green chili, diced (optional)
- 1¾ teaspoons Frontier Co-op Mexican Seasoning, or similar
- 1 tablespoon Celtic sea salt
- 1½ cups millet, soaked for at least 8 hours and rinsed
- ½ cup amaranth, soaked for at least 8 hours and rinsed
- 8 ears fresh corn, kernels removed, or 16 ounces frozen corn

6 cups filtered water or stock
1 large red bell pepper, seeded and diced
1 teaspoon A. Vogel Herbamare

1. Preheat the oven to 350 degrees. Butter a 3-quart casserole dish.

2. In a stockpot over medium-high heat, add the oil and cook the onion, green chili (if using), Mexican seasoning, and salt until the onion is translucent.*

3. Add the millet, amaranth, corn, and water and bring to a boil. Cover, lower the heat, and simmer for 30 minutes.

4. Fold in the bell pepper and Herbamare and adjust seasonings to taste.

5. Pour the mixture into the casserole dish. Dot with small amounts of ghee, if desired. Bake for 30 minutes.

* To make an Italian-flavored dish, use 1 tablespoon Italian seasoning instead of the Mexican blend, and exchange the corn and green chili for zucchini and shiitake mushrooms.

SOCKEYE SALMON COCONUT CURRY

BY RANDY HARTNELL

SERVES 2–4

1 tablespoon organic extra-virgin olive oil or organic macadamia nut oil
1 large shallot, minced (or substitute ½ white or yellow onion)
2 teaspoons grated fresh ginger
2 cloves garlic, minced
2–3 tablespoons Thai green curry paste
1 can unsweetened coconut milk
1 tablespoon brown sugar (optional)
1 cup chicken broth, vegetable broth, or water
2 heads baby bok choy, trimmed
2 fresh tomatoes, chopped
2–4 portions skinless-boneless Vital Choice Wild Alaskan Sockeye
    Salmon, thawed
Salt and pepper
Black rice or brown jasmine rice (optional)
Fresh cilantro leaves

1. Heat the oil over medium heat in a saucepan that's large enough to accommodate 2 to 4 salmon portions in a single layer. Add the shallot or onion, ginger, and garlic and cook, stirring often, for 5 minutes, or until the onion begins to soften.

2. Add the curry paste and cook for 1 minute, or until fragrant. Add the coconut milk (stir it first if the cream has separated from the thinner liquid), brown sugar (if using), and broth and bring to a boil. Reduce the heat to a simmer and add the bok choy and tomatoes. Cover and simmer for 2 minutes, or until the bok choy is tender.

3. Season the salmon with salt and pepper to taste and gently add them to the broth. Cover and gently simmer for 4 to 5 minutes, depending on your preference, until the salmon is just cooked through. The key to poaching salmon is slow and low—you don't want to boil the fish. Ideally it cooks at a bare simmer, allowing the salmon to stay whole and tender. The salmon is done once it just begins to flake.

4. Serve over rice (if using) and garnish with the cilantro.

MOROCCAN CHICKEN WITH GREENS

BY ANDREA NAKAYAMA

SERVES 4

> 1 tablespoon ghee
> ½ cup sliced shallots
> 1 tablespoon fresh ginger, peeled and chopped
> 1 teaspoon turmeric
> 1 teaspoon ground cinnamon
> 2 teaspoons paprika
> ½ teaspoon ground coriander
> ½ teaspoon ground cumin
> 1 teaspoon sea salt plus extra to taste
> 2 cups tomatoes, chopped
> 2 cups chicken stock
> 1 lemon, sliced, rind on and deseeded
> ½ cup chopped cilantro
> 6 boneless, skinless chicken thighs
> ½ bunch green kale, chard, or spinach, chopped

½ lemon, juiced
Pepper

1. Place a large saucepan or pot over medium heat. Add the ghee, shallots, and ginger and cook until soft. Add the turmeric, cinnamon, paprika, coriander, cumin, and salt and sauté for 1 minute. Add the tomatoes, stock, sliced lemon, and cilantro and simmer for 10 minutes.

2. Add the chicken, cover, and simmer for 30 minutes.

3. Add the greens and lemon juice. Cover and simmer for 5 to 10 minutes. Remove from the heat and add salt and pepper to taste.

BRAIN BENEFITS

Coriander contains the highest levels of beta-carotene, beta-cryptoxanthin, and lutein + zeaxanthin, which are thought to improve visual and cognitive function throughout the lifespan. These plant-based nutrients have anti-inflammatory properties, can improve brain structure and development (particularly in children), and may be protective against eye disease. In adults, a higher amount of lutein in the diet is related to better cognitive performance.[21]

CLEANSING CILANTRO AND OREGANO PESTO

BY CHRISTA ORECCHIO

MAKES ABOUT 1 CUP

1 bunch fresh cilantro, washed and dried, ends clipped
2 tablespoons fresh oregano
1 lime, juiced
¾ cup extra-virgin olive oil
⅓ cup pine nuts (optional)
2 cloves garlic, minced
Sea salt

Blend all the ingredients except the salt in a blender. Add the salt to taste. Use as a thicker salad dressing, a dip for vegetables, or a topping for cooked chicken or fish.

BRAIN BENEFITS

Pine nuts are not nuts at all, but seeds that show promise as possible dietary interventions for age-related brain dysfunction.[22]

CURRIED LENTIL-CASHEW BURGERS

BY CYNTHIA PASQUELLA

SERVES 6

1 cup water
½ cup red lentils, rinsed
Dash of salt
¾ cup raw cashews
1 small onion, chopped
6 teaspoons coconut oil
1 cup mushrooms, chopped
1 clove garlic, minced
2 teaspoons curry powder
½ cup old-fashioned oats
6 large lettuce leaves

1. Combine the water, lentils, and salt in a pot. Bring to a boil. Reduce the heat, cover partially, and simmer until the lentils are very tender. Drain in a colander and set aside to cool.

2. Meanwhile, place the cashews in a skillet over medium-high heat and toast for 4 minutes, or until fragrant. Remove from the skillet and set aside.

3. In the same skillet over medium heat, cook the onion in 1 teaspoon of the coconut oil until transparent. Add the mushrooms, garlic, curry powder, and 3 tablespoons water and cook for 2 minutes. Remove from the heat and set aside.

4. Place the cashews and lentils in a food processor and pulse until textured. Transfer to a bowl, add the mushroom mixture, and stir in the oats until mixed well.

5. Wet your hands and form 6 burger patties from the mixture. Cook the patties in the remaining 5 teaspoons coconut oil, or more as needed, over medium heat for 4 minutes on each side, or until brown and heated through.

6. Wrap the patties in the lettuce, add your favorite toppings, and enjoy!

SUBSTITUTIONS

This is a great recipe to make extra of and freeze for later. Just form into individual patties, wrap, and freeze for up to 30 days. You can also adjust the curry powder to suit your desired level of spiciness.

BRAIN BENEFITS

Lettuce—or a daily serving of green leafy vegetables that are rich in phylloqui-none, lutein, nitrate, folate, α-tocopherol, and kaempferol—may help to slow cognitive decline.[23]

QUINOA WITH WALNUTS

BY OCEAN ROBBINS

  1 tablespoon olive oil
  1 rib celery, chopped
  1 medium carrot, chopped
  1 medium onion, chopped
  6 button mushrooms, sliced thin
  2 cups water
  1 cup quinoa, soaked for 5 minutes, rinsed, and drained
  ½ teaspoon black pepper
  ½ teaspoon dried rosemary
  1–2 tablespoons organic or non-GMO-certified tamari or coconut
    aminos
  ½ cup chopped walnuts
  ¼ cup chopped fresh parsley

1. Heat the oil in a saucepan over medium-high heat. Add the celery, carrot, and onion and cook for 5 minutes, stirring.

2. Add the mushrooms and continue stirring for 1 minute. Stir in the water, qui-noa, pepper, rosemary, and tamari. Cover and bring to a boil, then reduce the heat and simmer for 25 minutes.

3. Place the cooked quinoa in a bowl and toss with the walnuts and parsley. Serve hot or cold.

ZUCCHINI PASTA WITH SALMON AND ARTICHOKES

BY LISA STIMMER

SERVES 4

> 6 zucchinis, medium to large, firm and straight, cut into "noodles"*
> 2 pounds fresh wild salmon fillets (skin removed)
> Sea salt and pepper
> 2 tablespoons high-heat cooking oil (avocado or grapeseed)
> 3 tablespoons olive oil
> 4 tablespoons shallots, minced
> 4 cloves garlic, minced
> 8 artichoke hearts (in water), quartered
> 1 lemon, zested and juiced
> 4 tablespoons chopped fresh parsley
> Pinch of cayenne
> 6 slices crumbled crispy turkey bacon, crispy bacon, or crispy pancetta

1. Salt the zucchini noodles, let sit for a few minutes, then massage and squeeze the water out of them. Make sure to drain any excess liquid.

2. Season the salmon with salt and pepper. In a large pan, heat the avocado oil over medium to high heat. Add the salmon top side down and sear till golden and crispy, then turn over to finish cooking. Cover only with a splatter screen, or it will not get crispy.

3. In a wok or large pan over medium heat, add the olive oil and shallots and cook until soft. Add the garlic and cook for 1 minute.

4. Add the zucchini noodles, increase the heat to medium-high, and cook for 2 minutes. Add the artichokes and lemon zest, stir to combine, and cook for 1 minute. Turn off the heat and add the parsley, lemon juice, and cayenne and stir to combine. Add the bacon and adjust seasonings to taste.

5. Distribute evenly on 4 plates or low bowls. Place the salmon on top and serve with extra lemon. Enjoy!

* ZUCCHINI NOODLE VARIETIES

To make zucchini "fettuccine": Use a potato peeler. The peeler method will give you long flat noodles or lengthwise ribbons. Peel off several from one side, then turn the zucchini and peel off more. Continue to turn and peel away ribbons until you get to the seeds at the core of the zucchini. Discard the core.

To make zucchini "spaghetti": Use a spiral slicer (spiralizer), mandolin slicer, or knife. If you have a spiralizer, this will be perfect for the job; if you don't have one, visit www.lisastimmer.com/store for my recommendation. If you have a mandolin, hook up the julienne attachment for perfectly formed noodles. If using a knife, cut the zucchini into thin slices, stack them up, and cut again lengthwise into thin strips. Discard the core.

BABY RACK OF LAMB WITH A RED WINE AND BALSAMIC REDUCTION

BY LISA STIMMER

SERVES 4

    2 (1.25 pounds each) baby racks of lamb, fat trimmed
    Rosemary, dried or fresh chopped
    Garlic granules or powder
    Sea salt and pepper
    ¼ cup sulfite-free red wine
    ¼ cup beef broth
    ½ cup balsamic vinegar
    1 tablespoon ghee
    Pureed yams (prepared with ghee and sea salt)
    Steamed broccoli or green beans (prepared with ghee and sea salt)

1. Preheat the broiler to 450 degrees.

2. Dust both sides of the lamb racks with the rosemary, garlic, and salt and pepper. Wrap the bones with foil to prevent charring. Place them, thick flesh sides down, on a baking sheet. Broil 8" to 10" from the flame for 8 minutes. Turn the racks over and broil for 7 minutes (for medium-rare). Remove from the oven and let rest 3 minutes. Remove the foil from the bones and cut between the bones to evenly separate.

3. In a pan, add the wine, broth, and vinegar. Bring to a simmer and let reduce to a thin syrup. Then add the ghee and salt and pepper to taste.

4. To serve, put a large dollop of pureed yams in the center of a plate to lean the ribs up against. Pour some sauce in front of the yams and arrange 3 to 4 ribs on top of the sauce. Arrange the broccoli or green beans nicely around the other side of the plate.

BRAIN BENEFITS

Balsamic vinegar has been hypothesized to improve cognitive function.[24]

PAN-SEARED SALMON OVER
TRI-COLOR SALAD WITH DIJON DRESSING

BY JJ VIRGIN

MAKES 2 SERVINGS

SALAD

2 teaspoons lemon juice

1 tablespoon finely chopped shallots

2 teaspoons Dijon mustard

⅛ teaspoon sea salt

⅛ teaspoon freshly ground black pepper

4 teaspoons extra-virgin olive oil

½ small head of radicchio, thinly sliced (about 2 cups)

1 Belgian endive, thinly sliced (about 1 cup)

3 cups baby arugula

SALMON

1 teaspoon olive oil

2 (6-ounce) wild salmon fillets, such as king or sockeye

⅛ teaspoon sea salt

⅛ teaspoon freshly ground black pepper

1. To make the salad: Combine the lemon juice, shallots, mustard, salt, and pepper in a small bowl. Slowly whisk in the oil until well-combined and set aside. In a separate bowl, combine the radicchio, endive, and arugula and set aside.

2. To make the salmon: Heat the oil in a small nonstick skillet over medium heat. Sprinkle the salmon with the salt and pepper and place in the skillet flesh side down. Cook for 4 to 5 minutes per side, or until the fish flakes easily with a fork. Remove from the skillet.

3. Toss the dressing with the salad and divide it between 2 plates. Top each with a salmon fillet.

BRAIN BENEFITS

Arugula is a green leafy vegetable that is rich in phylloquinone, lutein, nitrate, folate, α-tocopherol, and kaempferol, all of which may help to slow cognitive decline.[25]

ON THE SIDE:
ROASTED ASPARAGUS WITH LEMON ZEST

MAKES 4 SERVINGS

1½ pounds asparagus, trimmed
1 tablespoon palm fruit oil
¼ teaspoon sea salt
⅛ teaspoon freshly ground black pepper
2 teaspoons grated fresh lemon zest
2 teaspoons chopped fresh parsley

1. Preheat the oven to 425 degrees. Lightly oil a large baking sheet.

2. Combine the asparagus, oil, salt, and pepper in a medium bowl. Arrange the asparagus in a single layer on the baking sheet.

3. Roast the asparagus for 10 to 12 minutes, or until tender, shaking the pan once or twice. Remove from the oven and toss with the lemon zest and parsley. Serve warm, at room temperature, or chilled.

BLUEBERRY PORK TENDERLOIN AND
STIR-FRIED BABY SPINACH WITH TOASTED WALNUTS

BY IZABELLA WENTZ

SERVES 2

PORK TENDERLOIN
1 medium onion, diced
2 cups frozen blueberries, thawed
½ cup apple cider vinegar
2 teaspoons raw honey
1 teaspoon dried thyme
¼ cup coconut oil, for brushing the grill grate
½ pound pork tenderloin
1 teaspoon garlic powder
Sea salt and freshly ground black pepper

SPINACH
1 tablespoon olive oil
1 clove garlic, minced
10 ounces baby spinach
1 tablespoon balsamic vinegar
Sea salt and freshly ground black pepper
¼ cup toasted walnut halves

1. To make the pork tenderloin: In a large bowl, add the onion, blueberries, apple cider vinegar, honey, and thyme and mix well. Cover the bowl and let sit overnight in the refrigerator, or at room temperature for 1 hour.

2. Preheat the grill to medium-high. Brush the grill grate with the coconut oil. Season the tenderloin with garlic powder and salt and pepper. Grill 4 to 5 minutes per side, or until the juices run clear. Remove from the grill, pour the marinade over, and serve right away.

3. To make the spinach: Heat the olive oil in a large skillet over medium heat. Add the minced garlic and cook for 1 minute. Gradually add the spinach. Cook, turning with tongs, until slightly wilted. Drizzle with the balsamic vinegar, season with salt and pepper, and top with the walnuts.

DESSERTS

CHOCOLATE COCONUT CRÈME AND FRUIT

BY NANETTE ACHZIGER

SERVES 2

> 1 can full-fat coconut milk, refrigerated overnight
> ¼ cup raw cacao powder
> 1 tablespoon maple syrup
> 2 kiwis, sliced in half-moons
> 1 cup berries
> ⅔ cup nuts (almonds, walnuts, pecans, pistachios, etc.)

1. Scoop the solid cream from the can of coconut milk into a large bowl. Using a hand mixer, beat for 1 minute, then add the cacao powder and maple syrup. Beat for another minute or two to incorporate the mixture.

2. Split between 2 bowls and add the kiwis, berries, and nuts. Note: The crème can be made the night before and refrigerated.

BRAIN BENEFITS

Berries and **cocoa** contain dietary flavonoids that are thought to protect the brain in many ways, including the potential to protect neurons against injury induced by neurotoxins, an ability to suppress brain inflammation, and the potential to promote memory, learning, and cognitive function. Therefore, the consumption of flavonoid-rich foods, such as berries and cocoa, throughout life holds the potential to limit the neurodegeneration associated with a variety of neurological disorders and to prevent or reverse normal or abnormal deteriorations in cognitive performance.[26]

BONE BROTH PROTEIN
COCONUT CHOCOLATE PUDDING

BY JOSH AXE

SERVES 4

> 3 cans (14 ounces each) coconut milk, refrigerated overnight
> ½ cup coconut sugar
> 4 ounces unsweetened chocolate (70% or darker)
> 3 scoops Ancient Nutrition Bone Broth Protein powder
> 2 tablespoons cocoa powder
> Handful of raspberries

1. Open the cans of coconut milk and scoop the cream from the top of each into a medium mixing bowl. Using a handheld mixer, whip the cream until fluffy, then refrigerate. Reserve the coconut water.

2. In a small pan over medium-low heat, add the coconut sugar, chocolate, and the reserved coconut water. Stir gently until well combined.

3. Increase the heat to medium. Add the bone broth protein and cocoa powder. Mix well and refrigerate for 30 minutes, or until cool.

4. Remove the whipped coconut cream from the fridge and pour in the cooled chocolate mixture. Whip until well-combined. Return to the fridge and chill for 2 hours, or until set.

5. Serve topped with fresh raspberries.

LEMON TART WITH COCONUT FLOUR CRUST

BY DONNA GATES

MAKES 1 TART

CRUST
¾ cup coconut flour
1 tablespoon ghee, melted
3 tablespoons coconut oil
1 tablespoon MCT oil
1 tablespoon Lakanto Classic Monkfruit Sugar Substitute
2 eggs

FILLING

¾ cup lemon juice plus zest of 1 lemon*

2 tablespoons Body Ecology Stevia liquid concentrate

4 tablespoons Lakanto Classic Monkfruit Sugar Substitute

2 tablespoons MCT oil

2 whole eggs plus 2 yolks

2 tablespoons ghee

To make the crust: Preheat the oven to 350 degrees.

In a medium bowl, mix together the flour, ghee, oils, sugar substitute, and eggs with a fork. The mixture will be crumbly.

Oil a 9″ springform pan and press the crust tightly into the bottom of pan. Bake for 10 minutes. Remove from the oven and cool before adding the filling.

To make the filling: In a blender, place the lemon juice and zest, stevia, sugar substitute, oil, and eggs. Blend on high speed. Pour the mixture into a medium saucepan over low heat and add the ghee. Stir frequently until the mixture thickens.

Pour the custard-like filling into the crust and bake for 10 minutes. Remove, cool to room temperature, and refrigerate for several hours, or until chilled.

* You may not want to use the lemon zest if you are sensitive to oxalates. Lemon zest and zest from citrus fruits are very high in oxalates. But lemons also contain citric acid, which protects the body against oxalates.

CASHEW CAKE BATTER PUDDING

BY CHRISTA ORECCHIO

SERVES 6

1 heaping cup raw cashews, soaked for 1 hour and then drained

1 cup pure water, or unsweetened almond milk or coconut water

1 teaspoon vanilla extract

3 tablespoons coconut butter

½ teaspoon dark-liquid stevia

½ teaspoon sea salt

Blend all the ingredients together in a food processor. Refrigerate and serve cool. For added pleasure, mix in carob or chocolate chips before refrigerating.

BRAIN BENEFITS

Stevia, although an accepted sugar substitute that can contribute to improved caloric management and weight control, may enhance other aspects of human health. Stevia leaf extract has been associated with antiviral, antimicrobial, anti-inflammatory, and immunostimulatory responses.[27]

BLUEBERRY SORBET

BY LISA STIMMER

SERVES 8

> 4 cups fresh or frozen blueberries
> 1 cup frozen banana pieces (optional; gives a smoother consistency and
>   some sweetness)
> ¼ cup agave syrup, or to taste*
> 1 tablespoon lemon juice
> Pinch of sea salt

Put all the ingredients into a food processor and blend until smooth. (Alternatively, you can use a food mill.) Serve immediately or, for a harder consistency, place in small serving bowls and freeze for 20 minutes. If desired, serve with fresh blueberries and a sprig of mint.

* To make this sugar-free, use a few drops of stevia to taste, or omit the sweetener if using the banana.

CHOCOLATE MOUSSE

BY LISA STIMMER

SERVES 2

> ½ cup avocado, mashed (about 1 avocado)
> 2 tablespoons unsweetened coconut milk or almond milk
> 1 tablespoon coconut oil, melted
> 2½ tablespoons agave (or a few drops of stevia), or to taste
> ½ tablespoon nonalcoholic vanilla extract
> 3 tablespoons raw unsweetened cocoa powder
> ⅛ teaspoon sea salt
> ⅛ teaspoon ground cinnamon

1. In a small food processor, blend the avocado, scraping down the sides of the bowl as needed.

2. Add the milk, oil, agave, vanilla, cocoa powder, salt, and cinnamon. Purée until fully blended.

3. Transfer the mousse to individual bowls and store in the fridge until ready to eat. Optional topping: So Delicious CocoWhip (coconut whipped cream) and fresh raspberries. Garnish with a mint leaf.

ALMOND DARK CHOCOLATE BARK WITH SEA SALT

BY JJ VIRGIN

SERVES 12

> ⅓ cup raw almonds
> 4 ounces 70% dark chocolate or higher, chopped
> ⅛ teaspoon coarse sea salt

1. Preheat the oven to 350 degrees.

2. Place the nuts on a large baking sheet in a single layer. Bake for 6 to 7 minutes, or until lightly toasted. Remove from the oven and cool for 10 minutes. Coarsely chop and set aside.

3. Place three-quarters of the chocolate in a microwavable bowl and microwave in 15-second intervals, stirring between each, until just melted. Stir in the remaining chocolate until melted. Add the chopped nuts and pour the mixture onto a parchment-covered baking sheet. Spread into a thin 12″-diameter circle.

4. Sprinkle with the salt and refrigerate for 20 to 25 minutes, or until the chocolate is set. Break into smaller pieces and store in an airtight container in a cool place.

BRAIN BENEFITS

Almonds are a tree nut that is showing promise as possible dietary interventions for age-related brain dysfunction. Tree nuts are an important source of essential nutrients, such as vitamin E, folate, and fiber. Tree nuts also contain a variety of components, such as phytochemicals like flavonoids, proanthocyanidins, and phenolic acids, as well as monounsaturated and omega-3 and omega-6 polyunsaturated fatty acids that have the potential to combat age-related brain dysfunction. Evidence is accumulating that suggests that tree nuts have the ability to mitigate cognitive decline associated with aging.[28]

CASHEW BUTTER PROTEIN BALLS

BY MAGDALENA WSZELAKI

SERVES 12

¾ cup raw cashews
2 tablespoons coconut oil, melted, plus extra if necessary
⅓ cup almond flour
⅓ cup unsweetened shredded coconut
½ teaspoon ground cinnamon
1 teaspoon pure vanilla extract
2 tablespoons water
½ cup chopped dried cranberries (or cherries)

1. Place the cashews in a large bowl and cover them with hot water. Soak for 15 minutes, then drain thoroughly.

2. Place the cashews in the bowl of a high-speed blender and process for a few minutes until a very thick paste forms, stopping to scrape down the sides of the blender every once in a while. Add the oil and process until you get a thick but smooth cashew butter. If needed, add a bit more oil until you get the texture required.

3. In a large bowl, combine the cashew butter, almond flour, shredded coconut, cinnamon, vanilla, and water. Mix until you get a homogeneous mixture, much like the texture of cookie dough. Gently fold in the cranberries until they are evenly distributed.

4. Scoop 1 tablespoon of dough and roll it into a small ball between your palms. Repeat until all the mixture is used up. You should get 12 protein balls.

5. Eat immediately, or store in an airtight container in the refrigerator for up to a week or in the freezer for up to a month.

SMOOTHIES, SHAKES, AND TONICS

BONE BROTH PROTEIN
MOCHA FUDGE SMOOTHIE RECIPE

BY JOSH AXE

SERVES 1–2

- 1 cup frozen bananas
- ¼ cup raw cashews
- 2 tablespoons cocoa powder
- 1 teaspoon carob powder
- 1 teaspoon instant coffee
- 12 ounces coconut milk
- 1 teaspoon raw honey
- 1 scoop Ancient Nutrition Bone Broth Protein Powder, "pure" or chocolate

Place all the ingredients in a blender and purée until smooth. Add water and ice to blend as necessary.

BLUEBERRY ALMOND CHIA SHAKE

BY HYLA CASS

SERVES 1

- 1 serving protein powder
- 1 cup almond milk or coconut milk (or mix half of each)
- 2 tablespoons almond butter
- 1 tablespoon chia seeds
- 4 ice cubes
- ½ cup blueberries
- Stevia, as desired

Place all the ingredients in a blender and process until smooth, adding water as desired for consistency. Enjoy!

GREEN IS EASY SMOOTHIE

BY TREVOR CATES

SERVES 1

- 1 cup organic fresh spinach
- ¼ medium green apple, cored and peeled
- 1 cup filtered water or herbal tea
- 1 serving high-quality pea protein powder
- 1 teaspoon chopped fresh cilantro
- 1 teaspoon lime juice (or to taste)

In a blender, combine all the ingredients and blend until smooth. Pour into a tall glass and enjoy cold.

CITRUS WATER INFUSED WITH GINGER AND ROSEMARY

BY ALAN CHRISTIANSON

SERVES 6–8

- 2 quarts purified water
- 1 quart ice
- 2 tablespoons thinly sliced organic fresh ginger
- 2 sprigs organic rosemary, 4"–7" long
- 1 organic lemon, sliced into ½"-thick rounds

Add all the ingredients to a large glass decanter and stir lightly. Serve and enjoy.

AVOCADO BERRY PICK-ME-UP

BY SHANNON GARRETT

- 1 cup full-fat coconut milk
- ½ ripe avocado, seed and skin removed
- ¼ cup frozen raspberries
- ¼ cup frozen wild blueberries
- 1 tablespoon organic unsweetened coconut flakes
- 1 teaspoon flax oil
- 1 teaspoon gluten-free vanilla extract

1 teaspoon raw local honey

Filtered water or ice cubes

Add the milk, avocado, berries, coconut flakes, flax oil, vanilla, and honey to a high-speed blender and blend well. Add water as needed to thin the consistency or ice cubes for a creamier smoothie. Enjoy!

CHERRY SPIRULINA SMOOTHIE

BY DONNA GATES

SERVES 2 (8-OUNCE SMOOTHIES)

1 cucumber, chopped

2 zucchinis, chopped

3 large romaine lettuce leaves, torn into pieces

¼ cup mint, leaves only

½ cup coconut meat

6 ounces frozen dark cherries

1 teaspoon Body Ecology Super Spirulina Plus

12 drops stevia, or to taste

1 cup Body Ecology Innergy Biotic, or sparkling mineral water

1 cup filtered water

Place all the ingredients in a blender and puree, adding more water if needed.

BLENDED MATCHA FRAPPE

BY ANDREA NAKAYAMA

SERVES 2

2 teaspoons matcha green tea powder

2 cups nut or hemp milk, or 1 cup full-fat coconut milk with 1 cup water

1 pear, peeled and chopped

4 dates, pitted

1 generous dash ground cinnamon

Place all the ingredients in a blender and blend until well incorporated.

BRAIN BENEFITS

Green tea powder: Tea, one of the most consumed beverages in the world, presents benefits to human health that have been associated to its abundance in polyphenols. Although these compounds reach the brain in small quantities, accumulated evidence seems to indicate that tea can help prevent neurodegeneration and delay brain function decline.[29]

BREAKFAST

LEMONY LOW-GLYCEMIC SMOOTHIE

BY ANDREA NAKAYAMA

SERVES 2

- 2 cups water
- 2 cups wild blueberries
- 1 large handful parsley
- Zest of 1 lemon
- Squeeze of half a lemon
- 1 tablespoon flax meal
- 1 knob fresh ginger, about the size of a small adult thumbnail
- 1 teaspoon ground cinnamon
- 1 teaspoon vanilla extract
- 20 drops liquid vanilla stevia
- ¼ cup Brazil nuts
- 1 tablespoon maca root powder (optional)
- Ice (optional)

In a high-speed blender, such as a Vitamix or Blendtec, add all the ingredients and blend on high until creamy and smooth. This smoothie is more on the liquid side, so be sure to add the ice if you like it a bit more slushy. With a less powerful blender, be sure to chop the parsley and add the ingredients one at a time, blending until all the ingredients are liquefied.

BRAIN BENEFITS

Flax meal: Flaxseed possesses antioxidant properties that may play a major role in reducing depression symptoms.[30]

Maca root powder: Maca is a Peruvian plant that has nutritional and energizing properties and may enhance memory and learning.[31]

TURMERIC GINGER LEMONADE

BY CHRISTA ORECCHIO

SERVES 4

- 4 cups water
- 1 teaspoon organic turmeric powder (or a 3" strip fresh turmeric root, peeled
- 1 teaspoon organic ginger powder (or a 4" strip fresh ginger, peeled)
- Honey or dark-liquid stevia
- Lemon slices, or the juice of a full lemon

1. Put the water in a medium pot over high heat and bring it to a full boil. Add the turmeric and ginger and simmer for 8 to 10 minutes. This will extract the beneficial compounds from the turmeric and ginger.

2. Remove the pot from the stove. Strain the liquid into a cup through a fine-mesh strainer to filter out the spice particles. Add the stevia and lemon to taste.

GREEN AND LEAN SMOOTHIE

BY CYNTHIA PASQUELLA

SERVES 2

- 2 handfuls spinach
- 1 handful kale
- 1 fresh mango, peeled and pitted
- 1 cucumber, chopped
- 1 cup water
- ½ cup ice

Place all the ingredients in a Vitamix, or other high-speed blender, and blend until smooth. Enjoy!

SUBSTITUTIONS

Trade out the mango for 2 cups pineapple and feel free to add any leafy greens in place of the spinach and kale. For even more green power, add 1 tablespoon spirulina or ½ teaspoon chlorophyll. For an added energy boost, add 1 teaspoon maca. If you'll be enjoying this drink after a workout, use coconut water in place of water to rehydrate. Toss in a few sprigs of cilantro for a detoxifying bonus!

BLUEBERRY-PEACH SHAKE

BY JJ VIRGIN

SERVES 1

    1–2 scoops vanilla protein blend
    1 scoop fiber blend
    ½ cup fresh or frozen blueberries
    ½ medium peach, peeled, pitted, and sliced
    ⅛ teaspoon almond extract
    8–10 ounces unsweetened coconut milk
    5 or 6 ice cubes

In a blender, combine all the ingredients and blend on high until smooth. Thin with cold water, if desired.

CHOCOLATE, FLAX, AND AVOCADO SHAKE

BY JJ VIRGIN

SERVES 1

    1–2 scoops chocolate protein blend
    1 scoop fiber blend
    ¼ small avocado
    2 teaspoons freshly ground flaxseeds
    2 teaspoons almond butter
    8–10 ounces unsweetened coconut milk
    5 or 6 ice cubes

In a blender, combine all the ingredients and blend on high until smooth. Thin with cold water, if desired.

CARROT AND TURMERIC WATER KEFIR

BY MAGDALENA WSZELAKI

SERVES 2–4

    2 cups freshly squeezed carrot juice
    2 cups freshly squeezed orange juice
    3 coins (¼" thick) fresh ginger

1 tablespoon grated fresh turmeric root or 1½ teaspoons dried
1 packet Body Ecology Kefir Starter

1. In a clean 1-quart jar, combine the carrot juice, orange juice, ginger, and turmeric. Stir to combine. Add the kefir starter and stir.

2. Cover the top of the jar with a cloth or coffee filter and secure it with a rubber band or twine. Let sit at room temperature (72 to 74 degrees) for 24 hours.

3. Remove the cover and taste. For a fizzier drink, let sit for another 12 hours. When you are happy with the flavor, top with a lid and refrigerate. Use within 1 week.

ACTION STEP WEEK 10: TRACK YOUR PROGRESS

This week, as you start using these recipes and cutting out gluten, dairy, and sugar, begin keeping a record of how you are thinking and feeling, and if you notice changes and improvements. Track your sleep, your daytime productivity, and your general sense of calm on your smartphone. You may notice that you are less anxious when you take out the foods you might be sensitive to and let the underlying chronic inflammation subside. When this happens, you'll likely see that your brain fog clears and your memory returns. We have a world to save, and we need every one of your brains to do it.

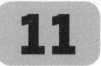

LIVING WITH ELECTROMAGNETIC POLLUTION

DOCTORS THE WORLD over are increasingly confronted with health problems with unidentified causes. As we dig deeper, these "causes" are frequently associated with accumulative toxic environments from all four quadrants of the Pyramid of Health (structure, mind-set, biochemistry, and electromagnetics), as opposed to one specific mechanism. While one or the other of the four quadrants may be more prominent, they all can play a role.

The last side of the Pyramid of Health is evaluating our risk of electromagnetic field (EMF) pollution. And it's our immune system, the armed forces of our bodies, trying to protect us, that is operating in a constant state of toxin-infiltration overload, whether it's structural toxins, emotional toxins, chemical toxins, or EMF toxins. Now, I know that some might read this and roll their eyes and say, "Really, Dr. Tom? You're going to tell me that my wired and wireless world is affecting my thinking?" Yes, I am. We have a collective history of not listening to the outliers, or the science that backs them up, when their message is inconvenient. My goal

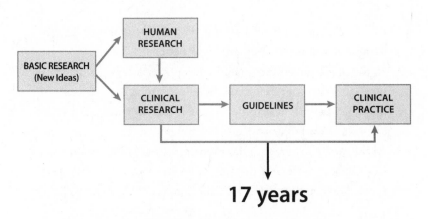

It takes an average of 17 years for basic science research to be used by your doctor.

is to bring their message about the dangers of EMFs to you in a way that makes sense and is embraceable.

This resistance to new ideas is a primary reason why the average length of time it takes for new, paradigm-shifting research to be implemented in everyday health practices is 17 years.[1] For example, it took on average 17 years from when scientists began saying there is something about cholesterol that may contribute to our pipes plugging up, and when the doctor down the street began checking cholesterol levels of patients.

Yet the facts speak for themselves:

- In the 1950s, newspapers across the western and southwestern United States carried front-page stories from government scientists telling us how "safe" the aftereffects of aboveground atomic blasts were. "Nothing to worry about" was the theme of the messaging. Now we know better.
- In the 1960s, government and industry scientists were telling us how "safe" cigarettes were. As a matter of fact, Camels were the brand of cigarettes "doctors recommended most." Now we know better.
- In the 1970s, government and industry scientists were telling us how safe it was to treat milking cows with human growth hormone. Now we know better.

- In the 1980s, government and industry panels told us how "healthy" margarine was for us. Now we know better.
- In the 1990s, government and industry scientists began telling us how safe cell phones are, even though common sense tells us that holding a battery next to our brains is probably not a good idea. Now we know better.
- At the turn of the century, the government was telling us how "safe" GMO foods were and that the extremely toxic chemicals being sprayed on our crops were "safe" for humans. Now we know better.

In 1979, I came across a research paper that identified the link between living within ¼ mile of high-power electrical wires and an increase of childhood leukemia.[2] This was my first exposure to the health risks of the electromagnetic field. Then, in 1982, I read another paper linking these same types of wires with adults and cancer in general.[3] In 1991, sleeping with an electric blanket all night long was found to increase the risk of breast cancer by 31 percent.[4] Since then, our world has only become more wired, and the electromagnetic pollution we all are exposed to has gone through the roof. Given the devastating numbers we're seeing now in the increase of all diseases and loss of life on the planet, we don't have time anymore to ignore the simple things we can do to reduce our toxic overload. But how can all of these small appliances and exposures create a big problem?

Electromagnetic radiation (EMR) delivers energy in waves, like light. It also travels at the same speed. This energy is both electric and magnetic. The waves alternate rapidly, from positive to negative in electrical terms, and from the North to South Poles in magnetic terms.

Electromagnetic radiation from any source penetrates the surrounding area, creating an electromagnetic field. This EMF is strongest at the source and weakens with increasing distance until it becomes too small to measure. However, a strong EMF can be due to either a powerful source of radiation far away or a weak radiation source close by. This is why the EMF from your smartphone next to your brain is much stronger than the EMF you experience from a cell phone tower ¼ mile away, but both have been associated with cancer development.

Penetration is a key issue when it comes to EMR health effects. Some forms of electromagnetic radiation are more penetrating than others. Electric light, for example, can penetrate air, water, and glass, but it cannot penetrate brick walls or metal sheets, and it can't penetrate far into human flesh. If you've ever done the experiment where you hold a flashlight up against your hand, you can see how far light can penetrate your skin. However, we know that x-rays easily penetrate human flesh—they wouldn't be useful otherwise.

Some common electromagnetic radiation found in our homes is very penetrating. Extremely low frequency (ELF) radiation (such as from an electrical appliance) will actually penetrate concrete pillars and metal sheets, and, of course, human flesh and bone. This radiation is relatively weak, so the measurable EMF extends for a short distance only, usually just a few feet.

Big exposures to electricity and radiation cause big problems: Think about an atomic bomb, for instance. Electricity travels across many different wavelengths and frequencies. The ones linked to poor health that we're most familiar with are x-rays: We know that too many x-rays put you at risk for cancer. Have you ever noticed how quickly dentists leave the room once they set you up for x-rays? They know how damaging accumulative small exposures can be over time.

Solar flares are another example of radiation that can affect your health. These huge explosions produce an electromagnetic field that gets projected out into space. This electromagnetic field then bombards the Earth with the radiation from the sun. The flares occur in cycles that peak every 11 years. This solar radiation is filtered by our atmosphere so that at ground level, it's not a problem for us. Have you ever noticed that when you are at the top of a mountain, hiking or skiing, you sunburn much easier than at ground level? There's a thinning of the protective atmosphere at higher elevations, so the radiation exposure is higher and we'll burn easier.

Likewise, when we are flying at 35,000 feet, the protective atmosphere is very thin, and given that the airplane is constructed of aluminum, and aluminum does not filter radiation the way that lead does, we are exposed to a substantially increased level of radiation. Which phase of the 11-year cycle we are in will determine the level of radiation exposure. If you are flying during the low part of the 11-year cycle, when you fly from New York to Los Angeles, you are exposed to radiation at the equivalent of less than one chest x-ray. However, if you are flying during the high peak of the 11-year cycle, when you fly from New York to Los Angeles, you are exposed to radiation at the equivalency of seven chest x-rays. Every time you fly. It's then no surprise that pilots have the highest incidence of lymphomas of any profession, and flight attendants have the highest incidence of hormone imbalances and pregnancy complications of any profession.[5] You don't see many pilots or flight attendants who have been flying for 30 years who have nice skin. They've aged prematurely from all of the EMF pollution. It's an environmental hazard of the job experts do not know how to compensate for, and the result is increased inflammation every day on the job and premature aging of cells.

When EMFs shine on you, their radiation actually shines *through* you. Some of it penetrates a few inches into your body. And some of it passes right through you. So it's not surprising that EMFs can affect every organ and every cell of your body. All of these exposures cause damage to us on the cellular level. Within every cell are tiny furnaces called *mitochondria*. As oxygen is taken into the body, the mitochondria use it to create the energy we need to keep the body functioning. During this process, part of the "exhaust" creates extra oxygen molecules called *free radicals*. These free radicals can damage the outer walls of our cells, and when enough damage accrues, it affects the function of tissues and organs. Usually, free radicals are neutralized by antioxidant vitamins and polyphenols that act like sponges, sopping up the free radicals. We get these vitamins from eating colorful fruits and vegetables; that's why I recommend eating different-colored vegetables every day. Every color contains a different family of vitamins, polyphenols, and antioxidants that are great for you.

However, if our diet is lacking in antioxidants and polyphenols, or we're overexposed to antigens (foods and environmental insults that stimulate an immune response), free radicals can pile up and create *oxidative stress,* a primary mechanism of inflammation and the resulting cellular damage, which accumulates and then progresses into tissue damage. When enough tissue damage has occurred, organ dysfunction begins and eventually progresses into organ disease. This is the point when you usually get a diagnosis.

Radiation and EMFs are one of the primary causes of unchecked oxidative stress. And if you keep throwing gasoline on the fire, creating inflammation by eating foods that you are sensitive to, or increasing your toxic load from other environmental pollutants, oxidative stress will fuel further inflammation, which then leads to more tissue damage, dysfunction, and eventually disease. Every exposure to EMFs increases oxidative stress. If you get damaged on one plane trip and then you go 3 weeks without flying, your body will heal itself, or the impact factor of the damage may be reduced. But if you're flying regularly, like I do, there is a cumulative effect. That's why I follow the same recommendation for radiation protection that I give to pilots and flight attendants: For 3 days before and 3 days after flying, take two to three times the antioxidant vitamins one would normally take for your weight and age.

Here's an example where I'm guesstimating the numbers, but you'll get my drift. When you have three trillion cells in your body, if you damage 100,000, you can't really tell that there's a problem. But if you destroy 100,000 cells once a week plus use your phone every day, damaging 5,000 cells a pop, and sleep next to your alarm clock, and work in a wireless office, over a couple of years, you've killed off a few hundred million cells and now have caused some damage.

EMFs AND YOUR BODY AND BRAIN

Symptoms due to EMF exposure generally get worse over time. After a long period (usually several years or even decades of EMF exposure), disease may become evident. And most startling of all, the EMF effects are now widely reported to occur at exposure levels significantly below most current national and international accepted safety limits. I imagine if we followed the discussions back before policies were set, we'd see the influence of corporate dollars, lobbyists, and scientists working to get those numbers elevated.

When an electromagnetic wave passes through your body, it induces an electric current inside you. Your body naturally uses electrical impulses for many purposes (e.g., thinking, conveying sensory information, initiating muscular movement, and controlling heartbeats). Even the chemical processes that go on in our cells, blood, body tissues, and organs, which we don't normally think of as being electrical in nature, all rely on electric charges inside the body for their proper function. An external EMF that creates electric currents within your body can, and does, interfere with many biological processes. Here are some of the more common symptoms of excessive EMF exposure in terms of brain health:

- Anxiety[6]
- Concentration difficulties[7]
- Depression[8]
- Fatigue[9]
- Headaches[10]
- Memory impairment[11]
- Nausea[12]
- Palpitations[13]
- Sleep disturbance[14]

Of course, all of these symptoms can be caused by many things, not just EMF exposure. But if you suffer from any of these symptoms, and you and your doctor do not know why, wouldn't it be sensible to assess your EMF exposure and reduce it if you can?

The most common health condition caused by EMF is electrohypersensitivity (EHS), which may already affect 3 percent of our population and is being recognized by health authorities, disability administrators and case workers, politicians, and courts of law.[15] EMFs disturb immune function through stimulation of various allergic and inflammatory responses, as well as by affecting the body's tissue repair processes. Just look at the title of an article in the journal *Pathophysiology:* "Disturbance of the Immune System by Electromagnetic Fields: A Potentially Underlying Cause for Cellular Damage and Tissue Repair Reduction Which Could Lead to

Disease and Impairment."[16] Remember, wherever the weak link in your chain is, pulling on the chain (in this case, excessive EMF exposure) can trigger the weak link to pull apart, producing symptoms. This can occur in your brain (which is common) or in any other tissue of the body.

For example, a 51-year-old diabetic man once tested his blood sugar when he was working at his computer; the test registered that his blood sugar was high. This was the weak link in his chain. When he walked away from his computer, within 10 minutes, his blood sugar dropped by more than 10 percent.[17] The effect of the electromagnetic toxicity of his computer showed up in his blood-sugar-regulating system. What made this case so interesting was the unusually quick change in blood sugar levels.

Here's another example: When filters are installed to block EMFs, such as when Graham-Stetzer (GS) filters have been installed in schools with sick building syndrome, both staff and students report improved health and more energy. In one study, the number of students needing inhalers for asthma was reduced in one school, and student behavior associated with ADD/ADHD improved in another. Blood sugar levels for some diabetics respond to the amount of dirty electricity in their environment, such as in the example of the diabetic man above. People with type 1 diabetes require less insulin and those with type 2 diabetes have lower blood sugar levels in an electromagnetically clean environment. Individuals diagnosed with multiple sclerosis have better balance and fewer tremors. Those requiring a cane walked unassisted within a few days to weeks after GS filters were installed in their homes.[18]

SOURCES OF EMF POLLUTION

Practically every new invention adds something to electromagnetic radiation pollution. Much of this is pulsed digital radio-frequency EMF from digital communications devices—probably the most dangerous kind for your health because of the sheer volume of exposure. In terms of electromagnetic exposure, we are literally swimming in a pool of EMF pollution, and one that gets bigger with each passing year. In the 1970s we were worried about color televisions and wristwatches with batteries. Then there were computers, the first mobile phones, then laptops and smartphones. The biggest television just 20 years ago was 19 inches, and today's 50-inch screens emit far more EMFs. So it's logical to assume that our children will experience greater EMF exposure than we did in the past. Today, we can find EMF pollution in the following:

- Batteries, of all shapes and sizes
- Cars, motorcycles, buses, trains, and planes
- Cell or mobile phones
- Cell phone masts
- Computers
- Digital phones and base stations
- Electrical appliances (including TVs)
- Electronic equipment
- High- and low-voltage power lines
- House wiring
- Microwave ovens
- Radio and TV transmitters
- Smart meters (electricity or gas meters that transmit radio signals)
- Wearable performance trackers (that monitor heart rate, sleep, and steps)
- Wireless baby monitors and base stations
- Wireless gaming consoles and base stations

YOU SHOULD BE SCARED OF YOUR MOBILE PHONE

Of the world's seven billion people, six billion have mobile phones. Children and teenagers are 500 percent more likely to get brain cancer if they use mobile phones. The research announced at the Royal Society of Medicine was reported at the first international conference on mobile phones and health. It came from a further analysis of data from one of the biggest studies carried out on the mobile phone/cancer link, headed by Professor Lennart Hardell, MD, PhD. Professor Hardell told the conference that people who started mobile phone use before the age of 20 had more than a fivefold increase in glioma, a malignant type of brain cancer.

Earlier we talked about the reduction in sperm count in men. Here's one of the reasons why: Mobile phone use not only causes a reduction in sperm motility and function, but it also damages the DNA (a man's blueprint of reproduction).[19]

Finally, an analysis of early unpublished data shows just how much higher the electromagnetic radiation absorption rates are in a 5- and 10-year-old's brain versus that of an adult. Electromagnetic radiation, the data shows, can penetrate almost straight through the entire brain of a 5-year-old child! A child's skull is much thinner than an adult's, so it provides less of a filter. Why is this so troublesome?

- Because more energy from a phone penetrates a child's skull, children will absorb more radiation.
- Children's cells are reproducing more quickly than adults'.
- Children's immune systems (their protection) are not as well developed as those of adults.
- Children have a longer potential for lifetime exposure, thus a higher risk.

Further, there is more than an 80 percent increased risk of a child having behavioral issues if his or her mother used a cell phone during pregnancy. When moms used a handset just two or three times a day during pregnancy, it was enough to raise the risk of their babies developing hyperactivity and difficulties with conduct, emotions, and relationships by the time they reached school age. Later on, when the children began using cell phones themselves, they were:

- 80 percent more likely to suffer from behavioral difficulties
- 25 percent more at risk to suffer from emotional problems

- 34 percent more likely to suffer from difficulties relating to their peers
- 35 percent more likely to be hyperactive
- 49 percent more prone to have problems with conduct[20]

The only good news, if there is any, is that the penetration capabilities of cell phones are relatively low in adults, but when you hold a battery to your head, it doesn't have to penetrate very far in the air to reach you. The electromagnetic penetration of a mobile phone drops by almost 50 percent if the phone is held ½ inch away from the body. The penetration power reduces by 66 percent if held 1 inch from the body.[21] When you put your phone in the pocket of your shirt, you are much more vulnerable to heart dysfunction.[22] If you put it in your pants pocket, you become more vulnerable to poor semen quality, infertility, prostate dysfunction, and prostate cancer.[23]

And, of course, the icing on the cake on this topic comes when you look at how the manufacturers protect themselves. Ever read the legal documents that come with an iPhone? Deep in the small print there is this statement: "Carry iPhone at least 10 millimeters away from your body to ensure exposure levels remain at or below the as-tested levels."

While it's extremely difficult for researchers to prove that cell phones and the electromagnetic radiation they produce cause disease, there are associations you should know about. Most of the reports conclude with a reasonable suspicion of mobile phone risk that exists based on clear evidence of a connection between prolonged exposures and these health problems:[24]

- **Overly excited brain cells.** Researchers from Italy found that the electromagnetic field emitted by cell phones can cause some cells in the brain's cortex (adjacent to the side of phone use) to become excited for about an hour, while others become inhibited.
- **DNA damage.** The German research group Verum studied the effect of radiation on human and animal cells. After being exposed to cell phone frequencies, the cells showed increased breaks in their DNA. These DNA breaks could not always be repaired,

and the damage would therefore be passed on to future cells and could predispose them to becoming cancerous.

- **Brain cell damage.** A study of the effects of cell phone frequencies on animal brains showed damage to the brain cells in various brain parts, including the cortex (the outermost or superficial layer of the brain), the hippocampus (which plays important roles in the consolidation of information from short-term memory to long-term memory, and in spatial memory that enables navigation), and the basal ganglia (which controls voluntary motor movements, procedural learning, routine behaviors or "habits" such as teeth grinding, eye movements, cognition, and emotion).
- **Increased risk of brain tumor.** Eleven different teams of researchers have published studies telling us that using a cell phone held against your ear for more than 10 years more than doubles your risk of developing a brain tumor.[25]
- **Increased risk of depression, anxiety, and cancer.** Eight of the 10 research papers studying the impact of living at distances less than 500 meters (the distance of five football fields) from cell tower base stations reported increased prevalence of adverse neurobehavioral symptoms (depression, anxiety) or cancer. None of the studies reported exposure above accepted international guidelines, suggesting that current guidelines may be inadequate in protecting our health.[26]

Obviously, this is a topic that none of us want to hear about; we all live on our smartphones. But isn't the inconvenience of using a corded headset instead of holding the phone directly to your head and avoiding a Bluetooth transmitter a minor one worth considering when you're trying to get healthier? Especially when you're working on enhancing your brain function and slowing down a degenerative, inflammatory condition in your brain, this "base hit" can give you big returns in the long run.

The following recommendations have been consistently made by panels of scientists from all over the world. I realize these recommendations can come across as harsh, and they may cost extra dollars. But what is every child's brain worth? Read these and be part of the solution, creating the change necessary so we can all lead healthier lives going forward. Remember what Albert Einstein said: "The problems we have created today cannot be solved with the same level of thinking that created the problem."

- Use a protective cell phone cover on your phone. I use one on my phone that reduces the radiation by more than 90 percent. Just google cell phone radiation covers; there are a number to choose from.
- Children of any age should not be using mobile and cordless phones.
- Whenever possible, pregnant women should avoid using mobile devices without a case, and they should avoid being in close proximity to people who are using their phones without a case.
- Avoid living near mobile towers or high-power electrical lines.
- Avoid schools installing wireless networks (keep computers hardwired).
- Avoid wireless (Bluetooth-type) headsets.
- Encourage auto-off switches for mobile phones when not in use.
- Use landline telephones whenever possible.
- Limit use of cordless phones and other wireless devices, wireless toys and baby monitors, wireless Internet, wireless security systems, etc.

"But wait. That's my whole life using these devices."
"That's my point."

GRAB ONTO THE LADDER: WHAT YOU CAN DO TO AVOID EMF POLLUTION

Most of the EMF pollution you are affected by is probably coming from something inside your house. What electrical equipment do you have in your house? What electronic equipment do you have nearby, or on your person? Are these devices having a subtle effect on you or a family member? If you know which is the strongest source of EMF in your environment, you can reduce your exposure by switching it off, whenever possible, and moving farther away from it. If it is a wireless device, replace it with a wired alternative.

TEST FOR EMF WITH A METER

I used to give my patients an EMF meter to take with them and test their homes overnight. An EMF meter tests for EMF leakage. Any leakage above 3.0 on this device is considered a problem. You can test your walls, electrical outlets, light switches, kitchen appliances, and any electrical or battery-powered devices. You can also check your car, especially if you have an electric car or hybrid. One of the potential problems with electric cars is the amount of EMF leakage. This doesn't mean that electric cars are worse than gas cars. The point is to figure out how to make electric cars safer.

THE CASE FOR GETTING A GREAT CASE FOR YOUR PHONE

I drive an Acura, and when I walk up within 10 feet of the car, the outside lights under the side-view mirrors and the internal dome lights automatically go on (so I can see a little clearer). How does that happen? My car key is emitting a frequency that's received by my car ("Heads up, here comes the owner"). It works only within 10 feet, but if I press on the alarm button to find the car from 20 feet away, that function will work. This means there are different degrees of frequencies the key can emit. When I'm holding my car key in my hand along with my cell phone, the car key will not turn on the lights as I walk up to the car and the car door does not unlock when I touch it. I have to take the car key out of the hand that's holding my cell phone. Why? The case I put on my phone is disrupting the electrical frequency of anything in its path, and thus it's also interrupting the key's "heads-up" message. There are many reasons to choose a case on your smartphone—appearance, protection when the phone is dropped, and/or reducing the EMFs emitted from the phone without disturbing reception. I vote for the last one.

The Pong brand makes a phone case that diffuses the electromagnetic broadcasting that's occurring from the car key. If I take the Pong device off and hold my car key in my hand with my cell phone, the car key works just fine. Once again, base hits win the ball game.

TAKE THE PHONE AWAY FROM YOUR HEAD

Whether you have a smartphone or a flip phone, everyone needs to be using a corded headset, corded earphones, or the speakerphone function when they make a call. This will keep the phone's battery away from your head. Bluetooth headsets are not an option, because you're still putting a little battery right near your brain.

WATCH YOUR WATCH

We started putting batteries in watches only around 1977. Now we think it's normal. No. It's common, but it's not normal. Nowadays, almost all watches have batteries. The smartphone watches also have EMF monitors, as well as fitness trackers, like FitBits. Check all watches for EMF pollution.

NIGHTTIME ROUTINES TO COMBAT EMFS

Turn off the wireless routers at home at night when you're going to sleep. You don't need them on, and turning them off will allow for better sleep.

Also, move your alarm clock and your cell phone away from your bed. Put them on the other side of the room so you're forced to get out of bed to shut them off. You won't hit the snooze button as often, and you'll be keeping the EMFs away from your head.

ACTION STEP WEEK 11: LEARN MORE ABOUT ELECTROMAGNETIC POLLUTION

Spend 1 hour a week learning more about electromagnetic pollution. Web sites like mercola.com and greenmedinfo.com post the most recent studies on EMFs. Approaching this issue from the idea that base hits win the ballgame, you'll be able to handle the "overwhelm factor" as you learn more about the dangers of cell phones and EMF leakage in general. Just like any other aspect of enhancing your health, within 6 months at 1 hour a week, you will have the knowledge to make your home much more EMF-friendly, for you and your family.

12

KEEP ASKING WHY, AND YOU'LL GET OUT OF THE POOL

DO YOU REMEMBER the prayer I included in Chapter 6, from my mentor, Dr. George Goodheart? He would always begin his Sunday morning lecture with that same prayer, and then he would talk about his philosophy of health care for an hour. He would continually drill it into us, every weekend, as if it were the first time he saw us, constantly saying, "Ask yourself, why. Why does the patient have these particular symptoms? Why do they have this complaint, or pain, or rash?"

As he said this, he would stomp his foot into the ground and take his right hand and make a fist and swing it through the air. He would do this every single time in exactly the same way, trying to bang his imperative into our heads, emphasizing how important it was to think outside the box and not rely on a cookie-cutter protocol that was supposed to work for every single patient who comes through our doors.

This investigative approach was an incredible part of my training. The consistency of his message from the prayer to the hour-long dialogue drilled his wisdom into our heads and set the stage for how I think about health care. You must ask why, or as we've been talking about in this book, get the best life jacket possible with the fewest side effects, and then get out of the water, walk up the hill, walk back upstream, and figure out what fell in the water that eventually went downstream and took you over the waterfall. My medical practice has always been an exploration in asking *why* is this patient's health affected, and then addressing and reversing the whys. In functional medicine, we call that going upstream.

I also realized early on in my career that whenever you have the opportunity to experience one of the great minds, in any field, it's critical to see what they do and how they do it, but more important, to capture how they think. My daughter learned this lesson as well. When she decided that she wanted to go to law school, she applied to a number of schools, some in the top tier, and others as well. She was accepted to all of them, and then she was faced with a difficult decision: how to choose the one that would be best for her. She had spent 8 years working in Washington, DC, so she called a friend who was very well respected in government circles. His advice was to read the research papers published by the professors whom she would be studying with at each school, and to see which ones resonated with her and how these people were able to express themselves.

My daughter took this advice, read all the research papers, and determined the professors whom she would most like to study with, based on their writings. She was so confident in her decision that she turned down the Ivy Leagues and accepted a spot at DePaul University in Chicago, where she eventually graduated cum laude. She came right out of school and applied for a job where there were 10,000 applicants. She got the job and clerked for the 7th Circuit Court of Appeals. She is now an Assistant US Attorney.

Just as my daughter chose whom she would learn to think from, my prayer is that you can embrace the thinking of the hundreds of research teams that tell us to go upstream. My goal has been to share what these researchers say about the science of regenerating your brain, so that you can see the bigger picture. I hope that you've gotten something out of this book that has spurred you on to learn more about the factors and mechanisms that are influencing the way you are thinking and feeling.

By now you see that my approach is not cookie-cutter at all. There is no single cure for many of the diseases and conditions that affect the brain. There is no one cure for Alzheimer's, and there never will be. There will never be a pill to resolve Alzheimer's, just as there is no one pill to address diabetes. Both of these diseases, and hundreds more, exist on the autoimmune spectrum and are influenced by a variety of factors. Now you know that you can address each of the factors, one by one, base hit by base hit. Eventually, you will win the ball game.

Do you know what my mentor Dr. George Goodheart would say after his Sunday morning prayer? "If anyone doesn't like it, it's too bad, it's my football." Well, your health journey is your football. Play hard. Give it your best. We're cheering for you.

WEEKLY BASE HITS FOR OPTIMAL BRAIN HEALTH

Week 1: Listen to your body so that you can notice changes that occur before they turn into bigger brain health problems. Even if you're having symptoms that just annoy you, like poor sleep, but aren't stopping your daily living, they still need to be taken seriously.

Week 2: Read more from Dr. Dale Bredesen. Download his landmark article from my Web site, or check out his new book, *The End of Alzheimer's,* to find out how his work validates what you've learned in this book.

Week 3: Start keeping track of what you are eating in terms of gluten, dairy, and sugar. Write down or enter into your smartphone every time you eat one of these three culprits. You'll have to start reading labels more carefully. The good news is that even after just a few days of cutting back, you'll notice a difference in your sleep, your productivity, and your memory.

Week 4: Review the Environmental Working Group's Web site, EWG.org, and learn more about healthy consumer products and the importance of organic food choices, so you can avoid the toxic ones.

Week 5: Set a baseline for great brain health by creating a completely comprehensive timeline with the free tools on my Web site.

Week 6: Find a functional medicine practitioner in your area who understands how to work with you and your timeline. Schedule a physical and talk to your doctor about these important supplements: folate (vitamin B_9), cobalamin (vitamin B_{12}), vitamin D_3, vitamin C, vitamin E, fish oils, the adaptogenic herbs, and plant foods high in phytochemicals, phytonutrients, and polyphenols.

Week 7: Work on strengthening your core—the muscles that support your spinal structure. Try the exercise outlined in Chapter 7, or add some abdominal work into your workout.

Week 8: Try Dr. Pedram Shojai's exercise in conscious breathing.

Week 9: Start following the instructions for eliminating gluten, dairy, and sugar. Stop throwing gasoline on the fire by avoiding gluten, dairy, and sugar, and choosing local and organic produce and meats/fish whenever possible. Add a cup of green tea to your daily regimen, and turn genes on to rebuild stronger, more vibrant, more resilient cells with adaptogenic herbs.

Week 10: As you start using the recipes and cutting out gluten, dairy, and sugar, keep a record of how you are thinking and feeling, and if you notice changes and improvements.

Week 11: Learn more about electromagnetic pollution. Web sites such as mercola.com and greenmedinfo.com post the most recent studies on EMFs.

Week 12: Recognize and identify all of the small wins, the base hits, you've been using to enhance your brain health. If you can remember them all, you're already making progress.

APPENDIX: RECIPE CONTRIBUTORS

Nanette Achziger is a healthy gut advocate, culinary explorer, author, and founder of an online gut health blog. She is passionate about sharing how easy it is to achieve gut health and well-being. Through tips and tools in her blog and in her book, *Kaizen*, Achziger shares ways to reduce toxic exposure and nourish your gut through food.

Dave Asprey is founder and CEO of Bulletproof, the world's first human performance and nutrition company. He is a Silicon Valley investor and technology entrepreneur who spent two decades and over $1 million to hack his own biology. Asprey is the creator of Bulletproof Coffee, host of the top-rated health podcast *Bulletproof Radio*, and author of the *New York Times* bestseller *The Bulletproof Diet*. He is also the founder of 40 Years of Zen, a $2.5 million brain-training and cognitive performance facility, and host of the largest biohacking conference in the world.

Asprey hacked his own health to lose 100 pounds and lower his biological age, all while increasing his IQ and learning how to gain more energy with less sleep. The *Financial Times* calls him a "bio-hacker who takes self-quantification to the extreme of self-experimentation."

Dr. Josh Axe is a doctor of natural medicine, chiropractic physician, and clinical nutritionist who operates one of the world's largest health Web sites. He is an expert in functional medicine, digestive health, and herbal remedies. He is also the bestselling author of *Eat Dirt* as well as *Essential Oils: Ancient Medicine*. Dr. Axe cofounded the Ancient Nutrition supplement company, which provides bone broth protein and certified organic herbal formulas.

Dr. Hyla Cass is a nationally acclaimed innovator and expert in the fields of integrative medicine, psychiatry, and addiction recovery. Dr. Cass helps individuals take charge of their health. One area is in withdrawing from both psychiatric medication and substances of abuse with the aid of natural supplements. Dr. Cass appears often as a guest on national radio and television, including *The Dr. Oz Show, E! Entertainment,* and *The View,* and in national print media. She has been quoted in many national magazines, blogs for the *Huffington Post,* and is the author of several bestselling books, including *Natural Highs; 8 Weeks to Vibrant Health; Supplement Your Prescription: What Your Doctor Doesn't Know About Nutrition;* and her ebook, *The Addicted Brain and How to Break Free.* She has created her own line of innovative nutritional supplements.

A member of the Medical Advisory Board of the Health Sciences Institute and *Taste for Life* magazine, Dr. Cass is also associate editor of *Total Health Magazine,* and she has served on the boards of California Citizens for Health and the American College for Advancement in Medicine. A native of Toronto, she graduated from the University of Toronto School of Medicine, interned at Los Angeles County–USC Medical Center, and completed a psychiatric residency at Cedars-Sinai Medical Center/UCLA. She is a Diplomate of the American Board of Psychiatry and Neurology and of the American Board of Integrative Holistic Medicine.

Dr. Trevor Cates is a nationally recognized naturopathic doctor. She is known as "The Spa Dr." and was the first woman licensed as a naturopathic doctor in the state of California. She was appointed by former governor Arnold Schwarzenegger to California's Bureau of Naturopathic Medicine Advisory Council. She has worked with world-renowned spas and sees patients in her private practice in Park City, Utah, with a focus on graceful aging and glowing skin. She has been featured on *The Doctors, Extra, First for Women,* and *Mind Body Green* and is host of *The Spa Dr.* podcast. Dr. Cates believes the key to healthy skin is inner *and* outer nourishment with nontoxic ingredients. Her book, *Clean Skin from Within,* was released in March 2017. Dr. Cates's The Spa Dr. skin care and supplement lines are formulated with natural and organic ingredients designed to help you achieve the clean and natural path to confidence and beautiful skin.

Alan Christianson is the *New York Times* bestselling author of *The Adrenal Reset Diet* and the founder of Integrative Health.

Heather Dubé, BA, INHC, CWC, CPT, and Damian Dubé, BS, FMP-P, FDN, CES, are Functional and Diagnostic Nutritionists. They empower individuals to take their body, mind, and spirit back naturally from thyroid imbalance, fatigue, and weight-related disorders. They are the cofounders of the e3 Energy Evolved System, a thyroid, autoimmune, and metabolism restoration methodology that helps people create natural wellness and fat loss even without exercise.

They began developing this system during their own healing journey. Heather was able to resolve her struggle with Hashimoto's thyroiditis, chronic fatigue, and autoimmune disease through individualized nutrition, movement, stress reduction, and lifestyle changes—and she returned to competitive athletics in just over two years. She did all this without Synthroid or other drugs.

Heather and Damian are expert contributors to *Experience Life* and *OnFitness* magazines and serve as nutrition science peer reviewers for TapouT XT.

Shannon Garrett, BS, RN, CNN, is a Certified Functional Nurse-Nutritionist and Autoimmune Thyroid Wellness Nurse Consultant for women. She serves on the advisory board of HeyHashi and is also a featured resource on the LDN Research Trust Web site as an LDN nurse educator. Garrett teaches women how to reverse the symptoms of Hashimoto's thyroiditis by incorporating lifestyle changes and customized nutrition. She is the author of *The Hashi's Sisters Guide to Low-Dose Naltrexone.*

Garrett is the founder of Holistic Thyroid Care and Shannon Garrett Wellness, Inc. She studied at the prestigious Aquinas College School of Nursing and Amridge University, and she continues her education in functional medicine and nutrition. She was one of the top graduates of the inaugural 12-week practitioner course at the Hashimoto's Institute.

Donna Gates, MEd, ABAAHP, is the international bestselling author of *The Body Ecology Diet: Recovering Your Health and Rebuilding Your Immunity; The Body Ecology Guide to Growing Younger: Anti-Aging Wisdom for Every Generation;* and *Stevia: Cooking with Nature's Calorie-Free Sweetener.* An Advanced Fellow with the American Academy of Anti-Aging Medicine, she is on a mission to change the way the world eats. The Body Ecology Diet was the first of its kind—sugar-free, gluten-free, casein-free, and probiotic rich. In 1994, Gates introduced the natural sweetener stevia to the United States, began teaching about fermented foods, and coined the phrase "inner ecosystem" to describe the network of microbes that maintains our basic physiological processes, from digestion to immunity. Over the past 25 years, she has become one of the most respected authorities in the field of digestive health, diet, and nutrition. A recognized host of *The Body Ecology Hour with Donna Gates* on Hay House radio, Gates regularly contributes to the *Huffington Post* and lectures at the "I Can Do It!" Conference, the Longevity Now Conference, and the Women's Wellness Conference.

Gates has been instrumental in transforming the natural foods industry. Stevia was approved as a "dietary supplement" and became a common item in every U.S. health food store. She educated society on the value of coconut oil, which had been demonized as a dangerous fat but is now promoted by holistic doctors. She also reintroduced kefir to the U.S. marketplace. Gates works with top doctors in the field of autism who view her diet as instrumental in changing the theory behind and treatment of the disorder. She founded Body Ecology Diet Recovering Our Kids (BEDROK), an active online community of over 2,000 parents, many of whom have seen their children in full recovery.

Randy Hartnell is president of Vital Choice Wild Seafood & Organics, the leading online seafood company that he and wife, Carla, founded in 2001. He is responsible for guiding the company on its mission of helping consumers source high-quality sustainable seafood, while educating them about the impact of food choices on their health, the environment, and the commercial fishing community. Hartnell is the public face of Vital Choice, fostering relationships with environmentally minded, health-conscious consumers and nutrition-oriented health and wellness advocates. Prior to founding Vital Choice, he spent more than 20 years as a commercial salmon fisherman in Alaska. He is a Washington State native and holds a degree in English literature from the University of California, Berkeley.

Andrea Nakayama is a Functional Nutritionist and Educator who is leading patients and practitioners around the world on a revolution to reclaim ownership of their health. Her passion for food as personalized medicine was born from the loss of her young husband to a brain tumor in 2002. Through her work at Replenish PDX, Nakayama is now regularly consulted as the nutrition expert for the toughest clinical cases in the practices of many world-renowned doctors, and she trains a thousand practitioners each year in her methodologies at Holistic Nutrition Lab.

Christa Orecchio, founder of The Whole Journey, is a clinical and holistic nutritionist with a passion for helping people to heal and achieve vibrant health. After healing herself from chronic candida, brain fog, and thyroid and adrenal problems, Orecchio was able to access a new level of health and happiness she previously did not think was possible. This inspired her to leave the business world to study holistic nutrition in 2003 so that she could "pay it forward" and help others experience the same powerful shifts.

Orecchio combines her holistic and scientific knowledge to help people heal, using food as their medicine, with a mind-body-spirit approach to wholeness. She has 10 years of private practice experience, is a local and national health TV show host, is the bestselling author of *How to Conceive Naturally*, and created Kick Candida for Good and the revolutionary Gut Thrive in 5 microbiome rejuvenation program.

Cynthia Pasquella is a celebrity nutritionist, spiritual leader, media personality, bestselling author, and the founder and director of the Institute of Transformational Nutrition. Pasquella is famous for inspiring millions of women to discover what they're really hungry for so they can make peace with food and themselves. She is the creator and host of "What You're Really Hungry For," a Web series that goes beyond food and examines why you know what to do to get healthy but still won't do it, as well as the secrets behind having the body, health, and life you've always wanted. Pasquella is a nutrition expert for *The Doctors*, *The Dr. Phil Show*, and *The Today Show* and has been featured in popular media outlets such as *Access Hollywood*, *E! News Live*, *Harper's Bazaar*, *Fitness* magazine, *Shape* magazine, and *Marie Claire*.

Ocean Robbins is cofounder and CEO of the Food Revolution Network, adjunct professor in Chapman University's Peace Studies Department, and coauthor with his dad, bestselling author John Robbins, of *Voices of the Food Revolution*. He launched Youth for Environmental Sanity (YES!) at age 16 and directed the organization for 20 years. Ocean Robbins has spoken in person to more than 200,000 people and facilitated hundreds of gatherings for leaders from over 65 nations. He is a recipient of many awards, including the Freedom's Flame Award and the national Jefferson Award for Outstanding Public Service.

Elaine De Santos was a frustrated stay-at-home mom who became a family health revolutionary and a certified transformational nutrition coach after dealing with the health issues of her family members. She experienced an immune system breakdown of her own that was a result of being overstressed and overtired from caring for her kids with allergies and her husband, Michael, who had a life-changing brain scare. Together, Elaine and Michael founded Family for Health with a mission to help families get healthier one meal at a time so that they grow better together and stay healthy for life.

Lisa Stimmer is the author of *Gluten-Free Vitality Diet* and *Eating for Vitality Diet*. Her programs provide step-by-step guidance for busy people to easily maintain a healthy gluten-free lifestyle with confidence. Through Stimmer's own journey from sickness to health, she has made it her goal to help others with health issues continue to enjoy tasty food. She has lived and thrived on this lifestyle for 30-plus years. She is a Certified Gluten Practitioner, Certified Natural Gourmet Chef, Certified Nutritionist, and Healthy Lifestyle Coach.

JJ Virgin is a celebrity nutrition and fitness expert who teaches clients how to lose weight and master their mind-set so they can lead bigger, better lives. She is the author of four *New York Times* bestsellers: *The Virgin Diet, The Virgin Diet Cookbook, JJ Virgin's Sugar Impact Diet*, and *JJ Virgin's Sugar Impact Diet Cookbook*. Her memoir, *Miracle Mindset: A Mother, Her Son, and Life's Hardest Lessons,* explores the powerful lessons in strength and positivity that she learned after her son Grant was the victim of a brutal hit-and-run accident. Virgin hosts the popular *JJ Virgin Lifestyle Show* podcast and regularly writes for *Huffington Post, Rodale Wellness,* and other major blogs and magazines. She's also a frequent guest on TV and radio and speaks at major events. In addition to her work with nutrition and fitness, Virgin is a business coach and founded the premier health entrepreneur event and community, The Mindshare Summit.

Izabella Wentz, PharmD, FASCP, is an internationally acclaimed thyroid specialist and licensed pharmacist who dedicated her career to addressing the root causes of autoimmune thyroid disease after being diagnosed with Hashimoto's thyroiditis in 2009. Dr. Wentz is the author of the *New York Times* bestselling patient guide *Hashimoto's Thyroiditis: Lifestyle Interventions for Finding and Treating the Root Cause* and the protocol-based book *Hashimoto's Protocol: A 90-Day Plan for Reversing Thyroid Symptoms and Getting Your Life Back*. As a patient advocate, researcher, clinician, and educator, she is committed to raising awareness on how to overcome autoimmune thyroid disease through *The Thyroid Secret* documentary series, the Hashimoto's Institute practitioner training, and her international consulting and speaking services, offered to both patients and health-care professionals.

Magdalena Wszelaki is the founder of Hormones Balance, a nutrition practice dedicated to helping women rebalance their hormones with nutritional and lifestyle changes. Wszelaki is a certified nutrition coach, speaker, educator, and soon-to-be-published cookbook author with a long history of hormonal challenges. Her health crisis was the direct result of a highly stressful life in advertising—starting with Graves' disease and later Hashimoto's disease (autoimmune conditions causing thyroid failure), adrenal fatigue, and estrogen dominance. Today she is in full remission, lives a symptoms-free, awesome life, and teaches women how to accomplish the same in her online programs and education.

NOTES

INTRODUCTION

1. Calderón-Garcidueñas L, Franco-Lira M, Mora-Tiscareño A, Medina-Cortina H, Torres-Jardón R, Kavanaugh M. Early Alzheimer's and Parkinson's disease pathology in urban children: Friend versus Foe responses—it is time to face the evidence. *BioMed Research International* 2013;2013:161687. doi: 10.1155/2013/161687. Epub 2013 Feb 7.

1: AUTOIMMUNITY: HOW IT AFFECTS BRAIN FUNCTION

1. Dobbs SM, Dobbs RJ, Weller C, Charlett A, Augustin A, Taylor D, Ibrahim MA, Bjarnason I. Peripheral aetiopathogenic drivers and mediators of Parkinson's disease and co-morbidities: role of gastrointestinal microbiota. *Journal of Neurovirology* 2016 Feb;22(1):22–32.
2. Mez J, Daneshvar DH, Kiernan PT et al. Clinicopathological evaluation of chronic traumatic encephalopathy in players of American football. *JAMA* 2017;318(4):360–70. doi:10.1001/jama.2017.8334.
3. Dantzer R, O'Connor JC, Freund GG, Johnson RW, Kelley KW. From inflammation to sickness and depression: when the immune system subjugates the brain. *Nature Reviews. Neuroscience* 2008 Jan;9(1):46–56.

4. http://www.alz.org/facts.

5. Eisenmann A, Murr C, Fuchs D, Ledochowski M. Gliadin IgG antibodies and circulating immune complexes. *Scandinavian Journal of Gastroenterology* 2009;44(2):168–71.

6. Watad A, Bragazzi NL, Adawi M, Amital H, Kivity S, Mahroum N, Blank M, Shoenfeld Y. Is autoimmunology a discipline of its own? A big data–based bibliometric and scientometric analyses. *Autoimmunity* 2017 Jun;50(4):269–74. doi: 10.1080/08916934.2017.1305361. Epub 2017 Mar 23.

2: THE LEAKY BRAIN

1. Schubert CR, Fischer ME, Pinto AA, Klein BEK, Klein R, Tweed TS, Cruickshanks KJ. Sensory impairments and risk of mortality in older adults. *The Journals of Gerontology. Series A, Biological Sciences and Medical Sciences* 2017 May 1;72(5):710–5. doi:10.1093/gerona/glw036.

2. Lafaille-Magnan ME, Poirier J, Etienne P, Tremblay-Mercier J, Frenette J, Rosa-Neto P, Breitner JCS; PREVENT-AD Research Group. Odor identification as a biomarker of preclinical AD in older adults at risk. *Neurology* 2017 Jul 25;89(4): 327–35.

3. Vojdani A. Brain-reactive antibodies in traumatic brain injury. *Functional Neurology, Rehabilitation, and Ergonomics* 2013;3(2–3):173–81.

4. Koh SX, Lee JK. S100B as a marker for brain damage and blood-brain barrier disruption following exercise. *Sports Medicine* 2014 Mar;44(3):369–85. doi: 10.1007/s40279-013-0119-9. Review. Erratum in: *Sports Medicine* 2014 Jun;44(6):867.

5. Wolff G, Davidson SJ, Wrobel JK, Toborek M. Exercise maintains blood-brain barrier integrity during early stages of brain metastasis formation. *Biochemical and Biophysical Research Communications* 2015 Aug 7;463(4):811–7.

6. Hemmings WA. The entry into the brain of large molecules derived from dietary protein. *Proceedings of the Royal Society of London. Series B, Biological Sciences* 1978 Feb 23;200(1139):175–92.

7. Wan W, Chen H, Li Y. The potential mechanisms of Aβ-receptor for advanced glycation end-products interaction disrupting tight junctions of the blood-brain barrier in Alzheimer's disease. *International Journal of Neuroscience* 2014 Feb;124(2):75–81.

8. Varatharaj A, Galea I. The blood-brain barrier in systemic inflammation. *Brain, Behavior, and Immunity* 2017 Feb;60:1–12.

9. Thelin EP, Nelson DW, Bellander BM. A review of the clinical utility of serum S100B protein levels in the assessment of traumatic brain injury. *Acta Neurochirurgica (Wien)* 2017 Feb;159(2):209–25.

10. Cheng F, Yuan Q, Yang J, Wang W, Liu H. The prognostic value of serum neuron-specific enolase in traumatic brain injury: systematic review and meta-analysis. *PLoS One* 2014 Sep 4;9(9):e106680.

11. Hadjivassiliou M, Sanders DD, Aeschlimann DP. Gluten-related disorders: gluten ataxia. *Digestive Diseases* 2015;33(2):264–8.

12. Kharrazian D, Vojdani A. Correlation between antibodies to bisphenol A, its target enzyme protein disulfide isomerase and antibodies to neuron-specific antigens. *Journal of Applied Toxicology* 2017 Apr;37(4):479–84.

13. Vojdani A, Mukherjee PS, Berookhim J, Kharrazian D. Detection of antibodies against human and plant aquaporins in patients with multiple sclerosis. *Autoimmune Diseases* 2015;2015.

14. Chen X, Threlkeld SW, Cummings EE, Juan I, Makeyev O, Besio WG, Gaitanis J, Banks WA, Sadowska GB, Stonestreet BS. Ischemia-reperfusion impairs blood-brain barrier function and alters tight junction protein expression in the ovine fetus. *Neuroscience* 2012 Dec 13;226:89–100.

15. Niederhofer H, Pittschieler K. A preliminary investigation of ADHD symptoms in persons with celiac disease. *Journal of Attention Disorders* 2006 Nov;10(2):200–4.

16. Rossignol DA, Rossignol LW, Smith S et al. Hyperbaric treatment for children with autism: a multicenter, randomized, double-blind, controlled trial. *BMC Pediatrics* 2009;9:21.

17. Addolorato G, Di Giuda D, De Rossi G, Valenza V, Domenicali M, Caputo F, Gasbarrini A, Capristo E, Gasbarrini G. Regional cerebral hypoperfusion in patients with celiac disease. *American Journal of Medicine* 2004 Mar 1;116(5):312–7.

18. Ballabh P, Braun A, Nedergaard M. The blood-brain barrier: an overview: structure, regulation, and clinical implications. *Neurobiology of Disease* 2004 Jun;16(1):1–13.

19. Lerner A, Aminov R, Matthias T. Transglutaminases in dysbiosis as potential environmental drivers of autoimmunity. *Frontiers in Microbiology* 2017 Jan 24;8:66.

20. Vojdani A. Lectins, agglutinins, and their roles in autoimmune reactivities. *Alternative Therapies in Health and Medicine* 2015;21 (Suppl) 1:46–51.

21. Ravnskov U, McCully KS. How macrophages are converted to foam cells. *Journal of Atherosclerosis and Thrombosis* 2012;19(10):949–50.

22. Ravnskov U, McCully KS. Review and hypothesis: vulnerable plaque formation from obstruction of Vasa vasorum by homocysteinylated and oxidized lipoprotein aggregates complexed with microbial remnants and LDL autoantibodies. *Annals of Clinical and Laboratory Science* 2009 Winter;39(1):3–16.

23. Marinho AC, Martinho FC, Zaia AA, Ferraz CC, Gomes BP. Monitoring the effectiveness of root canal procedures on endotoxin levels found in teeth with chronic apical periodontitis. *Journal of Applied Oral Science* 2014 Nov–Dec;22(6):490–5.

24. Silverman MH, Ostro MJ. Bacterial endotoxin in human disease. Princeton, NJ: KPMG 35 (1999).

25. Banks WA, Gray AM, Erickson MA et al. Lipopolysaccharide-induced blood-brain barrier disruption: roles of cyclooxygenase, oxidative stress, neuroinflammation, and elements of the neurovascular unit. *Journal of Neuroinflammation* 2015 Nov 25;12:223. doi: 10.1186/s12974-015-0434-1.

26. Klatt NR, Harris LD, Vinton CL et al. Compromised gastrointestinal integrity in pigtail macaques is associated with increased microbial translocation, immune activation, and IL-17 production in the absence of SIV infection. *Mucosal Immunology* 2010 Jul;3(4):387–98.

27. Bredesen DE. Reversal of cognitive decline: a novel therapeutic program. *Aging* (Albany, NY), 2014 Sep;6(9):707–17.

28. D'Andrea MR. Add Alzheimer's disease to the list of autoimmune diseases. *Medical Hypotheses* 2005;64(3):458–63.

29. Harris SA, Harris EA. Herpes simplex virus type 1 and other pathogens are key causative factors in sporadic Alzheimer's disease. *Journal of Alzheimer's Disease* 2015;48(2):319–53.

30. Bredesen DE. Reversal of cognitive decline.

3: A GREAT BRAIN BEGINS IN YOUR GUT

1. Flowers SA, Ellingrod VL. The microbiome in mental health: potential contribution of gut microbiota in disease and pharmacotherapy management. *Pharmacotherapy* 2015 Oct;35(10):910–6.

2. König J, Wells J, Cani PD, García-Ródenas CL, MacDonald T, Mercenier A, Whyte J, Troost F, Brummer RJ. Human intestinal barrier function in health and disease. *Clinical and Translational Gastroenterology* 2016 Oct 20;7(10):e196.

3. Marlicz W, Loniewski I, Grimes DS, Quigley EM. Nonsteroidal anti-inflammatory drugs, proton pump inhibitors, and gastrointestinal injury: contrasting interactions in the stomach and small intestine. *Mayo Clinic Proceedings* 2014 Dec;89(12):1699–709.

4. Round JL, Mazmanian SK. The gut microbiota shapes intestinal immune responses during health and disease. *Nature Reviews: Immunology* 2009 May;9(5): 313–23.

5. Kelly JR, Kennedy PJ, Cryan JF, Dinan TG, Clarke G, Hyland NP. Breaking down the barriers: the gut microbiome, intestinal permeability and stress-related psychiatric disorders. *Frontiers in Cellular Neuroscience* 2015 Oct 14;9:392.

6. Smythies LE, Smythies JR. Microbiota, the immune system, black moods and the brain-melancholia updated. *Frontiers in Human Neuroscience* 2014 Sep 15;8:720.

7. Maes M, Coucke F, Leunis JC. Normalization of the increased translocation of endotoxin from gram negative enterobacteria (leaky gut) is accompanied by a remission of chronic fatigue syndrome. *Neuroendocrinology Letters* 2007 Dec;28(6):739–44.

8. Vojdani A, Kharrazian D, Mukherjee P. The prevalence of antibodies against wheat and milk proteins in blood donors and their contribution to neuroimmune reactivities. *Nutrients* 2014 Jan;6(1):15–36.

9. Vojdani A, O'Bryan T, Green JA, McCandless J, Woeller KN, Vojdani E, Nourian AA, Cooper EL. Immune response to dietary proteins, gliadin and cerebellar peptides in children with autism. *Nutritional Neuroscience* 2004 Jun; 7(3):151–61.

10. https://www.nimh.nih.gov/health/statistics/prevalence/any-mental-illness-ami -among-us-adults.shtml.

11. Wildmann J, Vetter W, Ranalder UB, Schmidt K, Maurer R, Möhler H. Occurrence of pharmacologically active benzodiazepines in trace amounts in wheat and potato. *Biochemical Pharmacology* 1988 Oct 1;37(19):3549–59.

12. Hollon J, Puppa EL, Greenwald B, Goldberg E, Guerrerio A, Fasano A. Effect of gliadin on permeability of intestinal biopsy explants from celiac disease patients and patients with non-celiac gluten sensitivity. *Nutrients* 2015 Feb 27;7(3):1565–76.

13. Rodrigò L, Hernández-Lahoz C, Lauret E, Rodriguez-Peláez M, Soucek M, Ciccocioppo R, Kruzliak P. Gluten ataxia is better classified as non-celiac gluten sensitivity than as celiac disease: a comparative clinical study. *Immunologic Research* 2016 Apr;64(2):558–64.

14. Volta U, Bardella MT, Calabrò A, Troncone R, Corazza GR; Study Group for Non-Celiac Gluten Sensitivity. An Italian prospective multicenter survey on patients suspected of having non-celiac gluten sensitivity. *BMC Medicine* 2014 May 23;12:85. doi: 10.1186/1741-7015-12-85.

15. Van Hees NJM, Giltay EJ, Tielemans SMAJ, Geleijnse JM, Puvill T, Janssen N, van der Does W. Essential amino acids in the gluten-free diet and serum in relation to depression in patients with celiac disease. *PLOS One* 2015;10(4): n. pag. Web.

16. M. Finizio, Quaremba G, Mazzacca G, Ciacci C. Large forehead: a novel sign of undiagnosed coeliac disease. *Digestive and Liver Disease* 2005 Sep;37(9):659–64.

17. Lionetti E, Leonardi S, Franzonello C, Mancardi M, Ruggieri M, Catassi C. Gluten psychosis: confirmation of a new clinical entity. *Nutrients* 2015 Jul 8;7(7): 5532–9.

18. Bressan P, Kramer P. Bread and other edible agents of mental disease. *Frontiers in Human Neuroscience* 2016 Mar 29;10:130.

19. Sun Z, Zhang Z, Wang X, Cade R, Elmir Z, Fregly M. Relation of beta-

casomorphin to apnea in sudden infant death syndrome. *Peptides* 2003 Jun;24(6): 937–43.

20. Ramabadran K, Bansinath M. Opioid peptides from milk as a possible cause of sudden infant death syndrome. *Medical Hypotheses* 1988 Nov;27(3):181–7.

21. Bell SJ, Grochoski GT, Clarke AJ. Health implications of milk containing β-casein with the A2 genetic variant. *Critical Reviews in Food Science and Nutrition* 2006;46(1):93–100.

22. Wasilewska J, Sienkiewicz-Szlapka E, Kuzbida E, Jarmolowska B, Kaczmarski M, Kostyra E. The exogenous opioid peptides and DPPIV serum activity in infants with apnoea expressed as apparent life threatening events (ALTE). *Neuropeptides* 2011 Jun;45(3):189–95. doi:10.1016/j.npep.2011.01.005.

23. de la Monte SM, Wands JR. Alzheimer's disease is type 3 diabetes—evidence reviewed. *Journal of Diabetes Science and Technology* 2008 Nov;2(6):1101–13.

24. Wang D, Ho L, Faith J et al. Role of intestinal microbiota in the generation of polyphenol-derived phenolic acid mediated attenuation of Alzheimer's disease β-amyloid oligomerization. *Molecular Nutrition & Food Research* 2015 Jun; 59(6):1025–40.

25. Pistollato F, Sumalla Cano S, Elio I, Masias Vergara M, Giampieri F, Battino M. Role of gut microbiota and nutrients in amyloid formation and pathogenesis of Alzheimer disease. *Nutrition Reviews* 2016 Oct;74(10):624–34.

4: GARBAGE IN, GARBAGE OUT: HOW OUR TOXIC ENVIRONMENT AFFECTS THE BRAIN

1. Light TD, Choi KC, Thomsen TA et al. Long-term outcomes of patients with necrotizing fasciitis. *Journal of Burn Care & Research* 2010 Jan-Feb;31(1):93–9. doi: 10.1097/BCR.0b013e3181cb8cea.

2. Høgsberg T, Saunte DM, Frimodt-Møller N, Serup J. Microbial status and product labelling of 58 original tattoo inks. *Journal of the European Academy of Dermatology and Venereology* 2013 Jan;27(1):73–80.

3. Serup J. Individual risk and prevention of complications: doctors' advice to persons wishing a new tattoo. *Current Problems in Dermatology* 2017;52:18–29. Novel Agents and Drug Targets to Meet the Challenges of Resistant Fungi. McCarthy MW, Kontoyiannis DP, Cornely OA, Perfect JR, Walsh TJ. *J Infect Dis.* 2017 Aug 15;216(suppl 3):S474–S483

4. Sepehri M, Sejersen T, Qvortrup K, Lerche CM, Serup J. Tattoo pigments are observed in the Kupffer cells of the liver indicating blood-borne distribution of tattoo ink. *Dermatology* 2017;233(1):86–93. doi: 10.1159/000468149. Epub 2017 May 10.

5. Adler BL, Kim GH, Haden AD. Ulcerating nodules within tattoos revealing pulmonary sarcoidosis. *Arthritis & Rheumatology* 2017 Sep 7.

6. Jafari S, Buxton JA, Afshar K, Copes R, Baharlou S. Tattooing and risk of hepatitis B: a systematic review and meta-analysis. *Canadian Journal of Public Health* 2012 May-Jun;103(3):207–12.

7. Fray J, Lekieffre A, Parry F, Huguier V, Guillet G. Rose necrosis: necrotizing granulomatous reaction with infected node at red pigment of a tattoo. *Annales de Chirurgie Plastique et Esthetique* 2014 Apr;59(2):144–9.

8. Lehner K, Santarelli F, Vasold R, König B, Landthaler M, Bäumler W. Black tattoo inks are a source of problematic substances such as dibutyl phthalate. *Contact Dermatitis* 2011 Oct;65(4):231–8.

9. https://www.worldwildlife.org/pages/living-planet-report-2014.

10. Levine H, Jørgensen N, Martino-Andrade A, Mendiola J, Weksler-Derri D, Mindlis I, Pinotti R, Swan SH. Temporal trends in sperm count: a systematic review and meta-regression analysis. *Human Reproduction Update* 2017 Nov 1; 23(6):646–59. https://doi.org/10.1093/humupd/dmx022

11. UCL Institute for Global Health. UCL-Lancet Commission on managing the health effects of climate change. 2014. www.ucl.ac.uk/igh/research/projects/all -projects/lancet-1.

12. Intergovernmental Panel on Climate Change. Working Group I contribution to the IPCC fifth assessment report climate change 2013: the physical science basis summary for policymakers. 2013. www.ipcc.ch/report/ar5/wg1/#.UlJ6rNI3vTo.

13. American Association for the Advancement of Science. What we know: the reality, risks, and response to climate change. 2014. http://whatweknow.aaas.org/.

14. McCoy D, Montgomery H, Arulkumaran S, Godlee F. Climate change and human survival. *BMJ* 2014 Mar 26;348:g2351.

15. Olshansky SJ, Passaro DJ, Hershow RC, Layden J, Carnes BA, Brody J, Hayflick L, Butler RN, Allison DB, Ludwig DS. A potential decline in life expectancy in the United States in the 21st century. *New England Journal of Medicine* 2005 Mar 17;352(11):1138–45.

16. Environmental Working Group analysis of tests of 10 umbilical cord blood samples conducted by AXYS Analytical Services (Sydney, BC) and Flett Research Ltd. (Winnipeg, MB). https://www.ewg.org/research/body-burden-pollution -newborns#.Wixct7pFxtQ.

17. Bredesen DE. Inhalational Alzheimer's disease: an unrecognized—and treatable—epidemic. *Aging* 2016;8(2):304–13. Web.

18. https://www.cdc.gov/ncbddd/autism/data.html, accessed Oct 2, 2017.

19. http://themindunleashed.com/2014/10/mit-researchers-new-warning-todays -rate-half-u-s-children-will-autistic-2025.html.

20. Song P, Wu L, Guan W. Dietary nitrates, nitrites, and nitrosamines intake and the risk of gastric cancer: a meta-analysis. *Nutrients* 2015 Dec 1;7(12):9872–95.

21. Park KA, Kweon S, Choi H. Anticarcinogenic effect and modification of cytochrome P450 2E1 by dietary garlic powder in diethylnitrosamine-initiated rat hepatocarcinogenesis. *Journal of Biochemistry and Molecular Biology* 2002;35(6): 615–22.

22. Farombi EO, Shrotriya S, Na HK, Kim SH, Surh YJ. Curcumin attenuates dimethylnitrosamine-induced liver injury in rats through Nrf2-mediated induction of heme oxygenase-1. *Food and Chemical Toxicology* 2008;46(4):1279–87.

23. Hwang YP, Choi JH, Yun HJ et al. Anthocyanins from purple sweet potato attenuate dimethylnitrosamine-induced liver injury in rats by inducing Nrf2-mediated antioxidant enzymes and reducing COX-2 and iNOS expression. *Food and Chemical Toxicology*, 2011 Jan;49(1):93–9.

24. Hodges RE, Minich DM. Modulation of metabolic detoxification pathways using foods and food-derived components: a scientific review with clinical application. *Journal of Nutrition and Metabolism* 2015;2015:760689.

25. Vojdani A, O'Bryan T. The immunology of immediate and delayed hypersensitivity reaction to gluten. *European Journal of Inflammation* 2008 Jan;6(1):1–10.

26. Toppari J, Larsen JC, Christiansen P et al. Male reproductive health and environmental xenoestrogens. *Environmental Health Perspectives* 1996 Aug;104 (Suppl) 4:741–803.

27. Horan TS, Marre A, Hassold T, Lawson C, Hunt PA. Germline and reproductive tract effects intensify in male mice with successive generations of estrogenic exposure. *PLOS Genetics* 2017 Jul 20;13(7):e1006885. doi: 10.1371/journal.pgen.1006885. eCollection 2017 Jul.

28. Ohlsson C, Barrett-Connor E, Bhasin S, Orwoll E, Labrie F, Karlsson MK, Ljunggren O, Vandenput L, Mellström D, Tivesten A. High serum testosterone is associated with reduced risk of cardiovascular events in elderly men. The MrOS (Osteoporotic Fractures in Men) study in Sweden. *Journal of the American College of Cardiology* 2011 Oct 11;58(16):1674–81.

29. Longnecker MP, Rogan WJ. Persistent organic pollutants in children. *Pediatric Research* 2001 Sep;50(3):322–3.

30. Ohtani N, Iwano H, Suda K, Tsuji E, Tanemura K, Inoue H, Yokota H. Adverse effects of maternal exposure to bisphenol F on the anxiety- and depression-like behavior of offspring. *Journal of Veterinary Medical Science* 2017 Feb 28;79(2): 432–9.

31. Ritter R, Scheringer M, MacLeod M, Moeckel C, Jones KC, Hungerbühler K. Intrinsic human elimination half-lives of polychlorinated biphenyls derived from the temporal evolution of cross-sectional biomonitoring data from the United

Kingdom. *Environmental Health Perspectives* 2011 Feb;119(2):225–31. doi: 10.1289/ehp.1002211. Epub 2010 Oct 7.

32. Cheek AO, Kow K, Chen J, McLachlan JA. Potential mechanisms of thyroid disruption in humans: interaction of organochlorine compounds with thyroid receptor, transthyretin, and thyroid-binding globulin. *Environmental Health Perspectives* 1999 Apr;107(4):273–8.

33. Saal FS, Myers JP. Bisphenol A and risk of metabolic disorders. *JAMA* 2008 Sep 17;300(11):1353–5.

34. Kharrazian D, Vojdani A. Correlation between antibodies to bisphenol A, its target enzyme protein disulfide isomerase and antibodies to neuron-specific antigens. *Journal of Applied Toxicology* 2017 Apr;37(4):479–84.

35. Tiwari SK, Agarwal S, Chauhan LK, Mishra VN, Chaturvedi RK. Bisphenol-A impairs myelination potential during development in the hippocampus of the rat brain. *Molecular Neurobiology* 2015;51(3):1395–416. doi: 10.1007/s12035-014-8817-3. Epub 2014 Aug 2.

36. Bielefeldt AØ, Danborg PB, Gøtzsche PC. Precursors to suicidality and violence on antidepressants: systematic review of trials in adult healthy volunteers. *Journal of the Royal Society of Medicine* 2016 Oct;109(10):381–92.

37. Biedermann S, Tschudin P, Grob K. Transfer of bisphenol A from thermal printer paper to the skin. *Analytical and Bioanalytical Chemistry* 2010 Sep;398(1):571–6. doi: 10.1007/s00216-010-3936-9. Epub 2010 Jul 11.

38. Adapted from American Academy of Pediatrics, Shelov SP, ed. *Caring for Your Baby and Young Child: Birth to Age Five* (Bantam, 2009).

39. Kang KW, Park WJ. Lead poisoning at an indoor firing range. *Journal of Korean Medical Science* 2017 Oct;32(10):1713–6.

40. WHO, 2002; Prüss-Ustün et al., 2004.

41. World Health Organization fact sheet. "Mercury and Health," March 2017, http://www.who.int/mediacentre/factsheets/fs361/en/.

42. Vimy MJ, Lorscheider FL. Dental amalgam mercury daily dose estimated from intra-oral vapor measurements: a predictor of mercury accumulation in human tissues. *Journal of Trace Elements in Experimental Medicine* 1990 Jan;3:111–23.

43. Goniewicz ML, Knysak J, Gawron M et al. Levels of selected carcinogens and toxicants in vapour from electronic cigarettes. *Tobacco Control* 2014 Mar;23(2):133–9.

44. Hecht EM, Arheart K, Lee DJ, Hennekens CH, Hlaing WM. A cross-sectional survey of cadmium biomarkers and cigarette smoking. *Biomarkers* 2016 Jul;21(5):429–35.

45. Barton H. Predicted intake of trace elements and minerals via household drinking water by 6-year-old children from Kraków, Poland. Part 2: Cadmium, 1997–2001. *Food Additives and Contaminants* 2005 Sep;22(9):816–28.

46. Viala Y, Laurette J, Denaix L, Gourdain E, Méléard B, Nguyen C, Schneider A, Sappin-Didier V. Predictive statistical modelling of cadmium content in durum wheat grain based on soil parameters. *Environmental Science and Pollution Research International* 2017 Sep;24(25):20641–54. doi: 10.1007/s11356-017-9712-z. Epub 2017 Jul 15.

47. Xie LH, Tang SQ, Wei XJ, Shao GN, Jiao GA, Sheng ZH, Luo J, Hu PS. The cadmium and lead content of the grain produced by leading Chinese rice cultivars. *Food Chemistry* 2017 Feb 15;217:217–24.

48. Kumar P, Mahato DK, Kamle M, Mohanta TK, Kang SG. Aflatoxins: a global concern for food safety, human health and their management. *Frontiers in Microbiology* 2017 Jan 17;7:2170.

49. McCarthy MW, Kontoyiannis DP, Cornely OA, Perfect JR, Walsh TJ. Novel agents and drug targets to meet the challenges of resistant fungi. *Journal of Infectious Diseases* 2017 Aug 15;216(suppl 3):S474–83.

50. Murakami A, Tutumi T, Watanabe K. Middle ear effusion and fungi. *Annals of Otology, Rhinology, and Laryngology* 2012 Sep;121(9):609–14.

51. Brewer J, Thrasher JD, Hooper D. Reply to comment on detection of mycotoxins in patients with chronic fatigue syndrome. *Toxins* 2013;5:605–17 by John W. Osterman, MD. *Toxins* (Basel). 2016 Nov 7;8(11).

52. Gratz SW, Duncan G, Richardson AJ. The human fecal microbiota metabolizes deoxynivalenol and deoxynivalenol-3-glucoside and may be responsible for urinary deepoxy-deoxynivalenol. *Applied and Environmental Microbiology* 2013 Mar;79(6):1821–5.

53. Francino MP. Antibiotics and the human gut microbiome: dysbioses and accumulation of resistances. *Frontiers in Microbiology* 2016 Jan 12;6:1543.

54. Costelloe C, Metcalfe C, Lovering A, Mant D, Hay AD. Effect of antibiotic prescribing in primary care on antimicrobial resistance in individual patients: systematic review and meta-analysis. *BMJ* 2010 May 18;340:c2096. doi: 10.1136/bmj.c2096.

55. https://www.cdc.gov/drugresistance/threat-report-2013/pdf/ar-threats-2013-508.pdf.

56. Stensballe LG, Simonsen J, Jensen SM, Bønnelykke K, Bisgaard H. Use of antibiotics during pregnancy increases the risk of asthma in early childhood. *Journal of Pediatrics* 2013 Apr;162(4):832–8.

57. Slykerman RF, Thompson J, Waldie KE, Murphy R, Wall C, Mitchell EA. Antibiotics in the first year of life and subsequent neurocognitive outcomes. *Acta Paediatrica* 2017 Jan;106(1):87–94.

58. Zhang C, Li S, Yang L et al. Structural modulation of gut microbiota in life-long calorie-restricted mice. *Nature Communications* 2013;4:2163.

59. Kim JA, Kim JY, Kang SW. Effects of the dietary detoxification program on serum γ-glutamyltransferase, anthropometric data and metabolic biomarkers in adults. *Journal of Lifestyle Medicine* 2016 Sep;6(2):49–57. Epub 2016 Sep 30.

60. Horne BD, Muhlestein JB, Anderson JL. Health effects of intermittent fasting: hormesis or harm? A systematic review. *American Journal of Clinical Nutrition* 2015 Aug;102(2):464–70.

61. Chaix A, Zarrinpar A, Miu P, Panda S. Time-restricted feeding is a preventative and therapeutic intervention against diverse nutritional challenges. *Cell Metabolism* 2014 Dec 2;20(6):991–1005.

62. Heurung AR. Adverse reactions to sunscreen agents: epidemiology, responsible irritants and allergens, clinical characteristics, and management. *Dermatitis* 2014 Nov–Dec;25(6): 289–326.

63. http://www.ewg.org/sunscreen/report/executive-summary/#.WdO3KLpFxtQ.

64. Factor-Litvak P, Insel B, Calafat AM, Liu X, Perera F, Rauh VA, Whyatt RM. Persistent associations between maternal prenatal exposure to phthalates on child IQ at age 7 years. *PLOS One* 2014 Dec 10;9(12):e114003. doi: 10.1371/journal.pone.0114003. eCollection 2014.

65. Scherf KA, Brockow K, Biedermann T, Koehler P, Wieser H. Wheat-dependent exercise-induced anaphylaxis. *Clinical and Experimental Allergy* 2016 Jan; 46(1):10–20.

66. Thompson T, Grace T. Gluten in cosmetics: is there a reason for concern? *Journal of the Academy of Nutrition and Dietetics* 2012 Sep;112(23):1316–23.

67. Teshima R. Food allergen in cosmetics. *Yakugaku Zasshi* 2014;134(1):33–8.

68. Kwangmi K. Influences of environmental chemicals on atopic dermatitis. *Toxicological Research* 2015 Jun;31(2):89–96.

5: KNOW YOUR BIOMARKERS

1. Hauser PS, Ryan RO. Impact of apolipoprotein E on Alzheimer's disease. *Current Alzheimer Research* 2013 Oct;10(8):809–17.

2. Sepehrnia B, Kamboh MI, Adams-Campbell LL, Bunker CH, Nwankwo M, Majumder PP, Ferrell RE. Genetic studies of human apolipoproteins. X. The effect of the apolipoprotein E polymorphism on quantitative levels of lipoproteins in Nigerian blacks. *American Journal of Human Genetics* 1989 Oct;45(4):586–91.

3. Boscolo S, Passoni M, Baldas V, Cancelli I, Hadjivassiliou M, Ventura A, Tongiorgi E. Detection of anti-brain serum antibodies using a semi-quantitative immunohistological method. *Journal of Immunological Methods* 2006 Feb 20;309 (1–2):139–49.

4. Lanzini A, Lanzarotto F, Villanacci V et al. Complete recovery of intestinal

mucosa occurs very rarely in adult coeliac patients despite adherence to gluten-free diet. *Alimentary Pharmacology and Therapeutics* 2009 Jun 15;29(12):1299–308. doi: 10.1111/j.1365-2036.2009.03992.x. Epub 2009 Mar 3.

5. Hadjivassiliou M, Sanders DS, Grünewald RA, Woodroofe N, Boscolo S, Aeschlimann D. Gluten sensitivity: from gut to brain. *Lancet Neurology* 2010 Mar; 9(3):318–30.

6. Fasano A, Catassi C. Current approaches to diagnosis and treatment of celiac disease: an evolving spectrum. *Gastroenterology* 2001 Feb;120(3):636–51.

7. Addolorato G, Mirijello A, D'Angelo C, Leggio L, Ferrulli A, Vonghia L, Cardone S, Leso V, Miceli A, Gasbarrini G. Social phobia in coeliac disease. *Scandinavian Journal of Gastroenterology* 2008;43(4):410–5.

8. Zelnik N, Pacht A, Obeid R, Lerner A. Range of neurologic disorders in patients with celiac disease. *Pediatrics* 2004 Jun;113(6):1672–6.

9. Ibid.

10. Lichtwark IT, Newnham ED, Robinson SR, Shepherd SJ, Hosking P, Gibson PR, Yelland GW. Cognitive impairment in coeliac disease improves on a gluten-free diet and correlates with histological and serological indices of disease severity. *Alimentary Pharmacology & Therapeutics* 2014;40:160–70.

11. Skowera A, Peakman M, Cleare A, Davies E, Deale A, Wessely S. High prevalence of serum markers of coeliac disease in patients with chronic fatigue syndrome. *Journal of Clinical Pathology* 2001 Apr;54(4):335–6.

12. Yelland GW. Gluten-induced cognitive impairment ("brain fog") in coeliac disease. *Journal of Gastroenterology and Hepatology* 2017 Mar;32 (Suppl 1):90–3.

13. Delvecchio M, De Bellis A, Francavilla R et al. Italian Autoimmune Hypophysitis Network Study. Anti-pituitary antibodies in children with newly diagnosed celiac disease: a novel finding contributing to linear-growth impairment. *American Journal of Gastroenterology* 2010 Mar;105(3):691–6. doi: 10.1038/ajg.2009.642. Epub 2009 Nov 10.

14. Daulatzai MA. Non-celiac gluten sensitivity triggers gut dysbiosis, neuroinflammation, gut-brain axis dysfunction, and vulnerability for dementia. *CNS & Neurological Disorders—Drug Targets* 2015;14(1):110–31.

15. Challacombe DN, Wheeler EE. Are the changes of mood in children with coeliac disease due to abnormal serotonin metabolism? *Nutrition and Health* 1987; 5(3–4):145–52.

16. Salur L, Uibo O, Talvik I, Justus I, Metsküla K, Talvik T, Uibo R. The high frequency of coeliac disease among children with neurological disorders. *European Journal of Neurology* 2000 Nov;7(6):707–11.

17. Gobbi G. Coeliac disease, epilepsy and cerebral calcifications. *Brain & Development* 2005 Apr;27(3):189–200. Review.

18. Iughetti L, De Bellis A, Predieri B, Bizzarro A, De Simone M, Balli F, Bellastella A, Bernasconi S. Growth hormone impaired secretion and antipituitary antibodies in patients with coeliac disease and poor catch-up growth after a long gluten-free diet period: a causal association? *European Journal of Pediatrics* 2006 Dec;165(12):897–903. Epub 2006 Aug 3.

19. Perlmutter D, Vodjani A. Association between headache and sensitivities to gluten and dairy. *Integrative Medicine* 2013 Apr;12(2):18–23.

20. Zelnik N et al. Range of neurologic disorders. *Pediatrics*.

21. Niederhofer H. Association of attention-deficit/hyperactivity disorder and celiac disease: a brief report. *Primary Care Companion for CNS Disorders* 2011;13(3).

22. Gibbons CH, Freeman R. Autonomic neuropathy and coeliac disease. *Journal of Neurology, Neurosurgery, and Psychiatry* 2005 Apr;76(4):579–81.

23. Lionetti E, Leonardi S, Franzonello C, Mancardi M, Ruggieri M, Catassi C. Gluten psychosis: confirmation of a new clinical entity. *Nutrients* 2015 Jul 8; 7(7):5532–9. doi: 10.3390/nu7075235.

24. Isasi C, Tejerina E, Morán LM. Non-celiac gluten sensitivity and rheumatic diseases. *Reumatologia Clinica* 2016 Jan–Feb;12(1):4–10.

25. Lichtwark IT, Newnham ED, Robinson SR, Shepherd SJ, Hosking P, Gibson PR, Yelland GW. Cognitive impairment in coeliac disease improves on a gluten-free diet and correlates with histological and serological indices of disease severity. *Alimentary Pharmacology & Therapeutics* 2014 Jul;40(2):160–70.

26. Zylberberg HM, Demmer RT, Murray JA, Green PHR, Lebwohl B. Depression and insomnia among individuals with celiac disease or on a gluten-free diet in the USA: results from a national survey. *European Journal of Gastroenterology & Hepatology* 2017 Sep;29(9):1091–6.

27. Al Nimer F, Thelin E, Nyström H, Dring AM, Svenningsson A, Piehl F, Nelson DW, Bellander BM. Comparative assessment of the prognostic value of biomarkers in traumatic brain injury reveals an independent role for serum levels of neurofilament light. *PLOS One* 2015 Jul 2;10(7):e0132177.

28. Kobeissy F, Moshourab RA. Autoantibodies in CNS trauma and neuropsychiatric disorders: a new generation of biomarkers. In: Kobeissy FH, editor. *Brain Neurotrauma: Molecular, Neuropsychological, and Rehabilitation Aspects* (Boca Raton, FL: CRC Press/Taylor & Francis, 2015). Chapter 29.

29. Pollak TA, Drndarski S, Stone JM, David AS, McGuire P, Abbott NJ. The blood-brain barrier in psychosis. *Lancet Psychiatry* 2017 Aug 3. pii: S2215-0366(17)30293–6.

30. Lionetti E, Leonardi S, Franzonello C, Mancardi M, Ruggieri M, Catassi C. Gluten psychosis: confirmation of a new clinical entity. *Nutrients* 2015 Jul 8; 7(7):5532–9.

31. Blyth BJ, Farahvar A, He H, Nayak A, Yang C, Shaw G, Bazarian JJ. Elevated

serum ubiquitin carboxy-terminal hydrolase L1 is associated with abnormal blood-brain barrier function after traumatic brain injury. *Journal of Neurotrauma* 2011 Dec;28(12):2453–62.

32. Vojdani A. Brain-reactive antibodies in traumatic brain injury. *Functional Neurology, Rehabilitation, and Ergonomics* 2013;3(2–3):173–81.

33. Mercier E, Boutin A, Shemilt M et al. Predictive value of neuron-specific enolase for prognosis in patients with moderate or severe traumatic brain injury: a systematic review and meta-analysis. *CMAJ Open* 2016 Jul 22;4(3):E371–82.

34. Cascella NG, Santora D, Gregory P, Kelly DL, Fasano A, Eaton WW. Increased prevalence of transglutaminase 6 antibodies in sera from schizophrenia patients. *Schizophrenia Bulletin* 2013 Jul;39(4):867–71.

35. Baba H, Daune GC, Ilyas AA, Pestronk A, Cornblath DR, Chaudhry V, Griffin JW, Quarles RH. Anti-GM1 ganglioside antibodies with differing fine specificities in patients with multifocal motor neuropathy. *Journal of Neuroimmunology* 1989;25:143–50.

36. Jamieson GA, Maitland NJ, Wilcock GK, Yates CM, Itzhaki RF. Herpes simplex virus type 1 DNA is present in specific regions of brain from aged people with and without senile dementia of the Alzheimer type. *Journal of Pathology* 1992 Aug;167(4):365–8.

37. Berger T, Rubner P, Schautzer F, Egg R, Ulmer H, Mayringer I, Dilitz E, Deisenhammer F, Reindl M. Antimyelin antibodies as a predictor of clinically definite multiple sclerosis after a first demyelinating event. *New England Journal of Medicine* 2003 Jul 10;349(2):139–45.

38. Ashwood P, Van de Water J. Is autism an autoimmune disease? *Autoimmunity Reviews* 2004 Nov;3(7–8):557–62.

39. Gorgan JL, Kramer A, Nogai A, Dong L, Ohde M, Schneider-Mergener J, Kamradt T. Cross-reactivity of myelin basic protein-specific T cells with multiple microbial peptides: experimental autoimmune encephalomyelitis induction in TCR transgenic mice. *Journal of Immunology* 1999 Oct 1;163(7):3764–70.

40. Roy A, Hooper DC. Lethal silver-haired bat rabies virus infection can be prevented by opening the blood-brain barrier. *Journal of Virology* 2007 Aug;81(15):7993–8.

41. Vojdani A, Vojdani E, Cooper E. Antibodies to myelin basic protein, myelin oligodendrocytes peptides, alpha-beta-crystallin, lymphocyte activation and cytokine production in patients with multiple sclerosis. *Journal of Internal Medicine* 2003 Oct;254(4):363–74.

42. Gobbi G, Bouquet F, Greco L, Lambertini A, Tassinari CA, Ventura A, Zaniboni MG. Coeliac disease, epilepsy and cerebral calcifications. *Lancet* 1992 Aug 22;340(8817):439–43.

7: THE BASE OF THE PYRAMID: ADDRESSING YOUR STRUCTURE

1. Ormos G, Mehrishi JN, Bakács T. Reduction in high blood tumor necrosis factor-alpha levels after manipulative therapy in 2 cervicogenic headache patients. *Journal of Manipulative and Physiological Therapeutics* 2009 Sep;32(7):586–91.

2. Kolberg C, Horst A, Moraes MS, Kolberg A, Belló-Klein A, Partata WA. Effect of high-velocity, low-amplitude treatment on superoxide dismutase and glutathione peroxidase activities in erythrocytes from men with neck pain. *Journal of Manipulative and Physiological Therapeutics* 2012 May;35(4):295–300.

3. Kolberg C, Horst A, Moraes MS, Duarte FC, Riffel AP, Scheid T, Kolberg A, Partata WA. Peripheral oxidative stress blood markers in patients with chronic back or neck pain treated with high-velocity, low-amplitude manipulation. *Journal of Manipulative and Physiological Therapeutics* 2015 Feb;38(2):119–29.

4. Lambert GP, Schmidt A, Schwarzkopf K, Lanspa S. Effect of aspirin dose on gastrointestinal permeability. *International Journal of Sports Medicine* 2012 Jun;33(6):421–5. doi: 10.1055/s-0032-1301892. Epub 2012 Feb 29.

5. Bakhtadze MA, Vernon H, Karalkin AV, Pasha SP, Tomashevskiy IO, Soave D. Cerebral perfusion in patients with chronic neck and upper back pain: preliminary observations. *Journal of Manipulative and Physiological Therapeutics* 2012 Feb;35(2):76–85. doi: 10.1016/j.jmpt.2011.12.006. Epub 2012 Jan 16.

6. Browning JE. Mechanically induced pelvic pain and organic dysfunction in a patient without low back pain. *Journal of Manipulative and Physiological Therapeutics* 1990 Sep;13(7):406–11.

7. Spielman LJ, Little JP, Klegeris A. Physical activity and exercise attenuate neuroinflammation in neurological diseases. *Brain Research Bulletin* 2016;125:19–29.

8. Nijs J, Clark J, Malfliet A et al. In the spine or in the brain? Recent advances in pain neuroscience applied in the intervention for low back pain. *Clinical and Experimental Rheumatology* 2017 Sep–Oct;35 Suppl 107(5):108–15. Epub 2017 Sep 29.

9. Grant LK, Cain SW, Chang AM, Saxena R, Czeisler CA, Anderson C. Impaired cognitive flexibility during sleep deprivation among carriers of the Brain Derived Neurotrophic Factor (BDNF) Val66Met allele. *Behavioural Brain Research* 2017 Sep 22. pii: S0166-4328(17)30807-0. doi: 10.1016/j.bbr.2017.09.025. [Epub ahead of print]

10. Grob D, Frauenfelder H, Mannion AF. The association between cervical spine curvature and neck pain. *European Spine Journal* 2007 May;16(5):669–78.

11. Gracia MC. Exposure to nicotine is probably a major cause of inflammatory diseases among non-smokers. *Medical Hypotheses* 2005;65(2):253–8.

12. Bakhtadze MA, Vernon H, Karalkin AV, Pasha SP, Tomashevskiy IO, Soave

DJ. Cerebral perfusion in patients with chronic neck and upper back pain: preliminary observations. *Journal of Manipulative and Physiological Therapeutics* 2012 Feb;35(2):76–85.

13. García DV, Doorduin J, Willemsen AT, Dierckx RA, Otte A. Altered regional cerebral blood flow in chronic whiplash associated disorders. *EBioMedicine* 2016 Aug;10:249–57.

14. Linnman C, Appel L, Söderlund A, Frans O, Engler H, Furmark T, Gordh T, Långström B, Fredrikson M. Chronic whiplash symptoms are related to altered regional cerebral blood flow in the resting state. *European Journal of Pain* 2009 Jan;13(1):65–70.

15. Colcombe S, Kramer AF. (2003) Fitness effects on the cognitive function of older adults: a meta-analytic study. *Psychological Science* 2003 Mar;14(2):125–30.

16. Weuve J, Kang JH, Manson JE, Breteler MM, Ware JH, Grodstein F. Physical activity, including walking, and cognitive function in older women. *JAMA* 2004 Sep 22;292(12):1454–61.

17. Heyn P, Abreu BC, Ottenbacher KJ. The effects of exercise training on elderly persons with cognitive impairment and dementia: a meta-analysis. *Archives of Physical Medicine and Rehabilitation* 2004 Oct;85(10):1694–704.

18. Larson EB, Wang L, Bowen JD, McCormick WC, Teri L, Crane P, Kukull W. Exercise is associated with reduced risk for incident dementia among persons 65 years of age and older. *Annals of Internal Medicine* 2006 Jan 17;144(2):73–81.

19. Podewils LJ, Guallar E, Kuller LH, Fried LP, Lopez OL, Carlson M, Lyketsos CG. Physical activity, APOE genotype, and dementia risk: findings from the Cardiovascular Health Cognition Study. *American Journal of Epidemiology* 2005 Apr 1;161(7):639–51.

20. Rovio S, Kareholt I, Helkala EL, Viitanen M, Winblad B, Tuomilehto J, Soininen H, Nissinen A, Kivipelto M. Leisure-time physical activity at midlife and the risk of dementia and Alzheimer's disease. *Lancet. Neurology* 2005 Nov;4(11):705–11.

21. Trejo JL, Carro E, Torres-Aleman I. Circulating insulin-like growth factor I mediates exercise-induced increases in the number of new neurons in the adult hippocampus. *Journal of Neuroscience* 2001 Mar 1;21(5):1628–34.

22. Sugai E, Pedreira SC, Smecuol EG, Vazquez H, Niveloni SI, Mazure R, Kogan Z, Maurino E, Bai JC. High titers of anti-bone autoantibody are associated with osteoporosis of patients with celiac disease. *Gastroenterology* 2000 Apr;118(4, Pt 2).

8: THE POWER OF MIND-SET

1. National Academies of Sciences, Engineering, and Medicine; Health and Medicine Division; Board on Health Sciences Policy; Forum on Neurosciences and

Nervous System Disorders. Therapeutic Development in the Absence of Predictive Animal Models of Nervous System Disorders: Proceedings of a Workshop. Washington (DC): National Academies Press (US); 2017 Mar.

2. Sudo N. Role of microbiome in regulating the HPA axis and its relevance to allergy. *Chemical Immunology and Allergy* 2012;98:163–75. doi: 10.1159/000336510. Epub 2012 Jun 26.

3. Booth C. The rod of Aesculapios: John Haygarth (1740–1827) and Perkins' metallic tractors. *Journal of Medical Biography* 2005 Aug;13(3):155–61. doi:10.1258/j.jmb .2005.04-01.

4. Wootton David. *Bad Medicine: Doctors Doing Harm Since Hippocrates* (Oxford University Press, 2006).

5. Yapko Michael D. *Trancework: An Introduction to the Practice of Clinical Hypnosis* (Routledge, 2012).

6. Kaptchuk TJ, Miller FG. Placebo effects in medicine. *New England Journal of Medicine* 2015;373:8–9.

7. Crum AJ, Langer EJ. Mind-set matters: exercise and the placebo effect. *Psychological Science* 2007;18(2):165–71.

8. Kirsch I, Deacon BJ, Huedo-Medina TB, Scoboria A, Moore TJ, Johnson BT. Initial severity and antidepressant benefits: a meta-analysis of data submitted to the Food and Drug Administration. *PLOS Medicine* 2008 Feb;5(2):e45.

9. https://www.health.harvard.edu/newsletter_article/what-are-the-real-risks-of -antidepressants.

10. Grossman P, Niemann L, Schmidt S, Walach H. Mindfulness-based stress reduction and health benefits. A meta-analysis. *Journal of Psychosomatic Research* 2004 Jul;57(1):35–43.

11. Rosenkranz MA, Davidson RJ, Maccoon DG, Sheridan JF, Kalin NH, Lutz A. A comparison of mindfulness-based stress reduction and an active control in modulation of neurogenic inflammation. *Brain, Behavior, and Immunity* 2013 Jan; 27(1):174–84. doi: 10.1016/j.bbi.2012.10.013. Epub 2012 Oct 22.

12. Gerbarg PL, Jacob VE, Stevens L et al. The effect of breathing, movement, and meditation on psychological and physical symptoms and inflammatory biomarkers in inflammatory bowel disease: a randomized controlled trial. *Inflammatory Bowel Diseases* 2015 Dec;21(12):2886–96.

9: BIOCHEMISTRY: FOOD AS MEDICINE

1. Wang Y, Mao L-H, Jia E-Z et al. Relationship between diagonal earlobe creases and coronary artery disease as determined via angiography. *BMJ Open* 2016;6(2):e008558.

2. Mercola J. 8 sickening facts about flame retardants. Mercola.com, articles.mercola .com/sites/articles/archive/2013/12/11/8-flame-retardant-facts.aspx.

3. Rittirsch D, Flierl MA, Nadeau BA, Day DE, Huber-Lang MS, Grailer JJ, Zetoune FS, Andjelkovic AV, Fasano A, Ward PA. Zonulin as prehaptoglobin2 regulates lung permeability and activates the complement system. *American Journal of Physiology. Lung Cellular and Molecular Physiology* 2013 Jun 15;304(12):L863–72. doi: 10.1152/ajplung.00196.2012. Epub 2013 Apr 5.

4. Calderón-Garcidueñas L, Vojdani A, Blaurock-Busch E et al. Air pollution and children: neural and tight junction antibodies and combustion metals, the role of barrier breakdown and brain immunity in neurodegeneration. *Journal of Alzheimer's Disease* 2015;43(3):1039–58. doi: 10.3233/JAD-141365.

5. Hoffman JB, Hennig B. Protective influence of healthful nutrition on mechanisms of environmental pollutant toxicity and disease risks. *Annals of the New York Academy of Sciences* 2017 Jun;1398(1):99–107. doi: 10.1111/nyas.13365. Epub 2017 Jun 2.

6. Egner PA, Chen JG, Zarth AT et al. Rapid and sustainable detoxication of airborne pollutants by broccoli sprout beverage: results of a randomized clinical trial in China. *Cancer Prevention Research* (Philadelphia, Pa.) 2014 Aug;7(8):813–23. doi: 10.1158/1940-6207.CAPR-14-0103. Epub 2014 Jun 9.

7. Tong H, Rappold AG, Diaz-Sanchez D, Steck SE, Berntsen J, Cascio WE, Devlin RB, Samet JM. Omega-3 fatty acid supplementation appears to attenuate particulate air pollution–induced cardiac effects and lipid changes in healthy middle-aged adults. *Environmental Health Perspectives* 2012 Jul;120(7):952–7. doi: 10.1289/ehp.1104472. Epub 2012 Apr 19.

8. Zhong J, Karlsson O, Wang G et al. B vitamins attenuate the epigenetic effects of ambient fine particles in a pilot human intervention trial. *Proceedings of the National Academy of Sciences of the United States of America* 2017 Mar 28;114(13):-3503–8.

9. Romieu I, Sienra-Monge JJ, Ramírez-Aquilar M et al. Antioxidant supplementation and lung functions among children with asthma exposed to high levels of air pollutants. *American Journal of Respiratory and Critical Care Medicine* 2002 Sep 1;166(5):703–9.

10. Trayhurn P, Beattie JH. Physiological role of adipose tissue: white adipose tissue as an endocrine and secretory organ. *Proceedings of the Nutrition Society* 2001 Aug;60(3):329–39.

11. Costantini LC. Hypometabolism as a therapeutic target in Alzheimer's disease. *BMC Neuroscience* 2008 Dec 3;9 Suppl 2:S16. doi: 10.1186/1471-2202-9-S2-S16.

12. McCarty MF, DiNicolantonio JJ, O'Keefe JH. Ketosis may promote brain mac-

roautophagy by activating Sirt1 and hypoxia-inducible factor-1. *Medical Hypotheses* 2015 Nov;85(5):631–9. doi: 10.1016/j.mehy.2015.08.002. Epub 2015 Aug 10.

13. Xu K, Ye L, Sharma K, Jin Y, Harrison MM, Caldwell T, Berthiaume JM, Luo Y, LaManna JC, Puchowicz MA. Diet-induced ketosis protects against focal cerebral ischemia in mouse. *Advances in Experimental Medicine and Biology* 2017;977:205–13.

14. VanItallie TB. Biomarkers, ketone bodies, and the prevention of Alzheimer's disease. *Metabolism* 2015 Mar;64(3 Suppl 1):S51–7. doi: 10.1016/j.metabol.2014.10.033. Epub 2014 Oct 30.

15. Henderson ST. Study of the ketogenic agent AC-1202 in mild to moderate Alzheimer's disease: a randomized, double-blind, placebo-controlled, multicenter trial. *Nutrition & Metabolism (London)* 2009 Aug 10;6:31. doi: 10.1186/1743-7075-6-31.

16. USDA Economic Research Service. Recent trends in GE Adoption. http://www.ers.usda.gov/data-products/adoption-of-genetically-engineered-crops-in-the-us/recent-trends-in-ge-adoption.aspx.

17. Mesnage R, Clair E, Gress S, Then C, Székács A, Séralini GE. Cytotoxicity on human cells of cry1Ab and cry1Ac Bt insecticidal toxins alone or with a glyphosate-based herbicide. *Journal of Applied Toxicology* 2013 Jul;33(7):695–9.

18. Cattani D, de Liz Oliveira Cavalli VL, Heinz Rieg CE, Domingues JT, Dal-Cim T, Tasca CI, Mena Barreto Silva FR, Zamoner A. Mechanisms underlying the neurotoxicity induced by glyphosate-based herbicide in immature rat hippocampus: involvement of glutamate excitotoxicity. *Toxicology* 2014 Jun 5;320:34–45. doi: 10.1016/j.tox.2014.03.001. Epub 2014 Mar 15.

19. Hugel HM. Brain food for Alzheimer-free ageing: focus on herbal medicines. *Advances in Experimental Medicine and Biology* 2015;863:95–116.

20. Subash S, Essa MM, Braidy N, Awlad-Thani K, Vaishnav R, Al-Adawi S, Al-Asmi A, Guillemin GJ. Diet rich in date palm fruits improves memory, learning and reduces beta amyloid in transgenic mouse model of Alzheimer's disease. *Journal of Ayurveda and Integrative Medicine* 2015;6:111–20.

21. https://www.ewg.org/foodnews/?gclid=CjoKCQjwvabPBRD5ARIsAIwFXBl QuUBwIFRWJcMMNdGsamiRR9BfYolIomS-m-nccnR6KEdoyWFSiKsa Al2uEALw_wcB#.WenmorpFxtQ.

22. Vidart d'Egurbide Bagazgoïtia N, Bailey HD, Orsi L et al. Maternal residential pesticide use during pregnancy and risk of malignant childhood brain tumors: a pooled analysis of the ESCALE and ESTELLE studies (SFCE). *International Journal of Cancer* 2017 Sep 26. doi: 10.1002/ijc.31073. [Epub ahead of print.]

23. Zacharasiewicz A. Maternal smoking in pregnancy and its influence on child-

hood asthma. *ERJ Open Research* 2016 Jul 29;2(3). pii: 00042-2016. eCollection 2016 Jul.

24. Svanes C, Koplin J, Skulstad SM et al. Father's environment before conception and asthma risk in his children: a multi-generation analysis of the Respiratory Health in Northern Europe study. *International Journal of Epidemiology* 2017 Feb 1;46(1): 235–45. doi: 10.1093/ije/dyw151.

25. Pizzorno J. *The Toxin Solution: How Hidden Poisons in the Air, Water, Food, and Products We Use Are Destroying Our Health—And What We Can Do to Fix It* (HarperCollins, 2017).

26. Bergamo P, Maurano F, D'Arienzo R, David C, Rossi M. Association between activation of phase 2 enzymes and down-regulation of dendritic cell maturation by c9,t11-conjugated linoleic acid. *Immunology Letters* 2008 May 15;117(2):181–90.

27. Bassaganya-Riera J, Hontecillas R, Horne WT, Sandridge M, Herfarth HH, Bloomfeld R, Isaacs KL. Conjugated linoleic acid modulates immune responses in patients with mild to moderately active Crohn's disease. *Clinical Nutrition* 2012 Oct;31(5):721–7.

28. Gaullier JM, Halse J, Høye K, Kristiansen K, Fagertun H, Vik H, Gudmundsen O. Conjugated linoleic acid supplementation for 1 y reduces body fat mass in healthy overweight humans. *American Journal of Clinical Nutrition* 2004 Jun;79(6):1118–25.

29. Kvalem HE, Knutsen HK, Thomsen C et al. Role of dietary patterns for dioxin and PCB exposure. *Molecular Nutrition & Food Research* 2009 Nov;53(11):1438–51.

30. Patandin S, Dagnelie PC, Mulder PG, Op de Coul E, van der Veen JE, Weisglas-Kuperus N, Sauer PJ. Dietary exposure to polychlorinated biphenyls and dioxins from infancy until adulthood: a comparison between breast-feeding, toddler, and long-term exposure. *Environmental Health Perspectives* 1999 Jan;107(1):45–51.

31. Caspersen IH, Aase H, Biele G et al. The influence of maternal dietary exposure to dioxins and PCBs during pregnancy on ADHD symptoms and cognitive functions in Norwegian preschool children. *Environment International* 2016 Sep;94:649–60.

32. Caspersen IH, Haugen M, Schjølberg S, Vejrup K, Knutsen HK, Brantsæter AL, Meltzer HM, Alexander J, Magnus P, Kvalem HE. Maternal dietary exposure to dioxins and polychlorinated biphenyls (PCBs) is associated with language delay in 3 year old Norwegian children. *Environment International* 2016 May;91:180–7.

33. Hites RA, Foran JA, Carpenter DO, Hamilton MC, Knuth BA, Schwager SJ. Global assessment of organic contaminants in farmed salmon. *Science* 2004 Jan 9;303(5655): 226–9.

34. Seierstad SL, Seljieflot I, Johansen O, Hansen R, Haugen M, Rosenlund G, Frøyland L, Arnesen H. Dietary intake of differently fed salmon: the influence on markers of human atherosclerosis. *European Journal of Clinical Investigation* 2005 Jan;35(1):52–9.

35. Foran JA, Good DH, Carpenter DO, Hamilton MC, Knuth BA, Schwager SJ. Quantitative analysis of the benefits and risks of consuming farmed and wild salmon. *Journal of Nutrition* 2005 Nov;135(11): 2639–43.

36. National Resources Defense Council. The Smart Seafood Buying Guide. August 25, 2015, https://www.nrdc.org/stories/smart-seafood-buying-guide.

37. Fernando WM, Martins IJ, Goozee KG, Brennan CS, Jayasena V, Martins RN. The role of dietary coconut for the prevention and treatment of Alzheimer's disease: potential mechanisms of action. *British Journal of Nutrition* 2015 Jul 14;114(1):1–14.

38. Jin JS, Touyama M, Hisada T, Benno Y. Effects of green tea consumption on human fecal microbiota with special reference to *Bifidobacterium* species. *Microbiology and Immunology* 2012 Nov;56(11):729–39.

39. Walker AW, Ince J, Duncan SH et al. Dominant and diet-responsive groups of bacteria within the human colonic microbiota. *ISME Journal* 2011 Feb;5(2): 220–30.

40. Thompson T. Gluten contamination of commercial oat products in the United States. *New England Journal of Medicine* 2004 Nov 4;351(19):2021–2.

41. Sharma GM, Pereira M, Williams KM. Gluten detection in foods available in the United States—a market survey. *Food Chemistry* 2015 Feb 15;169:120–6. [Epub 2014 Aug 5.]

42. Bellioni-Businco B, Paganelli R, Lucenti P, Giampietro PG, Perborn H, Businco L. Allergenicity of goat's milk in children with cow's milk allergy. *Journal of Allergy and Clinical Immunology* 1999 Jun;103(6):1191–4.

43. Jenkins J, Breiteneder H, Mills EN. Evolutionary distance from human homologs reflects allergenicity of animal food proteins. *Journal of Allergy and Clinical Immunology* 2007 Dec;120(6):1399–405.

44. Restani P, Gaiaschi A, Plebani A, Beretta B, Cavagni G, Fiocchi A, Poiesi C, Velonà T, Ugazio AG, Galli CL. Cross-reactivity between milk proteins from different animal species. *Clinical and Experimental Allergy* 1999 Jul;29(7):997–1004.

45. Suutari TJ, Valkonen KH, Karttunen TJ, Ehn BM, Ekstrand B, Bengtsson U, Virtanen V, Nieminen M, Kokkonen J. IgE cross reactivity between reindeer and bovine milk beta-lactoglobulins in cow's milk allergic patients. *Journal of Investigational Allergology and Clinical Immunology* 2006;16(5):296–302.

46. Iacono G, Carroccio A, Cavataio F, Montalto G, Soresi M, Balsamo V. Use of ass'

milk in multiple food allergy. *Journal of Pediatric Gastroenterology and Nutrition* 1992 Feb;14(2):177–81.

47. Vojdani A, Vojdani C. Immune reactivities against gums. *Alternative Therapies in Health and Medicine* 2015;21 Suppl 1:64–72.

48. Moneret-Vautrin DA, Morisset M, Flabbee J, Beaudouin E, Kanny G. Epidemiology of life-threatening and lethal anaphylaxis: a review. *Allergy* 2005 Apr;60(4):443–51.

49. Finkel AV, Yerry JA, Mann JD. Dietary considerations in migraine management: does a consistent diet improve migraine? *Current Pain and Headache Reports* 2013 Nov;17(11): 373. doi: 10.1007/s11916-013-0373-4.

50. Popkin BM, Hawkes C. The sweetening of the global diet, particularly beverages: patterns, trends, and policy responses. *Lancet Diabetes and Endocrinology* 2016 Feb;4(2): 174–86.

51. USDA. Profiling Food Consumption in America, http://www.usda.gov/factbook/chapter2.pdf.

52. Singh A, Lal UR, Mukhtar HM, Singh PS, Shah G, Dhawan RK. Phytochemical profile of sugarcane and its potential health aspects. *Pharmacognosy Reviews* 2015 Jan–Jun;9(17):45–54.

53. Bokulich NA, Blaser MJ. A bitter aftertaste: unintended effects of artificial sweeteners on the gut microbiome. *Cell Metabolism* 2014 Nov 4;20(5):701–3.

54. James J, Thomas P, Cavan D, Kerr D. Preventing childhood obesity by reducing consumption of carbonated drinks: cluster randomised controlled trial. *BMJ* 2004 May 22;328(7450): 1237. doi: 10.1136/bmj.38077.458438.EE.

55. Purohit V, Bode JC, Bode C et al. Alcohol, intestinal bacterial growth, intestinal permeability to endotoxin, and medical consequences: summary of a symposium. *Alcohol* 2008 Aug;42(5):349–61.

56. The Harvard Mahoney Neuroscience Institute Newsletter, 2017, Sugar and the Brain, On the Brain, http://neuro.hms.harvard.edu/harvard-mahoney-neuroscience-institute/brain-newsletter/and-brain-series/sugar-and-brain, accessed 2017 Oct 12.

57. Kaushik M, Reddy P, Sharma R, Udameshi P, Mehra N, Marwaha A. The effect of coconut oil pulling on *Streptococcus mutans* count in saliva in comparison with chlorhexidine mouthwash. *Journal of Contemporary Dental Practice* 2016 Jan 1;17(1):38–41.

58. Ogbolu DO, Oni AA, Daini OA, Oloko AP. In vitro antimicrobial properties of coconut oil on Candida species in Ibadan, Nigeria. *Journal of Medicinal Food* 2007 Jun;10(2):384–7.

59. Bieschke J, Russ J, Friedrich RP, Ehrnhoefer DE, Wobst H, Neugebauer K,

Wanker EE. EGCG remodels mature alpha-synuclein and amyloid-beta fibrils and reduces cellular toxicity. *Proceedings of the National Academy of Sciences of the United States of America* 2010 Apr 27;107(17):7710–5.

60. Ehrnhoefer DE, Bieschke J, Boeddrich A, Herbst M, Masino L, Lurz R, Engemann S, Pastore A, Wanker EE. EGCG redirects amyloidogenic polypeptides into unstructured, off-pathway oligomers. *Nature Structural & Molecular Biology* 2008 Jun;15(6):558–66.

61. Grelle G, Otto A, Lorenz M, Frank RF, Wanker EE, Bieschke J. Black tea theaflavins inhibit formation of toxic amyloid-beta and alpha-synuclein fibrils. *Biochemistry* 2011 Dec 13;50(49):10624–36.

62. Bastianetto S, Yao ZX, Papadopoulos V, Quirion R. Neuroprotective effects of green and black teas and their catechin gallate esters against beta-amyloid-induced toxicity. *European Journal of Neuroscience* 2006 Jan;23(1):55–64.

63. Panossian A. Understanding adaptogenic activity: specificity of the pharmacological action of adaptogens and other phytochemicals. *Annals of the New York Academy of Sciences* 2017 Aug;1401(1):49–64. Epub 2017 Jun 22.

64. Kongkeaw C, Dilokthornsakul P, Thanarangsarit P, Limpeanchob N, Norman Scholfield C. Meta-analysis of randomized controlled trials on cognitive effects of *Bacopa monnieri* extract. *Journal of Ethnopharmacology* 2014;151(1):528–35.

65. Calabrese C. Effects of a standardized *Bacopa monnieri* extract on cognitive performance, anxiety, and depression in the elderly: a randomized, double-blind, placebo-controlled trial. *Journal of Alternative and Complementary Medicine* 2008 Jul;14(6):707–13. doi: 10.1089/acm.2008.0018.

66. Hota SK, Barhwal K, Baitharu I, Prasad D, Singh SB, Ilavazhagan G. *Bacopa monniera* leaf extract ameliorates hypobaric hypoxia induced spatial memory impairment. *Neurobiology of Disease* 2009 Apr;34(1):23–39.

67. Zhou Y, Qu ZQ, Zeng YS, Lin YK, Li Y, Chung P, Wong R, Hägg U. Neuroprotective effect of preadministration with *Ganoderma lucidum* spore on rat hippocampus. *Experimental and Toxicologic Pathology* 2012 Nov;64(7–8):673–80.

68. Choudhary D, Bhattacharyya S, Bose S. Efficacy and safety of ashwagandha (*Withania somnifera* (L.) Dunal) root extract in improving memory and cognitive functions. *Journal of Dietary Supplements* 2017 Nov 2;14(6):599–612.

69. Manchanda S, Kaur G. *Withania somnifera* leaf alleviates cognitive dysfunction by enhancing hippocampal plasticity in high fat diet induced obesity model. *BMC Complementary and Alternative Medicine* 2017 Mar 3;17(1):136.

70. Jamshidi N, Cohen MM. The clinical efficacy and safety of tulsi in humans: a systematic review of the literature. *Evidence-Based Complementary and Alternative Medicine* 2017; 2017:9217567.

71. Gohil KJ, Patel JA, Gajjar AK. Pharmacological review on *Centella asiatica:* a potential herbal cure-all. *Indian Journal of Pharmaceutical Sciences* 2010 Sep;72(5):546–56.
72. Heo HJ, Kim DO, Choi SJ, Shin DH, Lee CY. Potent inhibitory effect of flavonoids in *Scutellaria baicalensis* on amyloid-beta-protein-induced neurotoxicity. *Journal of Agricultural and Food Chemistry* 2004 Jun 30; 52(13):4128–32.

10: THE FIX YOUR BRAIN RECIPES

1. https://www.ncbi.nlm.nih.gov/pubmed/21110905.
2. Ibid.
3. https://www.ncbi.nlm.nih.gov/pubmed/23748211.
4. https://academic.oup.com/nutritionreviews/article-abstract/72/9/605/1860232.
5. https://www.ncbi.nlm.nih.gov/pubmed/19685255.
6. https://www.ncbi.nlm.nih.gov/pmc/articles/PMC2782876/.
7. https://www.ncbi.nlm.nih.gov/pubmed/29263222.
8. https://academic.oup.com/jn/article/136/3/810S/4664377.
9. https://www.ncbi.nlm.nih.gov/pmc/articles/PMC5071963/.
10. https://www.ncbi.nlm.nih.gov/pubmed/28098514.
11. https://www.ncbi.nlm.nih.gov/pmc/articles/PMC1702408/.
12. https://www.ncbi.nlm.nih.gov/pubmed/15534434.
13. https://www.sciencedirect.com/science/article/pii/S0278691509005912?via%3Dihub.
14. https://www.hindawi.com/journals/ecam/2013/946298/.
15. https://link.springer.com/chapter/10.1007/978-3-319-28383-8_12.
16. Ibid.
17. https://www.ncbi.nlm.nih.gov/pubmed/?term=honey+brain+health+benefits.
18. http://onlinelibrary.wiley.com/doi/10.1111/j1541-4337.2008.00047.x/full.
19. https://www.sciencedirect.com/science/article/pii/S0273230003001004.
20. https://www.ncbi.nlm.nih.gov/pubmed/26092628.
21. https://www.ncbi.nlm.nih.gov/pubmed/20443063.
22. https://pdfs.semanticscholar.org/1044/1b1f37d7329ad57eed745fcd91fe14b76fae.pdf.
23. https://www.ncbi.nlm.nih.gov/pubmed/29263222.
24. http://onlinelibrary.wiley.com/doi/10.1111/1750-3841.12434/full.
25. https://www.ncbi.nlm.nih.gov/pubmed/29263222.
26. https://www.ncbi.nlm.nih.gov/pubmed/19685255.
27. https://benthamopen.com/contents/pdf/TOOBESJ/TOOBESJ-2-101.pdf.
28. https://pdfs.semanticscholar.org/1044/1b1f37d7329ad57eed745fcd91fe14b76fae.pdf.
29. https://www.ncbi.nlm.nih.gov/pubmed/25553449.
30. https://www.ncbi.nlm.nih.gov/pmc/articles/PMC4375225/.
31. https://www.hindawi.com/journals/ecam/2012/193496/abs/.

11: LIVING WITH ELECTROMAGNETIC POLLUTION

1. Morris ZS, Wooding S, Grant J. The answer is 17 years, what is the question: understanding time lags in translational research. *Journal of the Royal Society of Medicine* 2011 Dec;104(12):510–20.

2. Wertheimer N, Leeper E. Electrical wiring configurations and childhood cancer. *American Journal of Epidemiology* 1979 Mar;109(3):273–84.

3. Wertheimer N, Leeper E. Adult cancer related to electrical wires near the home. *International Journal of Epidemiology* 1982 Dec;11(4):345–55.

4. Vena JE, Graham S, Hellmann R, Swanson M, Brasure J. Use of electric blankets and risk of postmenopausal breast cancer. *American Journal of Epidemiology* 1991 Jul 15;134(2):180–5.

5. Gundestrup M, Storm HH. Radiation-induced acute myeloid leukemia and other cancers in commercial jet cockpit crew: a population-based cohort study. *Lancet* 1999 Dec 11;354(9195):2029–31.

6. Djordjevic NZ, Paunović MG, Peulić AS. Anxiety-like behavioural effects of extremely low-frequency electromagnetic field in rats. *Environmental Science and Pollution Research International* 2017 Sep;24(27):21693–9.

7. Sage C, Burgio E. Electromagnetic fields, pulsed radiofrequency radiation, and epigenetics: how wireless technologies may affect childhood development. *Child Development* 2017 May 15. [Epub ahead of print.]

8. Belyaev I, Dean A, Eger H et al. EUROPAEM EMF Guideline 2016 for the prevention, diagnosis and treatment of EMF-related health problems and illnesses. *Reviews on Environmental Health* 2016 Sep 1;31(3):363–97.

9. Schoeni A, Roser K, Bürgi A, Röösli M. Symptoms in Swiss adolescents in relation to exposure from fixed site transmitters: a prospective cohort study. *Environmental Health* 2016 Jul 16;15(1):77.

10. Mohammadianinejad SE, Babaei M, Nazari P. The effects of exposure to low-frequency electromagnetic fields in the treatment of migraine headache: a cohort study. *Electronic Physician* 2016 Dec 25;8(12):3445–9.

11. Heuser G, Heuser SA. Functional brain MRI in patients complaining of electro hypersensitivity after long-term exposure to electromagnetic fields. *Reviews on Environmental Health* 2017 Sep 26;32(3):291–9.

12. Pall ML. Microwave frequency electromagnetic fields (EMFs) produce widespread neuropsychiatric effects, including depression. *Journal of Chemical Neuroanatomy* 2016 Sep;75(Pt B):43–51.

13. Gobba F. Subjective non-specific symptoms related with electromagnetic fields: description of 2 cases. *Epidemiologia e Prevenzione* 2002 Jul–Aug;26(4):171–5.

14. Danker-Hopfe H, Dorn H, Bolz T, Peter A, Hansen ML, Eggert T, Sauter C.

Effects of mobile phone exposure (GSM 900 and WCDMA/UMTS) on poly-somnography based sleep quality: An intra- and inter-individual perspective. *Environmental Research* 2016 Feb;145:50–60.

15. Havas M. Radiation from wireless technology affects the blood, the heart, and the autonomic nervous system. *Reviews on Environmental Health* 2013;28(2–3):75–84. doi: 10.1515/reveh-2013-0004.

16. Johansson O. Disturbance of the immune system by electromagnetic fields: a potentially underlying cause for cellular damage and tissue repair reduction which could lead to disease and impairment. *Pathophysiology* 2009 Aug;16(2–3):157–77.

17. Havas M. Dirty electricity elevates blood sugar among electrically sensitive diabetics and may explain brittle diabetes. *Electromagnetic Biology and Medicine* 2008;27(2):135–46.

18. Havas M. Electromagnetic hypersensitivity: biological effects of dirty electricity with emphasis on diabetes and multiple sclerosis. *Electromagnetic Biology and Medicine* 2006;25(4):259–68.

19. De Iuliis GN, Newey RJ, King BV, Aitken RJ. Mobile phone radiation induces reactive oxygen species production and DNA damage in human spermatozoa in vitro. *PLOS One* 2009 Jul 31;4(7):e6446.

20. The Independent September 21, 2008: EMF & Health: A Global Issue. September 8-9, 2008, The Royal Society of London.

21. Gupta M, Khanna R, Rhangra K. Penetration of cell phone and cell tower radiation in human body: a comprehensive study. *International Journal of Recent Trends in Engineering & Research* 2017 Jul 1;3(7).

22. Roggeveen S, van Os J, Viechtbauer W, Lousberg R. EEG changes due to experimentally induced 3G mobile phone radiation. *PLOS One* 2015 Jun 8;10(6):e0129496.

23. Tas M, Dasdag S, Akdag MZ, Cirit U, Yegin K, Seker U, Ozmen MF, Eren LB. Long-term effects of 900 MHz radiofrequency radiation emitted from mobile phone on testicular tissue and epididymal semen quality. *Electromagnetic Biology and Medicine* 2014 Sep;33(3):216–22.

24. Kesari KK, Siddiqui MH, Meena R, Verma HN, Kumar S. Cell phone radiation exposure on brain and associated biological systems. *Indian Journal of Experimental Biology* 2013 Mar;51(3):187–200.

25. Khurana VG, Teo C, Kundi M, Hardell L, Carlberg M. Cell phones and brain tumors: a review including the long-term epidemiologic data. *Surgical Neurology* 2009 Sep;72(3):205–14.

26. Khurana VG, Hardell L, Everaert J, Bortkiewicz A, Carlberg M, Ahonen M. Epidemiological evidence for a health risk from mobile phone base stations. *International Journal of Occupational and Environmental Health* 2010 Jul–Sep;16(3):263–7.

ACKNOWLEDGMENTS

As I've dived deeper into the scientific principles and explanations behind functional medicine, I've made it a point to understand that the scientists who publish the vast majority of the research papers I've read are writing for a very targeted audience (other scientists), and they are not English majors. But without their research, this book, and its practical everyday applications for rejuvenating your brain, would not have been possible.

My publishing team has been extraordinary. My Rodale editor, Marisa Vigilante, and her assistant, Danielle Curtis, were integral to this book's progress. Alyse Diamond at Penguin Random House picked up the project and took it to the finish line. My agents, Celeste Fine and John Maas, have been exemplary. It's been great to know that I, and this book, are in the hands of pros.

I'd like to thank Pamela Liflander, whose editorial support goes way beyond just allowing my ideas to flow freely. Pam organized my flowing ideas, took my calls at every hour of any day, and translated my "geekiness" of segmented ideas into a smooth flowing line of thought, again and again. This body of knowledge would not have come through so clearly without Pam's patient, flowing pen (actually a keyboard, but you know what I mean).

And most important, I must thank my beautiful partner and wife, Marzena, who in the last two years of writing this book has tirelessly listened to me through excitement, confusion, excitement, frustration, excitement, despair, excitement, and everything in between. Thank you Marzi for supporting me in reading 93 research papers on the blood-brain barrier on our honeymoon! You made it so much fun to "geek out" and celebrate our marriage at the same time. There is no one like you in the world.

And of course, thanks to you, Dear Reader, for investing the time, and dollars, to read this book. My prayer is that you will see the path to clear the dust and cobwebs from your mind and help insure a long life with a vibrant, energized brain. God knows, we need every one of us thinking more clearly protecting our planet, our children, and our future. Love, peace, and happiness to us all.

INDEX

ABOUT THE AUTHOR

Tom O'Bryan, DC, CCN, DACBN, is an internationally recognized and sought-after speaker and workshop leader for professional educational conferences, events, and consumer health consortiums. His areas of expertise focus on brain health, food sensitivities, environmental toxins, and the development of autoimmune disease. He is the creative visionary behind a series of exclusive private retreats that deep dive to support an individual's journey out of pain and disease and into a life of vibrant health. He is a frequent contributor to online summits and programs, as well as several bestselling collaborative books and documentaries, including *Broken Brain*, by Dr. Mark Hyman.

Tom O'Bryan is the mind behind the *Betrayal* documentary series on autoimmune disease (BetrayalSeries.com) and the Gluten Summit (The GlutenSummit.com), and the author of the bestselling book *The Autoimmune Fix* (TheAutoimmuneFix.com). He has also created a vast library of content and health-related products on his website, theDr.com, and is the chief medical officer of SunHorseEnergy.com. He is also the founder of

the Certified Gluten Practitioner Program (CertifiedGlutenPractitioner
.com) and the Advanced Autoimmune Training Program.

Dr. O'Bryan also holds positions at the following organizations:

- Adjunct Faculty, The Institute for Functional Medicine
- Adjunct Faculty, The National University of Health Sciences
- Adjunct Faculty, Integrative and Functional Nutrition Academy
- Clinical Consultant on Functional Medicine, NuMedica
- Clinical Consultant on Functional Medicine, Vibrant America
- Editorial Review Board, *Alternative Therapies in Health and Medicine*
- Medical Advisory Board, Functional Medicine Coaching Academy
- Medical Advisory Board, Functional Medicine University
- Medical Advisory Board, The Institute for Functional Medicine
- Medical Advisory Board, Nutritional Therapy Association
- Medical Advisory Board, National Association of Nutrition Professionals
- Scientific Advisory Board, International and American Association of Clinical Nutritionists

To invite Dr. O'Bryan to speak at your event, please visit theDr.com/
Inquiries.